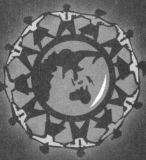

Series Editor: Richard Riegelman

EDITION

ESSENTIAL PUBLIC HEALTH

Essentials of
Public Health
Preparedness
and Emergency
Management

Edited by

Rebecca Katz, PhD, MPH

Associate Professor
Georgetown University
Washington, DC

James A. Banaski, Jr., MS, MEP, CEM

Senior Public Health Emergency Management Professional
Atlanta, Georgia

JONES & BARTLETT
LEARNING

World Headquarters
Jones & Bartlett Learning
5 Wall Street
Burlington, MA 01803
978-443-5000
info@jblearning.com
www.jblearning.com

Jones & Bartlett Learning books and products are available through most bookstores and online booksellers. To contact Jones & Bartlett Learning directly, call 1-800-832-0034, fax 978-443-8000, or visit our website, www.jblearning.com.

12154-4

Production Credits
VP, Product Management: David D. Cella
Director of Product Management: Michael Brown
Product Specialist: Danielle Bessette
Product Specialist: Carter McAlister
Editorial Intern: Alexia Demetroulakos
Production Manager: Carolyn Rogers Pershouse
Director of Vendor Management: Amy Rose
Vendor Manager: Juna Abrams
Senior Marketing Manager: Sophie Fleck Teague
Manufacturing and Inventory Control Supervisor: Amy Bacus
Composition: codeMantra U.S. LLC

Project Management: codeMantra U.S. LLC
Cover Design: Michael O'Donnell
Director of Rights & Media: Joanna Gallant
Rights & Media Specialist: Robert Boder
Media Development Editor: Troy Liston
Cover Image (Title Page, Part Opener, Chapter Opener):
 © f00sion/E+/Getty
Printing and Binding: Edwards Brothers Malloy
Cover Printing: Edwards Brothers Malloy

Library of Congress Cataloging-in-Publication Data
Names: Katz, Rebecca, 1973- author. | Banaski, James A., Jr., author.
Title: Essentials of public health preparedness and emergency management /
 Rebecca Katz, James A. Banaski, Jr.
Other titles: Essentials of public health preparedness. | Essential public health.
Description: Second edition. | Burlington, Massachusetts: Jones & Bartlett
 Learning, [2019] | Series: Essential public health | Preceded by:
 Essentials of public health preparedness / Rebecca Katz. c2013 | Includes
 bibliographical references and index.
Identifiers: LCCN 2017041818 | ISBN 9781284121476 (pbk.: alk. paper)
Subjects: | MESH: Civil Defense | Disaster Planning | Security Measures |
 Terrorism—prevention & control | Emergencies | Public Health
 Administration | United States
Classification: LCC RA445 | NLM WA 295 | DDC 363.34/8—dc23
LC record available at https://lccn.loc.gov/2017041818

6048

Printed in the United States of America
22 21 20 19 18   10 9 8 7 6 5 4 3 2

Contents

PART I Principles of Public Health Preparedness and Emergency Management 1

Chapter 1 Introduction to Public Health Preparedness 3

PART II Defining the Problem 11

Chapter 2 Threats from Biological, Chemical, Nuclear, and Radiological Weapons 13

Chapter 3 Threats from Naturally Occurring Disease and Natural Disaster 33

Prologue

From bioterrorism to environmental disasters and emerging communicable disease, threats to health now appear everywhere we look. *Essentials of Public Health Preparedness and Emergency Management, Second Edition* takes an all-hazards approach to public health preparedness and emergency management, providing broad perspectives on the local, national, and global threats.

Rebecca Katz, PhD, MPH, an associate professor of global health and the co-director of the Center for Global Health Science and Security at Georgetown University Medical Center, Washington, D.C., takes on the challenge of putting public health preparedness in the larger context of public policy and national security. She brings to this challenge a wealth of background in the policy aspects of public health preparedness, having worked at the intersection of infectious diseases and national security for the State Department and the Defense Intelligence Agency.

This second edition has added "emergency management" to its title and content and added a new author, James A. Banaski, Jr., MS, MEP, CEM, who brings hands-on emergency management experience as a team lead for the Global Response Preparedness Team in the Emergency Response and Recovery Branch of the Centers for Disease Control and Prevention (CDC), Atlanta, Georgia. He leads a team that works with the Ministries of Health to assist in the development of preparedness and response programs.

Essentials of Public Health Preparedness and Emergency Management, Second Edition also includes a series of case studies such as Ebola and Zika, which demonstrate approaches to addressing the treatment of emerging infectious diseases. Additional case studies focus on bioterrorism, environmental disasters, and the need for a coordinated approach, involving the full range of first responders, public health and clinical health professionals, and a range of other emergency response professionals. An impressive list of experts have contributed to these case studies.

Essentials of Public Health Preparedness and Emergency Management, Second Edition assumes no prior background in public health, yet it speaks to undergraduate students at community colleges and 4-year colleges, graduate students, as well as public health practitioners.

Public health preparedness has become a cornerstone of public health and a major undertaking of governmental public health.

Competencies have been developed by the Association of School and Programs of Public Health with support and encouragement from CDC. *Essentials of Public Health Preparedness and Emergency Management, Second Edition* will help students and practitioners achieve these competencies.

The second edition has added new materials plus new chapters and now consists of 14 chapters that comprehensively introduce the full range of topics in public health preparedness and emergency management. The 14 chapters, including an abundance of case studies, should make the second edition an ideal text for a wide range of undergraduate and graduate public health courses as well as courses for first responders, health administrators, nurses, and other clinical health professionals.

I am confident that you will find *Essentials of Public Health Preparedness and Emergency Management, Second Edition* engaging and enlightening. I am delighted that *Essentials of Public Health Preparedness and Emergency Management, Second Edition* is part of our Essential Public Health series.

Richard Riegelman, MD, MPH, PhD
Series Editor, Essential Public Health

Preface

The last 15 years have seen many changes in terms of how we view our security and the role of the public health community. Infectious diseases continue to emerge and reemerge around the world, and the globalization of our food supply and the speed and volume of international travel make us all vulnerable to the emergence of a new agent. There is mounting evidence that large-scale epidemics can dramatically affect the economic, social, and security foundations of a nation. There is an ever-evolving threat of the terrorist use of weapons of mass destruction against our population, particularly the use of biological weapons. We are constantly reminded of the devastating effects of natural disasters, particularly hurricanes and fire. All of these factors have led to the emergence of the subdiscipline within public health— public health preparedness. The public health community plays a vital role in identifying, responding to, containing, and recovering from emergencies. It is imperative that public health professionals develop an awareness of the emerging threats, the means of addressing those threats, security challenges inherent in these activities, and be able to identify and work with other sectors with similar responsibilities.

An essential component of effective public health preparedness and response is public health emergency management and emergency operations centers. Responding to large-scale public health events often requires coordination with multiple organizations and international entities through an emergency response plan, and emergency operations centers play an essential role in coordinating an effective response.

Public health preparedness and emergency management has been rapidly developing at the global, federal, state, and local levels. The CDC has an entire division devoted to emergency management and the world's gold standard public health emergency operations centers. The World Health Organization published a first-ever guidance and standards document for public health emergency operations centers, in a response to global demand from Ministries of Health. Academia is now acknowledging this as an essential area of expertise necessary for a fully developed public health workforce.

The first edition of *Essentials of Public Health Preparedness and Emergency Management* was designed based on a course that one of the authors (Rebecca Katz) had been teaching for 10 years. The additions of emergency management and other changes to the text are based on student feedback, feedback from faculty at other schools who have used the text, and colleagues working in this area.

The goal of this book is to introduce students to the field of public health preparedness and emergency management, and for the first time to combine all of the topics in this field into one single text. Public health preparedness and emergency management are new concepts for many students, from the undergraduate to doctoral students. As such, the text is written in a way that presupposes no previous exposure to the concepts, yet still provides enough depth for students who may have more advanced knowledge.

Essentials of Public Health Preparedness and Emergency Management, Second Edition is divided into five parts:

Part I: Principles of Public Health Preparedness and Emergency Management
Part II: Defining the Problem
Part III: Infrastructure
Part IV: Solving Problems
Part V: Practical Applications and Operations

Part I provides an overview and background to the field of public health preparedness. We look at how the field has evolved and how different entities have defined the discipline. We also review the definitions and evolution of national security and homeland security, with particular emphasis on how they relate to public health. Finally, we look at the role of the public health professional in emergency preparedness, from designing policy to participating in disaster response, and explore potential careers in the field.

Part II of the text begins to characterize the problems that require preparedness on the part of the public health community. Chapter 2 covers threats from biological, chemical, nuclear, and radiological weapons. We define these threats and review the history of use—both intentional and accidental. The chapter then looks at how the current threat from weapons of mass destruction (WMD) is evaluated and returns to the role of the public health community in responding to WMD. Chapter 3 discusses threats from naturally occurring disease and natural disasters: the historical impact of disease and natural disaster on homeland and national security, preparedness activities around the threat of naturally occurring diseases, evaluating the current threat from disease and disasters, and the public health and foreign policy response to these threats.

Part III moves from definitions and threat characterization to a review of the infrastructure, primarily on the federal level, that has emerged in the past 15 years to address public health preparedness. Chapter 4 focuses on national infrastructure for public health preparedness and planning. We review the creation of the National Strategy for Homeland Security and the offices and organizations that were created in the aftermath of 9/11. This chapter also introduces the reader to the Intelligence Community. We look at the National Response Framework, with particular emphasis on public health and medical response components, the National Incident Management System, and specific plans for public health emergencies. Finally, Chapter 5 presents the legislation, regulations, and policy guidance that have emerged to address public health preparedness and to mitigate the threats of WMD, naturally occurring disease, and other disasters.

Part IV of the book is generally categorized as solving problems and includes a variety of approaches the community has taken to address biological threats, along with the challenges of each approach. Chapter 6 explores biosecurity and biosafety: defining the dual use dilemma, how biosecurity is used to minimize the threat, the role of the life sciences community in establishing codes of conduct and self-policing scientific publications, reviewing pathogen security efforts, and examining emerging challenges in biosecurity. In Chapter 7, we look at the research agenda and the infrastructure that has been built to support research directly relating to biological threats. We also look

at the enterprise that has been built to support the development of medical countermeasures.

Chapter 8 focuses on the response—the systems that have been established to coordinate and govern the humanitarian response to emergencies. Chapter 9 describes the domestic and international surveillance programs, and concentrates on the challenges associated with investigating an alleged-use event and on making an attribution assessment. This chapter also explores the relationship between the Federal Bureau of Investigation and the public health community, particularly as it pertains to criminal and epidemiological investigations.

The last section of the book, Part V, focuses on the practical applications and operations associated with public health preparedness and emergency management. Chapter 10 introduces the idea of preparedness as a program through the preparedness cycle and the idea of a deliberate planning process for preparedness. Chapter 11 covers practical applications of public health emergency management, explaining the Incident Command System and the Threat and Hazard Identification and Risk Assessment process. In Chapter 12, we explore the development and use of an emergency operations center. Chapter 13 covers capacity development programs, such as training, exercises, and evaluation. Chapter 14 discusses a few of the most recent public health responses.

We are excited to introduce a series of case studies that appear throughout the book, written by experts from across the discipline. Our hope is that these case studies bring to life some of challenges and solutions offered to advance public health preparedness and emergency management.

This book is designed to give the reader an appreciation for the complexities of issues that must be considered by public health professionals in designing preparedness and response plans, policies, regulations and legislation, and emergency management. We hope readers will better understand the essential role of the public health community in preparing for and responding to security threats.

New to This Edition

As mentioned in the Preface, this edition reflects major changes that have evolved in the field of public health preparedness in the past 6 years and brings in the essentials of emergency management. These changes were made based on student feedback, feedback from faculty at other schools who have used the text, and colleagues working in this area. The most obvious changes are the addition of five chapters on emergency management (Chapters 10–14) written by James A. Banaski, Jr., an emergency management expert from the CDC. We have also added a series of case studies throughout the book, intended to provide in-depth review of issues directly related to the text. For these case studies, we have brought in guest contributors. We have updated each of the chapters that have remained from the previous edition to reflect new developments in the field, more recent outbreaks and challenges, and an ever-evolving national and international system to describe and address challenges in public health preparedness and emergency management.

Contributors

Jennifer Bryning Alton, MPP

Case Study: Passage of the Pandemic and All-Hazards Preparedness Act of 2006 (appears in Chapter 5)

Malaya Fletcher, MPH

Case Study: Risk Communications in a Time of Zika—Conducting Community Assessments During Public Health Emergencies (appears in Chapter 14)

Ellie Graeden, PhD

Case Study: Research Note on Data Integration for Effective Response to Public Health Emergencies (appears in Chapter 7)

Ami Patel, PhD, MPH

Case Study: Risk Communications in a Time of Zika—Conducting Community Assessments During Public Health Emergencies (appears in Chapter 14)

Erin M. Sorrell, PhD, MS

Case Study: The H5N1 Transmission Papers—Reinvigorating the Dual Use Dilemma (appears in Chapter 6)

Claire Standley, PhD, MSc

Case Study: Epidemics and Biobanking (appears in Chapter 7) and Case Study: Public Health Emergency Management in Guinea—Before and After the 2014 Ebola Outbreak (appears in Chapter 14)

Acknowledgments

From Rebecca Katz:

This book is based on a class I taught for many years at George Washington University's School of Public Health and Health Services (Washington, D.C.)—a class I inherited in 2006 from Brian Kamoie. So, I continue to thank Brian for his foresight and efforts in designing this class and for trusting me to build on the foundation he provided. I thank all of the students who have provided helpful comments on the text over the years. I thank my colleagues at Georgetown Center for Global Health Science and Security for their support while I worked on this book, specifically Claire Standley for research assistance on Chapter 5 and Aurelia Attal-Juncqua for research assistance on Chapter 4. Many, many thanks to Emily Harris, who provided exceptional, detailed assistance in making this book happen. I am also thankful to Jennifer Alton, Claire Standley, Erin M. Sorrell, Ellie Graeden, Malaya Fletcher, and Ami Patel for generously contributing case studies to this edition. And to Jim Banaski for being willing to come on board this project and share his fantastic expertise with us.

Most importantly, I thank my family—Matt, Olivia, and Benjamin—for their love and support.

From James A. Banaski, Jr.:

I would like to publicly thank my colleagues from the CDC for their kind input and encouragement as I wrote chapters for this book. Specifically, I would like to thank Kim Hanson, Luis Hernandez, Jennifer Brooks, Mike Gerber, and Mark Anderson, whose guidance and critiques have made this a better book. Thank you to Claire Standley and Erin M. Sorrell, true professionals that I have had the pleasure of working with in many different capacities. Thank you Emily Harris, who is the reason this book looks coherent. I would also like to thank my wife, Kim, and my children, Ashley and Avery, for allowing me to sacrifice family time in order to do something I have always wanted to do. And last, but certainly not least, Dr. Rebecca Katz. Thank you for inviting me to be a part of this project. I have always wanted to do something like this and you made it happen.

About the Authors

Rebecca Katz, PhD, MPH is an associate professor of global health and the co-director of the Center for Global Health Science and Security at Georgetown University Medical Center (Washington, D.C.). She is also an affiliate faculty in the Georgetown University School of Foreign Service and the McCourt School of Public Policy. Prior to joining Georgetown University in 2016, she spent 10 years in the Department of Health Policy and Management at the Milken Institute School of Public Health at George Washington University. She is trained in epidemiology, demography, economics, global health, and public policy. Since 2007, she has focused her research on the implementation of the International Health Regulations, health diplomacy, and public health preparedness policy. Since September 2004, she has been a public health scientist and expert consultant at the U.S. Department of State. She currently supports the Biological Policy Staff in the Bureau of International Security and Nonproliferation. She has been with this office since it was created in 2010, and works primarily on the Biological Weapons Convention and provides content and policy expertise on emerging and pandemic threats.

Dr. Katz has an undergraduate degree in political science and economics from Swarthmore College (Swarthmore, Pennsylvania), a master's in public health from Yale University (New Haven, Connecticut), and PhD from Princeton University (Princeton, New Jersey).

James A. Banaski, Jr., MS, MEP, CEM is the team lead for the Global Response Preparedness Team (GRPT) in the Emergency Response and Recovery Branch, Division of Global Health Protection, Center for Global Health at the Centers for Disease Control and Prevention (CDC) in Atlanta, Georgia. He leads a team that works with Ministries of Health to assist in the development of preparedness and response programs to help meet the requirements under the International Health Regulations (2005) to detect, respond to, and report public health threats of international concern. Before coming to the CDC, he worked with the U.S. Army North, conducting training and exercises for the Weapons of Mass Destruction Civil Support Teams. Before that, he served as a training specialist at the U.S. Army Chemical School at Fort Leonard Wood, Missouri. He has served in numerous public health emergencies, including H1N1, numerous hurricanes, the Deepwater Horizon oil spill, the American Samoa Tsunami response, the Japan Earthquake and Tsunami response, the Joplin, Missouri tornado relief, the worldwide Ebola response, and the international Zika Response.

Mr. Banaski is an 11-year veteran of the U.S. Army Chemical Corp and served in various locations in the United States, Europe, and the Middle East.

Mr. Banaski has a dual bachelor of science degree in environmental science and biology from Drury University (Springfield, Missouri) and a master of science degree in environmental management from Webster University (Webster Groves, Missouri). He also holds the Master Exercise Practitioner certification from the Department of Homeland Security and the Certified Emergency Manager designation from the International Association of Emergency Managers.

About the Contributors

Jennifer Bryning Alton, MPP leads Bavarian Nordic's U.S. public policy and government affairs activities, including policy development, lobbying, public affairs, alliance development, and trade association management. She is also a board member for the Alliance for Biosecurity, a coalition of biopharmaceutical companies and academic partners working to ensure medical countermeasures are available to protect public health and enhance national health security. She previously worked in the U.S. Senate as public health policy director for Senator Richard Burr on the Health, Education, Labor, and Pensions Committee, where she led the development and negotiation of policy and legislation on public health issues, and successfully shepherded the bipartisan Pandemic and All-Hazards Preparedness Act into law in 2006, transforming the country's preparedness for health security threats. She also worked at the U.S. Department of Health and Human Services, where she was selected as a presidential management fellow in the Office of the Assistant Secretary for Budget and received the Secretary's Distinguished Service Award. She holds a master of public policy degree from the Luskin School of Public Affairs (University of California, Los Angeles, CA) and a bachelor's degree from Whittier College (Whittier, CA).

Malaya Fletcher, MPH serves as the Global Migration & Monitoring Coordinator for the Philadelphia Department of Public Health (PDPH), where she focuses on emerging infectious disease surveillance and travel health. She currently oversees the agency's Zika education activities. In this capacity, she was the lead planner for Philadelphia's first Community Assessment for Public Health Emergency Response, which is used to evaluate the efficacy of the agency's Zika media campaign. Prior to her current position, she served as the public health preparedness planner at PDPH, where her primary responsibilities included regional coordination for the Philadelphia–Camden–Wilmington Metropolitan Statistical Area, radiological incident planning, and medical countermeasure procurement. Outside of Philadelphia, she has worked in pandemic flu planning for Washington State Schools, researched maternal–child health in India as a Boren

Scholar, and conducted capacity assessments at district hospitals in Ghana.

An epidemiologist and emergency planner, her interests include global health security, mixed methods research, and integrating emergency management with routine public health functions through trainings and exercises. Fletcher is committed to overcoming the traditional boundaries of public health and emergency management and translating findings into evidence-based policies. She is a member of the Advisory Board for the Systems-Level Mass Fatality Preparedness Study at the University of California's Philip R. Lee Institute for Health Policy Studies (San Francisco, CA). She is also an Emerging Leaders in Biosecurity Initiative fellow with the Johns Hopkins Center for Health Security (Baltimore, MD). She received an MPH in epidemiology and a Global Health Certificate from Columbia University (New York) in 2012. She also has a bachelor's in microbiology and Certificate in Health Care Organizations & Society from Arizona State University (Tempe, AZ).

Ellie Graeden, PhD is the founder and CEO of Talus Analytics, a small research and consulting firm that specializes in translating complex, computational, and scientific analysis into useful data for decision makers. She earned a doctorate in biology from the Massachusetts Institute of Technology (Cambridge, MA), where she held a National Science Foundation Graduate Research Fellowship. She has a bachelor of science in microbiology from Oregon State University (Corvallis, OR). Across her research and consulting career, she has built a unique approach to data analysis, visualization, and computational modeling that informs policy and practical decision-making. Her past projects have included efforts in support of Federal Emergency Management Agency to identify and characterize the models used for emergency management and in support of the White House National Security Council to coordinate data-driven decision-making for public health emergencies. She has, in addition, led teams funded by the Bill and Melinda Gates Foundation to develop and deploy public health models for local use in the developing world, built a data and analysis platform for the CDC pandemic flu response, and developed an integrated flood risk analysis and community resilience investment planning method funded by the Department of Homeland Security's Science and Technology Directorate.

Ami Patel, PhD, MPH is presently a senior epidemiologist at CSL Behring (King of Prussia, PA). She previously spent 9 years as a CDC career epidemiology officer (CEFO) for the PDPH. In her role as a CEFO, she managed PDPH's Acute Communicable Disease Program and its team of 15 epidemiologists, disease surveillance investigators, and program assistants in their conduct of routine surveillance, outbreak investigations, educational outreach efforts and training, and special studies for over 60 enteric, vaccine-preventable, vector-borne, respiratory virus and healthcare-associated viral hepatitis diseases/conditions along with emerging infections.

Dr. Patel began her career with the CDC in 2002 at the National Institute of Occupational Safety and Health (Pittsburgh, PA). She then joined the CDC's Epidemic Intelligence Service (EIS) in 2005, where she was assigned to the Virginia Department of Health. After completing EIS in 2007, she became a CEFO. She received her master of public health in 2002 and a doctorate in epidemiology in 2005 from the University of Pittsburgh's Graduate School of Public Health (Pittsburgh, PA). She maintains an active interest in teaching and mentoring students, and is an instructor at Thomas Jefferson University's School of Population Health and Philadelphia College of Osteopathic Medicine (Pittsburgh, PA).

Erin M. Sorrell, PhD, MS is an assistant research professor in the Department of Microbiology and Immunology and a member of the Center for Global Health Science and Security at Georgetown University (Washington, D.C.). Her work focuses on developing partnerships across the U.S. government, international organizations, and ministries around the world to identify elements required to support health systems strengthening and laboratory capacity building for disease detection, reporting, risk assessment, and response. Her research uses evidence-based approaches to determine gaps and identify capacities for effective global health programs and policies.

Previously, Dr. Sorrell was a senior research scientist at The George Washington University's Milken Institute School of Public Health in the Department of Health Policy and Management (Washington, D.C.). Prior to joining the cuniversity, she was a senior analyst

in the Office of Cooperative Threat Reduction's Biosecurity Engagement Program at the Department of State, where she also worked as an American Association for the Advancement of Science's science and technology policy fellow. She worked on foreign assistance activities in sub-Saharan Africa, the Middle East, and North Africa.

Dr. Sorrell was a postdoctoral fellow both at Erasmus Medical Center (Rotterdam, The Netherlands) and the University of Maryland (College Park, MD). Her research focused on the molecular mechanisms of interspecies transmission, primarily focusing on avian to human transmission of H2, H7, H9, and H5 influenza A viruses. She received her master's and doctorate in virology from the University of Maryland and a bachelor's in animal science from Cornell University (Ithaca, NY).

Claire Standley, PhD, MSc is an assistant research professor within the Center for Global Health Science and Security at Georgetown University, with a primary faculty appointment in the Department of International Health. Her research focuses on the analysis of health systems strengthening and international capacity building for public health, with an emphasis on prevention and control of infectious diseases in both humans and animals, as well as public health emergency preparedness and response.

Prior to joining Georgetown University, Dr. Standley was a senior research scientist at The George Washington University Milken Institute School of Public Health, and also served as an American Association for the Advancement of Science's science and technology policy fellow at the Department of State, where she supported programs for laboratory capacity building, disease surveillance, and cooperative research across the Middle East, sub-Saharan Africa, and the Lower Mekong.

Dr. Standley has broad and multidisciplinary training across the life sciences, including an undergraduate degree in natural sciences (zoology) from the University of Cambridge (Cambridge, UK); a master's in biodiversity, conservation, and management from the University of Oxford (Oxford, UK); a PhD in genetics (with a focus on biomedical parasitology) from the University of Nottingham (Nottingham, UK), as part of a joint program with the Natural History Museum of London. She served as a postdoctoral research associate at Princeton University (Princeton, NJ), where she examined the dynamics between disease, biodiversity, and public health, working at field sites in Tanzania and Costa Rica.

Abbreviations

AAR/IP	after action report/improvement plan
AI	avian influenza
AMR	antimicrobial resistance
ANSS	Agence National de Securité Sanitaire
AoR	Area of Responsibility
APHA	American Public Health Association
APHIS	Animal and Plant Health Inspection Service
APHL	Association of Public Health Laboratories
ARS	acute radiation syndrome
ASPPH	Association of Schools and Programs of Public Health
ASPR	Assistant Secretary for Preparedness and Response
ASTHO	Association of State and Territorial Health Officers
BAA	Broad Agency Announcement
BARDA	Biomedical Advanced Research and Development Authority
BSL	biosafety level
BSWG	Biosecurity Working Group
BT	bioterrorism
BW	biological warfare/biological weapons
BWC	Biological and Toxin Weapons Convention
CASPER	Community Assessment for Preparedness and Emergency Response
CBD	Convention on Biological Diversity
CBRN	chemical, biological, radiological, and nuclear
CDC	Centers for Disease Control and Prevention
CD-ROM	Compact Disk-Read Only Memory
CERT	Community Emergency Response Team
CIA	Central Intelligence Agency
CN	chloroacetophenone
CNLEB	Cellule de Coordination de la riposte contra la maladie à virus Ebola
COE	Centers of Excellence
COMINT	communications intelligence
CONOPs	concept of operations
COOP	Continuity of Operations
CPG	Community Preparedness Guide
CR	dibenzoxazepine
CRI	Cities Readiness Initiative
CS	chlorobenzylidenemalononitrile
CSTE	Council of State and Territorial Epidemiologists
CTICC	Cyber Threat Intelligence Integration Center
CTR	Cooperative Threat Reduction
CW	chemical warfare/chemical weapons
CWC	Chemical Weapons Convention
CWS	Chemical Warfare Service
CYBINT	Cyber Intelligence
DDII	Deputy Director of National Intelligence for Intelligence Integration
DDMA	District Disaster Management Agency
DEA	Drug Enforcement Administration
DHHS	Department of Health and Human Services
DHS	Department of Homeland Security
DIA	Defense Intelligence Agency
DNI	Director of National Intelligence
DOD	Department of Defense
DOE	Department of Energy
DOS	Department of State
DRC	Disaster Recovery Centers
DRR	Disaster Risk Reduction
DURC	Dual Use Research of Concern
ECDC	European Union Center for Disease Prevention and Control
EEE	Eastern equine encephalitis
EIS	Epidemic Intelligence Service
ELINT	Electronic Intelligence
EM	Emergency Management
EMC	Erasmus Medical Center
EMT	Emergency Medical Teams
EO	Executive Order
EOC	Emergency Operations Center

EOC-NET	Emergency Operations Centre Network		**HSPD**	Homeland Security Presidential Directive
EPA	Environmental Protection Agency		**HSS**	Health and Human Services
EPI-X	Epidemic Information Exchange		**HUMINT**	Human Intelligence
ERC	Emergency Relief Coordinator			
ERF	Emergency Response Framework		**IA**	Office of Intelligence and Analysis (DHS)
ESF	Emergency Support Function			
ESFLG	Emergency Support Function Leadership Group		**IAEA**	International Atomic Energy Agency
			IAP	Incident Action Plan
			IASC	Inter-Agency Standing Committee
FAA	Federal Aviation Administration		**IBC**	Institutional Biosafety Committee
FAO	Food and Agriculture Organization of the United Nations		**IC**	Intelligence Community
			ICS	Incident Command System
FBI	Federal Bureau of Investigation		**IDSR**	Integrated Disease Surveillance and Response
FDA	Food and Drug Administration			
FELTP	Field Epidemiology Laboratory Training Program		**IHR**	International Health Regulations
			IMS	Incident Management System
FEMA	Federal Emergency Management Agency		**INR**	Bureau of Intelligence and Research (DOS)
FESAP	Federal Experts Security Advisory Panel		**INTERPOL**	International Criminal Police Organization
FETP	Field Epidemiology Training Program		**IO**	international organization
FININT	Financial Intelligence		**IOM**	International Organization for Migration
FIRESCOPE	Firefighting Resources of California Organized for Potential Emergencies			
			IPAPI	International Partnership on Avian and Pandemic Influenza
FISINT	Foreign Instrumentation Signals Intelligence		**IRD**	Institut de recherche pour le développement
FSE	Full Scale Exercise		**IRF**	Integrated Research Facility
FSS	Federal Security Service		**IRFC**	International Federation of Red Cross and Red Crescent Societies
FY	Fiscal Year			
G8	Group of 8			
GEOINT	Geographic Intelligence		**JEE**	Joint External Evaluation Tool
GHSA	Global Health Security Agenda		**JIC**	Joint Information Center
GISN	Global Influenza Surveillance Network		**JIM**	Joint Investigative Mechanisms
GISRS	Global Influenza Surveillance and Response System			
			KGB	Komitet Gosudarstvennoy Bezopasnosti
GOARN	Global Outbreak Alert and Response Network			
GOF	gain-of-function			
GPHIN	Global Public Health Information Network		**LRN**	Laboratory Response Network
			LSD	Lysergic acid diethylamide
GPP	Global Partnership Program			
			MASINT	Measurement and Signature Intelligence
HAN	Health Alert Network			
HC	Humanitarian Coordinator		**MCM**	Medical Countermeasures
HELP	Senate Committee on Health, Education, Labor and Pensions		**MERS**	Middle East Respiratory Syndrome
			MIC	methyl isocyanate
HPAI	highly pathogenic avian influenza		**MOU**	Memorandum of Understanding
HPP	Hospital Preparedness Programs		**MPH**	Master of Public Health
HSEEP	Homeland Security Exercise and Evaluation Program		**MSEHPA**	Model State Emergency Health Powers Act

MTA	Material Transfer Agreement	OCHA	Office for Coordination of Humanitarian Affairs
NACCHO	National Association of County and City Health Officials	OFDA	Office of Foreign Disaster Assistance
NAM	National Academy of Medicine	OHCHR	Office of the High Commissioner for Human Rights
NAS	National Academies of Science	OIE	Organization for Animal Health
NATO	North Atlantic Treaty Organization	OPCW	Organization for the Prohibition of Chemical Weapons
NBACC	National Biodefense Analysis and Countermeasures Center	OPHPR	Office of Public Health Preparedness and Response
NBIC	National Biosurveillance Integration Center	OSINT	Open Source Intelligence
NCPC	National Counterproliferation Center	OTA	Office of Technology Assessment
NCSC	National Counterintelligence and Security Center	P3	Prevent 3
NCTC	National Counterterrorism Center	PAHPA	Pandemic and All Hazards Preparedness Act
NDAA	National Defense Authorization Act	PDD	Presidential Decision Directive
NDMA	National Disaster Management Authority	PDMA	Provincial Disaster Management Agency
NDMS	National Disaster Medical System	PDPH	Philadelphia Department of Public Health
NEP	National Exercise Program	PEPFAR	U.S. President's Emergency Plan for AIDS Relief
NGA	National Geospatial-Intelligence Agency	PETS	Pets Evacuation and Transportation Standards Act
NGO	nongovernmental organization	PHAC	Public Health Agency of Canada
NHSS	National Health Security Strategy	PHEIC	Public Health Emergency of International Concern
NIAID	National Institute of Allergy and Infectious Diseases	PHEM	Public Health Emergency Management
NIC	National Intelligence Council	PHEMCE	Public Health Emergency Medical Countermeasures Enterprise
NIH	National Institutes of Health	PHEOC	Public Health Emergency Operations Center
NIMS	National Incident Management System	PHEP	Public Health Emergency Preparedness
NOAA	National Oceanic and Atmospheric Association	PHPR	Public Health Preparedness and Response
NORAD	North American Aerospace Defense Command	PIO	Public Information Officer
NPS	National Pharmaceutical Stockpile	PIP Framework	Pandemic Influenza Preparedness Framework
NPT	Nuclear Non-proliferation Treaty	PNAS	Proceedings of the National Academy of Science
NRC	Norwegian Refugee Council	PREP	Public Readiness and Emergency Preparedness Act
NRF	National Response Framework	PPD	Presidential Policy Directive
NRO	National Reconnaissance Office	PS	chloropicrin
NRP	National Response Plan	RFC	Reconstruction Finance Corporation
NSA	National Security Agency		
NSABB	National Science Advisory Board for Biosecurity		
NSC	National Security Council		
NSD	National Security Directive		
NSDD	National Security Decision Directive		
NSPD	National Security Presidential Directive		
NSPM	National Security Presidential Memorandum		
NSS	National Security Strategy		

SARS	Severe Acute Respiratory Syndrome
SENAH	National Service for Humanitarian Action
SEPA	Smallpox Emergency Personnel Protection Act
SIGINT	Signals Intelligence
SITREP	Situation Report
SMART	Simple, Measurable, Achievable, Realistic, Task Oriented
SNS	Strategic National Stockpile
SOP	standard operation procedure
STD	sexually transmitted disease
T2	trichothecene mycotoxin
TB	tuberculosis
TCL	target capabilities list
TECHINT	Technical Intelligence
TFAH	Trust for America's Health
THIRA	Threat and Hazard Identification and Risk Assessment
TOPOFF	Top Officials
UNDP	U.N. Development Programme
UNHCR	United Nations High Commissioner for Refugees
UNICEF	U.N. Children's Fund
UNMAS	U.N. Mine Action Service
UNSCR	U.N. Security Council Resolution
UNSGM	U.N. Secretary-General's Mechanism

USA PATRIOT	Uniting and Strengthening America by Providing Appropriate Tools Required to Intercept and Obstruct Terrorism
USAID	U.S. Agency for International Development
USAMRIID	U.S. Army Medical Research Institute for Infectious Diseases
USC	United States Code
USDA	U.S. Department of Agriculture
USNORTHCOM	U.S. Northern Command
USG	U.S. Government
UTL	universal task list
UTMB	University of Texas Medical Branch
UW	University of Wisconsin
VECTOR	State Research Centre for Virology and Biotechnology
VEE	Venezuelan Equine Encephalitis
WASH	Water, Sanitation and Hygiene
WEE	Western Equine Encephalitis
WFP	World Food Programme
WHA	World Health Assembly
WHO	World Health Organization
WMD	Weapons of Mass Destruction
WRS	War Research Service
WWI	World War One
WWII	World War Two

© f00sion/E+/Getty

PART I
Principles of Public Health Preparedness and Emergency Management

CHAPTER 1

Introduction to Public Health Preparedness

LEARNING OBJECTIVES

By the end of this chapter, the reader will be able to:

- Define public health preparedness and understand the scope of events that can lead to a public health emergency
- Identify the difference between homeland security and national security
- Define and understand the evolution of public health emergency management
- Understand the role of the public health professional in emergency preparedness and response activities
- Be familiar with the types of careers available to public health professionals in preparedness
- Define core competencies for public health preparedness and emergency management

▶ Introduction

This chapter is all about definitions—understanding what public health preparedness means, what emergency management means, and how we think about national security, homeland security, and defense in the context of public health. We also begin to explore the role of public health professionals in emergency preparedness and response activities, articulate core competencies for public health professionals working in this space, and introduce readers to the types of careers available to public health professionals interested in preparedness and emergency management.

▶ Definitions

Promote General Welfare and Provide for the Common Defense

The Preamble to the Constitution of the United States lays the groundwork for creation of the nation and for basic responsibilities of the federal government (BOX 1-1). Among these responsibilities are to "promote the general welfare" and "provide for the common defense." Public health preparedness, as a subdiscipline of public health, strives to address these two fundamental components of a government's responsibility to its population.

We the People of the United States, in Order to form a more perfect Union, establish Justice, insure domestic Tranquility, provide for the common defense, promote the general Welfare, and secure the Blessings of Liberty to ourselves and our Posterity, do ordain and establish this Constitution for the United States of America.

The Constitution of the United States.

The notions of both homeland security and national security are paramount to public health preparedness. Before we define public health preparedness, let us start with what exactly "provide for the common defense" means.

National Security

Political scientists have long debated what exactly defines national security. The concept means different things to different people. Some see it as policies—including diplomatic, economic, and military power—enacted by governments in order to ensure the survival and safety of the state. Others define it as safeguarding territorial integrity and national independence—basically, the existence of the state.[1] George Kennan wrote that national security is "the continued ability of this country to pursue its internal life without serious interference."[1(pp52–53)] The reoccurring theme within all discussions of national security, however, is the extent to which an individual is willing to sacrifice freedom in exchange for security—the balance between security and liberty.

The most extreme position regarding national security is that it does not matter if the threat to security comes from within or from outside the nation. Citizens will look to the state for protection against all types of threats. In exchange, the state can ask anything of that citizen, short of his life (**BOX 1-2**). For most people, and particularly for those in the United States, there is a more balanced perspective of security and personal liberty. While U.S. citizens want to be protected from threats and support the government in doing so, they want it to be done in such a way that they are able to retain personal freedoms and liberties.

Homeland Security

The founding fathers penned the argument that the Constitution would protect U.S. citizens against conflict at home and that geography would protect the nation from conflict abroad.[2] The basic belief

Without security provided for by the state, there is a state of anarchy. Hobbes describes such a state as follows:

In such condition there is no place for industry, because the fruit thereof is uncertain: and consequently no culture of the earth; no navigation, nor use of the commodities that may be imported by sea; no commodious building; no instruments of moving and removing such things as require much force; no knowledge of the face of the earth; no account of time; no arts; no letters; no society; and which is worst of all, continual fear, and danger of violent death; and the life of man, solitary, poor, nasty, brutish, and short.

Hobbes, T. *Leviathan*. Edited by Richard Tuck. Cambridge University Press; 1991.

was that no threat would reach our borders, and the oceans would protect us from conflict on our shores. As history has proven, however, geography cannot protect us from all external threats, particularly from terrorist actors.

After the terrorist attacks on September 11, 2001, the nation, for the first time, began to speak collectively about "homeland security." The Department of Defense defined homeland security as "the prevention, preemption, deterrence of, and defense against aggression targeted at U.S. territory, sovereignty, domestic population, and infrastructure, as well as the management of the consequences of such aggression and other domestic emergencies."[3(p24)] Others definitions vary slightly, but, at the core, homeland security is about preventing attacks on the United States and minimizing damage through appropriate preparations and rapid recovery.[4(p2),5(p11)]

Homeland Defense

Homeland defense is a component of homeland security. "Defense" is "the protection of U.S. sovereignty, territory, domestic population, and critical defense infrastructure against external threats or aggression."[6] Broadly, this means everything from national missile defense to critical infrastructure protection. The concepts of preparedness and response, however, are typically included in "security" and not in "defense."

Public Health Preparedness

Public health preparedness, like homeland security, is a term that represents concerns and actions that have occurred throughout history. The term itself, however, and the field devoted to thinking about, preparing for, and mobilizing resources to respond to public health emergencies is relatively new.

The Association of Schools and Programs of Public Health (ASPPH) defined public health preparedness as "a combination of comprehensive planning, infrastructure building, capacity building, communication, training, and evaluation that increase public health response effectiveness and efficiency in response to infectious disease outbreaks, bioterrorism, and emerging health threats."[7(p5)] A group at the RAND Corporation, however, proposed a definition in 2007 that is a broader and better characterization of the field:

> "[P]ublic health emergency preparedness … is the capability of the public health and health care systems, communities, and individuals, to prevent, protect against, quickly respond to, and recover from health emergencies, particularly those whose scale, timing, or unpredictability threatens to overwhelm routine capabilities. Preparedness involves a coordinated and continuous process of planning and implementation that relies on measuring performance and taking corrective action."[8(s9)]

This definition raises the question: What exactly is a public health emergency? According to the RAND definition, it is an event "whose scale, timing, or unpredictability threatens to overwhelm routine capabilities." These types of events fit into the following four basic categories:

1. The intentional or accidental release of a chemical, biological, radiological, or nuclear (CBRN) agent
2. Natural epidemics or pandemics, which may involve a novel, emerging infectious disease, a reemerging agent, a previously controlled disease, or occur in areas with limited infrastructure or resources
3. Natural disasters such as hurricanes, earthquakes, floods, or fires
4. Man-made environmental disasters such as oil spills

For any of these categories of events to be classified as a public health emergency, it is not just enough for the event to occur, but it also must pose a high probability of large-scale morbidity, mortality, or a risk of future harm.

A Trust for America's Health (TFAH) report refers to public health preparedness as requiring the basic functions of a public health system, such as epidemiology, laboratory capacity, and event-based surveillance capacity.[9,10] These core functions need to be supplemented by specialized training, procedures, laws, regulations, and planning, so that all relevant sectors can operate effectively and in a coordinated fashion during a crisis. Doing this well also requires the development of systems for surge capacity, distribution of medical countermeasures, and detecting and managing a response to rapidly mitigate the consequences of the event and move toward recovery.

At the global level, the World Health Organization's Revised International Health Regulations, adopted in 2005, define a public health emergency of international concern (PHEIC) as "[A]n extraordinary event which is determined . . . to constitute a public health risk to other States through the international spread of disease and to potentially require a coordinated international response."[11] Such an emergency can involve any of the above four types of public health events, as long as it is unusual, unexpected, and has the potential to cross international borders.

Some public health concerns that have been called "emergencies" do not meet the criteria of any of the previous definitions. Public health preparedness refers to planning for and responding to acute events, as opposed to chronic conditions that evolve over time. The prevalence of breast cancer, for example, may be a "public health crisis," but it is not considered an emergency within the purview of public health preparedness.[12(pp2282-2283)]

Effective public health preparedness spans a wide range of activities. This text focuses primarily on the policy and legal actions to support preparedness and application of the principals of emergency management to public health operations, but a "prepared community" also entails the ability to do the following:

- Perform health risk assessments
- Establish an incident command system or related structure
- Actively engage and communicate effectively with the public
- Have functional epidemiologic and laboratory capacity to perform surveillance, detect emerging events, and appropriately diagnose patients
- Be able to deploy rapid response teams to investigate outbreaks
- Develop, stockpile, and distribute medical countermeasures (drugs and vaccines)
- Have "surge capacity" within the medical system to provide care for large populations during an emergency
- Maintain an appropriate workforce, financial resources, communication systems, and logistics to detect, respond to, and recover from events[8]

The responsibility of the public health community to prepare for and address acute health emergencies is thus extensive and can be a challenge, particularly in environments where the public health system is under-resourced.

Emergency Management

The Federal Emergency Management Agency defines emergency management as the managerial function charged with creating the framework within which communities reduce vulnerability to hazards and cope with disasters. The mission of emergency management is to protect communities by coordinating and integrating all activities necessary to build, sustain, and improve the capability to mitigate against, prepare for, respond to, and recover from threatened or actual natural disasters, acts of terrorism, or other man-made disasters.[13]

▶ Public Health Preparedness and Federalism

Public health preparedness requires cooperation among a variety of sectors at multiple levels of government. At the federal level, multiple agencies such as the Departments of Health and Human Services (including Centers for Disease Control and Prevention [CDC], National Institutes of Health, the Food and Drug Administration, and the other agencies within the department), Homeland Security, State, Defense, Justice, Transportation, Commerce, Energy and Treasury; the Environmental Protection Agency; and the Intelligence Community are all involved and are coordinated in the end by the National Security Council staff of the White House.

While a strong federal policy and infrastructure is essential, public health professionals recognize that most public health activities occur at the local and state levels. Clinical care is an essential component of public health, yet that care is not coordinated or delivered in Washington, DC. It is in every doctor's office, hospital, and clinic around the country. Disease surveillance is essential, but it starts with detection of an unusual event—for example, by an astute clinician or a capable laboratory, wherever the event emerges. Not only is this a reality in practice, it is codified by the 10th Amendment of the Constitution: "The powers not delegated to the United States by the Constitution, nor prohibited by it to the States, are reserved to the States respectively, or to the people."[14] This means that police powers, including the powers to regulate

health and safety, are the responsibility of the states. The federal government supports public health preparedness domestically, as it must build relations globally to ensure an effective worldwide system for preparedness, information sharing, and collaboration in preventing, detecting, reporting, and responding to public health threats. It is the state and local entities, however, that are relied upon to implement policies, build infrastructure, and interface with local populations to promote health security. This is the case in the United States, as it is throughout the world.

States have the responsibility for developing their own emergency preparedness plans, and all have some level of planning and preparedness training in place. Preparedness efforts at the state level have strived to meet national preparedness objectives, yet at the same time focus on the unique threats, challenges, assets, and populations specific to particular jurisdictions. States that are subject to relatively more frequent hurricanes may have well-developed plans to address that particular hazard, while landlocked states far from oceans may have better-developed plans for disasters such as tornadoes. States will also take into account the particular demographics of their region when planning how to address vulnerable populations, nursing homes, and schools in emergencies.

In carrying out their responsibilities, state and local public health professionals are supported by several professional associations, including the American Public Health Association (APHA), the Council of State and Territorial Epidemiologists (CSTE), the Association of Public Health Laboratories (APHL), the Association of State and Territorial Health Officers (ASTHO), and the National Association of County and City Health Officials (NACCHO). These associations play an active role in providing guidance, securing funding, and assisting the public health workforce in meeting the preparedness challenge.

▶ Developing the Public Health Preparedness Workforce: Charge and Careers

In December 2006, Congress passed the Pandemic and All-Hazards Preparedness Act (known as PAHPA, pronounced "papa"), which reauthorized and built upon the Public Health Security and Bioterrorism Preparedness and Response Act (also known as the Bioterrorism Act of 2002). Among other things,

BOX 1-3 Pandemic and All-Hazards Preparedness Act of 2006. Section 304: Core Education and Training

TITLE III—ALL-HAZARDS MEDICAL SURGE CAPACITY
SEC. 304. CORE EDUCATION AND TRAINING
(d) Centers for Public Health Preparedness; Core Curricula and Training—

1. IN GENERAL—The Secretary may establish at accredited schools of public health, Centers for Public Health Preparedness (hereafter referred to in this section as the "Centers").
2. ELIGIBILITY—To be eligible to receive an award under this subsection to establish a Center, an accredited school of public health shall agree to conduct activities consistent with the requirements of this subsection.
3. CORE CURRICULA—The Secretary, in collaboration with the Centers and other public or private entities shall establish core curricula based on established competencies leading to a 4-year bachelor's degree, a graduate degree, a combined bachelor and master's degree, or a certificate program, for use by each Center. The Secretary shall disseminate such curricula to other accredited schools of public health and other health professions schools determined appropriate by the Secretary, for voluntary use by such schools.
4. CORE COMPETENCY-BASED TRAINING PROGRAM—The Secretary, in collaboration with the Centers and other public or private entities shall facilitate the development of a competency-based training program to train public health practitioners. The Centers shall use such training program to train public health practitioners. The Secretary shall disseminate such training program to other accredited schools of public health, health professions schools, and other public or private entities as determined by the Secretary, for voluntary use by such entities.
5. CONTENT OF CORE CURRICULA AND TRAINING PROGRAM—The Secretary shall ensure that the core curricula and training program established pursuant to this subsection respond to the needs of State, local, and tribal public health authorities and integrate and emphasize essential public health security capabilities consistent with section 2802(b)(2).

Pandemic and All-Hazards Preparedness Act., P.L. 109–417 (2006).

PAHPA called for the development of a public health workforce versed in preparedness and public health security capabilities (**BOX 1-3**). It required curricula to be developed and called for the facilitation of competency-based training in public health preparedness within schools of public health and other institutions. It should be noted that the reauthorization of PAHPA in 2013 did not explicitly discuss training in schools of public health.

The ASPPH—with support from U.S. CDC—developed model core competencies in public health preparedness and response (PHPR). ASPPH efforts were targeted at public health workers who have 10 years of experience or 5 years with a master's in public health (MPH) or higher degree, and focused on four core areas (see **FIGURE 1-1**).[15]

In today's climate, it is important for many different types of public health professionals, at every level of government and the private sector with diverse knowledge and expertise, to be versed in public health preparedness. When a public health emergency occurs, it affects the entire public health and medical system. Everyone from laboratory technicians to clinicians to program managers may be affected. We hope this text provides important context for the next generation of leaders in public health preparedness and emergency management.

▶ Jobs in Public Health Preparedness

Trained professionals in public health preparedness and emergency management are now sought after by a multitude of organizations and agencies. This ranges from public health and healthcare organizations looking to be better positioned for public health emergencies to security communities broadening their scope to include public health. Below are some examples of areas in which public health preparedness and emergency management personnel are sought after:

■ *Private sector:* Think tanks, consulting firms, private industry, and government contractors hire public health professionals who specialize in preparedness. These jobs include operational planning for private companies, strategic planning for the pharmaceutical industry, and policy analysis and training to support both government entities and clinical operations.
■ *State and local government:* Just about every state and local health department now has dedicated staff for preparedness, and most jurisdictions have emergency management teams focused on public health. In addition, state and local departments of emergency management, agriculture, commerce, and transportation may also employ public health

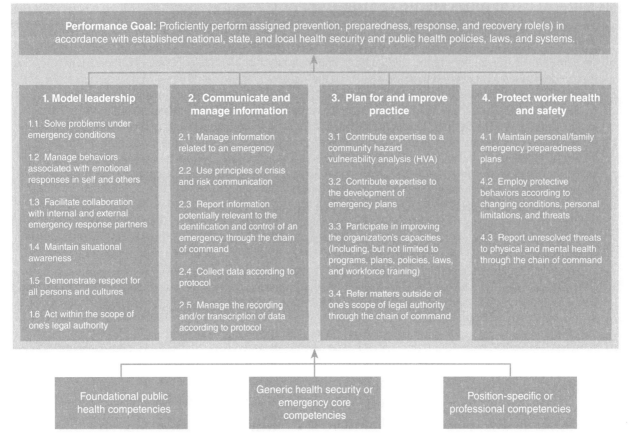

FIGURE 1-1 Public health preparedness and response competency map

preparedness experts, which again demonstrate the necessity of diverse expertise.

- *Academia:* Researchers are needed to further the field of preparedness, and informed professors are required for curriculum development and training of students and mid-career professionals.

- *Federal government:* As we will learn throughout this text, the federal government is heavily involved in public health preparedness, requiring skilled professionals to work not just at the Department of Health and Human Services, but also at the Departments of State, Agriculture, Defense, Treasury, Justice, Homeland Security,

and within the Intelligence Community and the U.S. Agency for International Development.

- *International organizations:* Nongovernmental organizations (NGO) and international organizations (IOs), such as those that are part of the United Nations, are engaged in public health preparedness activities. These include everything from disaster management to refugee health to law enforcement.

In all, there is a great deal of work to be accomplished and a need for smart, energetic, and enthusiastic people. The world can always use more strong public health professionals, and specifically public health professionals who can contribute to emergency preparedness and response.

Key Words

Community preparedness	Homeland defense	Pandemic and All-Hazards Preparedness Act
Core competencies	Homeland security	Public health preparedness
Emergency management	National security	Workforce

Discussion Questions

1. Is public health preparedness the same as national preparedness? Is public health preparedness well defined and can it be operationalized?
2. What types of emergency events require a public health role?
3. What types of public health emergencies require planning for underserved populations and how such planning might be incorporated into preparedness activities?
4. What is the difference between national and homeland security?
5. From the list of eleven components of public health preparedness, which three do you think are most important and should be prioritized? Why?
6. What is the role of public health officials in emergency management?

References

1. Bergen P, Garrett L. *The Princeton Project on National Security Report of the Working Group on State Security and Transnational Threats*. pp 41–56. Available at: http://www.princeton.edu/~ppns/conferences/reports/fall/SSTT.pdf. Accessed June 2017.
2. Hamilton A. *The Federalist No. 8, The Consequences of Hostilities Between the States*. November 20, 1787.
3. Advanced Materials and Processes Technology Information Analysis Center. Homeland Security vs. Homeland Defense. Is There a Difference? *The AMPTIAC Quarterly*. February 2003;6(4):24–29. Available at: https://www.dsiac.org/sites/default/files/journals/AMPQ6_4.pdf. Accessed June 2017.
4. Office of Homeland Security. *National Strategy for Homeland Security*. July 2002. Available at: https://www.dhs.gov/sites/default/files/publications/nat-strat-hls-2002.pdf. Accessed June 2017.
5. Kettl DF. The Century Foundation. *The States and Homeland Security, Building the Missing Link*. New York, NY: Century Foundation; 2003.
6. United States Department of Defense. *DoD 101, An Introductory Overview of the Department of Defense*. Available at: https://www.defense.gov/About/DoD-101/. Accessed June 2017.
7. Association of Schools of Public Health, Core Curricula Working Group. *Practical Implications, Approaches, Opportunities and Challenges of a Preparedness Core Curricula in Accredited Schools of Public Health*. 2012.
8. Nelson C, Lurie N, Wasserman J, et al. Conceptualizing and Defining Public Health Emergency Preparedness. *American Journal of Public Health*. 2007;97(S1):S9–S11.
9. This section comes from Katz R, Standley, C. Public health preparedness policy. In: Teitelbaum, JB, ed. *Essentials of Health Policy & Law*, 3rd ed. Burlington, MA: Jones & Bartlett; 2017:253–270.
10. Levi J, Segal LM, Lieberman DA, et al. *Outbreaks: Protecting Americans from Infectious Diseases*. Trust for America's Health. 2014. Available at: http://healthyamericans.org/assets/files/Final%20Outbreaks%202014%20Report.pdf. Accessed June 2017.
11. World Health Organization. *International Health Regulations (2005)*. 2nd ed. 2008. Article I. Available at: http://whqlibdoc.who.int/publications/2008/9789241580410_eng.pdf. Accessed June 2017.
12. Harford J, Azavedo E, Fischietto M, Breast Health Global Initiative Healthcare Systems Panel. Guideline Implementation for Breast Healthcare in Low- and Middle-Income Countries: Breast Healthcare Program Resource Allocation. *Cancer*. 2008;113(8 Suppl):2282–2296.
13. FEMA. *Emergency Management: Definition, Vision, Mission, Principles*. Available at: https://training.fema.gov/hiedu/docs/emprinciples/0907_176%20em%20principles12x18v2f%20johnson%20(w-o%20draft).pdf. Accessed June 2017.
14. Constitution of the United States of America. Tenth amendment.
15. Association of Schools of Public Health Preparedness and Response, Core Competency Development Project Leadership Group. *Public Health Preparedness and Response Core Competency Development Project Tenets, Target Audience, and Performance Level*. 2010.

© f00sion/E+/Getty

PART II
Defining the Problem

CHAPTER 2

Threats from Biological, Chemical, Nuclear, and Radiological Weapons

By the end of this chapter, the reader will be able to:

- Define biological, chemical, radiological, and nuclear weapons
- Understand the threats from and history of use of weapons of mass destruction
- Characterize the current threat from weapons of mass destruction, specifically biological weapons, used by both state and non state actors
- Identify the public health community's role in responding to weapons of mass destruction

▶ Introduction

In this chapter, we begin to explore and define the threats the public health community should be prepared to address. We begin with a focus on weapons of mass destruction (WMD), including chemical, biological, radiological, and nuclear (CBRN) weapons. While we look at all of these types of weapons, our main focus will be predominately on biological weapons, as they are most directly linked to the public health and medical communities through detection, response, and recovery. Public health, though, is responsible for managing the health consequences of all threats, regardless of origin.

For the public health and medical communities to be prepared for and to respond appropriately to CBRN threats, they must work closely with a wide range of communities. Many of these groups, such as law enforcement, military entities, and the intelligence community, are not traditional public health partners. These communities and the specific interactions are discussed in more detail later in the text. Here, we present the WMD threats. We look first at chemical, then nuclear and radiological threats, and then focus on the details of biological weapons more extensively. The majority of this chapter, and the rest of this text, centers on the biological threat, as this threat has the strongest links to public health preparedness.

▶ Chemical Threats

Article II, paragraph 1 of the Chemical Weapons Convention (CWC) defines chemical weapons as one of the following, either in combination or separately:

(a) Toxic chemicals and their precursors, except where intended for purposes not prohibited under this convention, as long as the types and quantities are consistent with such purposes

(b) Munitions and devices, specifically designed to cause death or other harm through the toxic properties of those toxic chemicals specified in subparagraph (c), which would be released as a result of the employment of such munitions and devices

(c) Any equipment specifically designed for use directly in connection with the employment of munitions and devices specified in subparagraph (b)[1]

In general, chemical warfare is the use of a chemical substance to directly harm or kill human, plants, or animals. (It is worth noting that the CWC does not include chemicals that harm plants. The Geneva Protocol of 1925, however, does incorporate anti-plant agents. There is some debate over whether defoliants and other chemicals used against plants should be considered chemical weapons under international legal regimes.[2]) Chemical agents are nonliving, manufactured chemicals. They tend to be highly toxic and can enter the body through inhalation or through the skin. Adding to the complexity of treatment, illness or death can come within minutes of exposure, or take as long as several hours.[3] As described in **BOX 2-1** and **2-2**, there are several main categories of chemical warfare agents: blister (e.g., mustard gas), blood (e.g., cyanide), choking (e.g., chlorine), and nerve (e.g., sarin). Toxins (discussed in the next subhead) are also a major category of agents, as are psychotomimetic agents, which can alter mental status. In addition, there is a class termed "riot control agents," which produce temporary, usually nonfatal irritation of the skin, eyes, and respiratory tract. Riot control agents, often known as "tear gas," include chloroacetophenone (CN), chlorobenzylidene-malononitrile (CS), and chloropicrin (PS). The CWC and the U.S. government do not consider this class of agents to be chemical weapons. Other nations, however, disagree.[4]

The public health response to chemical events will range depending on the event itself, its origin, and the location. Possible activities may include the following:

- Issuing shelter-in-place orders
- Evacuating populations
- Organizing decontamination efforts
- Restricting entry to particular areas
- Ensuring food and water are safe
- Immediate and long-term monitoring of health effects[5]

Toxins

Toxins are nonliving poisons produced by living entities, such as plants, fungi, insects, and animals. Because they are chemical by-products of biological agents, they occupy a conceptual gray area between chemical and biological weapons. The Biological Weapons Convention covers toxins, and the CWC covers a discrete list of toxins, including ricin. This is another area where for the purposes of arms control and legal international obligations, countries do not always agree on how toxins should be categorized.

BOX 2-1 Types of Chemical Agents

- **Nerve agents**—primarily act on the nervous system, causing seizures and death. Examples of this category include sarin, VX, tabun, and soman. This category also includes fourth-generation chemical weapons, known as novichok agents, which are thought to be much more lethal than VX.
- **Blister agents or vesicants**—primarily cause irritation of the skin and mucous membrane. Examples of this category include mustard gas and arsenical lewisite.
- **Choking agents or pulmonary toxicants**—primarily cause damage to the lungs, including pulmonary edema and hemorrhage. Examples include phosgene, diphosgene, and chlorine.
- **Blood agents**—primarily cause seizures and respiratory and cardiac failure in high doses. Examples include hydrogen cyanide and cyanogen cyanide.
- **Riot control agents**—cause incapacitation due to irritation of eyes and respiratory system. Examples include CN, CS, and dibenzoxazepine (CR).
- **Psychotomimetic agents**—in low doses, these cause psychiatric effects. An example is lysergic acid diethylamide (LSD).
- **Toxins**—symptoms range from death to incapacitation depending on the agent. Examples include ricin and saxitoxin.

Data from Ganesan K, Raza SK, Vijayaraghavan R. Chemical Warfare Agents. *Journal of Pharmacy and BioAllied Sciences*. 2010;2(3): 166–178. 10.4103/0975-7406.68498; Organisation for the Prohibition of Chemical Weapons. Types of Chemical Agents. *About Chemical Weapons*. Available at: https://www.opcw.org/about-chemical-weapons/types-of-chemical-agent/. Accessed April 2017.

BOX 2-2 Schedule 1 of the Chemical Weapons Convention

The CWC maintains a list of chemicals and precursors for monitoring purposes. Schedule 1 chemicals and precursors are for those chemicals that can most easily be used as weapons and there is very little use for them otherwise. Below is a list of the Schedule 1 chemicals:

1. *O*-Alkyl (<C_{10}, including cycloalkyl) alkyl (Me, Et, *n*-Pr, or *i*-Pr)-phosphonofluoridates, for example,
   Sarin: *O*-isopropyl methylphosphonofluoridate
   Soman: *O*-pinacolyl methylphosphonofluoridate
   Schedule 1 phosphoramidocyanidates, where R_1 = (cyclo)alkyl with C < C_{10} and R_2/R_3 = Me, Et, *i*-Pr, or *n*-Pr
   Schedule 1 phosphonothiolate, where R_1 = *H* or (cyclo)alkyl with C < C_{10} and $R_2/R_3/R_4$ = Me, Et, *i*-Pr, or *n*-Pr
2. *O*-Alkyl (<C_{10}, including cycloalkyl) *N,N*-dialkyl (Me, Et, *n*-Pr, or i-Pr) phosphoramidocyanidates, for example,
   Tabun: *O*-ethyl *N,N*-dimethylphosphoramidocyanidate
3. *O*-Alkyl (*H* or <C_{10}, including cycloalkyl) *S*-2-dialkyl (Me, Et, *n*-Pr, or *i*-Pr)-aminoethyl alkyl (Me, Et, *n*-Pr, or *i*-Pr) phosphonothiolates and corresponding alkylated or protonated salts, for example,
   VX: *O*-ethyl *S*-2-diisopropylaminoethyl methylphosphonothiolate
4. Sulfur mustards:
   2-Chloroethylchloromethylsulfide
   Mustard gas: bis(2-chloroethyl)sulfide
   Bis(2-chloroethylthio)methane
   Sesquimustard: 1,2-bis(2-chloroethylthio)ethane
   1,3-Bis(2-chloroethylthio)-*n*-propane
   1,4-Bis(2-chloroethylthio)-*n*-butane
   1,5-Bis(2-chloroethylthio)-*n*-pentane
   Bis(2-chloroethylthiomethyl)ether
   O-Mustard: bis(2-chloroethylthioethyl)ether
5. Lewisites:
   Lewisite 1: 2-chlorovinyldichloroarsine
   Lewisite 2: bis(2-chlorovinyl)chloroarsine
   Lewisite 3: tris(2-chlorovinyl)arsine
6. Nitrogen mustards:
   HN1: bis(2-chloroethyl)ethylamine
   HN2: bis(2-chloroethyl)methylamine
   HN3: tris(2-chloroethyl)amine
7. Saxitoxin
8. Ricin

Reproduced from Organisation for the Prohibition of Chemical Weapons. *Annex on Chemicals Schedule 1.* Available at: https://www.opcw.org/chemical-weapons-convention/annexes/annex-on-chemicals/. Accessed April 2017.

History

In April 1915, during World War I, the German army attacked the French with chlorine gas in Ypres, Belgium, marking the first large-scale use of chemical weapons during warfare. Several months later, in September 1915, the British used chlorine gas against the Germans at the Battle of Loos. This was followed in June 1918 by the first use of chemical warfare by the United States. It was clear that by the end of World War I, all sides were actively using the chemical weapons in their arsenals.[6] **FIGURE 2-1** shows soldiers in World War I suffering from the effects of chemical warfare.

Many nations continued to utilize chemical warfare throughout the 20th century, including the British use of adamsite (a vomiting agent) against the Bolsheviks during the Russian Civil War, Spanish use of chemical weapons against rebels in Morocco in the 1920s, Italian use of mustard gas against Ethiopians in 1936, and Nazi German use of hydrocyanic acid for the mass extermination of Jews and other concentration camp prisoners.[7]

During the Vietnam War, the United States used defoliants such as dioxin, also known as "Agent Orange," as well as other normally nonlethal agents. The United States does not consider defoliants to be chemical weapons, therefore it does not consider this use to be chemical warfare. High levels of morbidity and mortality from those exposed to the agents, though, have led to large research efforts and calls by many that this was, in fact, chemical warfare.[8,9]

Other examples of chemical warfare include the use of phosgene and mustard gas by Egypt against

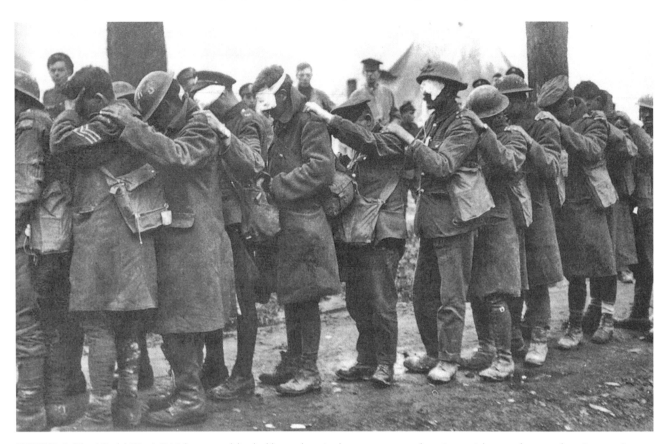

FIGURE 2-1 The World War I: British troops blinded by a chemical weapons attack wait outside an advance dressing station, near Bethune, France. Each man has his hand on the shoulder of the man in front of him. Battle of Estaires.
(An image reminiscent of John Singer Sargent's famous painting "Gassed.")
© Photo 12/Universal Images Group/Getty.

Yemen (1963–1967), and the use of chemical weapons by Iraq during the Iran–Iraq War (primarily in 1983 and 1984), initially with riot control agents and eventually using mustard gas.[10,11] One particular use of chemical weapons by Iraq was repeatedly cited as part of the U.S. rationale in 2002 for invading the country.[12] In 1988, in a campaign against the Kurds, Saddam Hussein used what was most likely to be mustard gas, possibly mixed with sarin, against the town of Halabja, killing thousands.[13]

More recently, Syria, under President Bashar Al-Assad, was accused of using chemical weapons in the civil war that started in 2012.[14–16] Almost immediately, there were concerns about the implications for Syria's suspected stockpile of chemical weapons, with subsequent reports (verified by the Organization for the Prohibition of Chemical Weapons (OPCW) and the United Nations) of use of mustard and chlorine gases.[17] A 2016 report found that the Islamic State terrorist organization had used chemical weapons at least 52 times in Syria and Iraq since 2014. Most of those attacks were tied to chlorine or sulfur mustard agents.[18]

Another example of the offensive use of chemical agents comes from the doomsday cult Aum Shinrikyo, based in Japan. On March 20, 1995, Aum Shinrikyo released sarin gas into the Tokyo subway system. Twelve people died, approximately 50 were severely injured, and almost 1000 suffered temporary vision problems.[19] Over 5500 people, however, sought medical attention, swarming area hospitals and testing public health capacities. This chemical weapons use event highlighted the importance of emergency preparedness, especially in the area of hospital surge capacity and triage.

While most of the cited examples of chemical weapons use have been large-scale warfare incidents, these agents have also been used throughout history as assassination tools (**TABLE 2-1**).[20] One particularly illustrative example was the 1979 assassination of a Bulgarian exile named Georgi Markov (**BOX 2-3**).

In addition to intentional releases of chemical agents, the accidental releases of agents have also posed significant challenges to public health and medical systems worldwide, and have adversely affected the health of populations. (See **FIGURE 2-2** for numbers of persons evacuated from chemical events in select areas of the United States.) For example, in 1981, cooking oil was accidentally

TABLE 2-1 Select Chemical Incidents Since 1976

Year	Location	Description of Incident	Consequences
1976	Seveso, Italy	Airborne release of dioxin from an industrial plant	▪ No immediate human deaths ▪ 3,300 animal deaths ▪ 80,000 animals slaughtered
1984	Bhopal, India	Methyl isocyanate (MIC) leak from tank	▪ 3,800 immediate deaths ▪ 15,000–20,000 premature deaths ▪ 500,000 exposed to the gas
1984	Mexico City, Mexico	Explosion of liquefied petroleum gas (LPG) terminal	▪ 500 deaths ▪ 6,400 injuries
1995	Tokyo, Japan	Deliberate release of warfare agent	▪ 12 deaths ▪ 54 critical casualties ▪ Thousands of people affected
2000	Enschede, The Netherlands	Explosion of a fireworks factory	▪ 20 deaths ▪ 562 casualties ▪ Hundreds of houses destroyed ▪ 2,000 people evacuated
2001	Toulouse, France	Explosion of 300–400 tons of ammonium nitrate in a fertilizer facility	▪ 30 deaths ▪ 2,500 casualties ▪ 500 homes uninhabitable
2002	Galicia, Spain	Shipwreck of the *Prestige*, causing the release of 77,000 tons of fuel	▪ Estimated cleanup costs of U.S. $2.8 billion
2002	Jabalpur, India	Mass poisoning due to the use of pesticide containers as kitchen utensils	▪ 3 deaths ▪ At least 10 hospitalizations
2003	Baton Rouge, USA	Release of chlorine gas from a facility	▪ No human deaths
2004	Neyshabur, Iran	Train explosion due to mixing of incompatible chemicals	▪ Hundreds of deaths and casualties among emergency responders and onlookers
2005	Songhua River, China	Plant explosion releasing 100 tons of pollutants in the Songhua River	▪ 5 deaths ▪ Millions of people without water for several days
2005	Bohol, The Philippines	Inadvertent use of an insecticide in the preparation of sweets	▪ 29 deaths ▪ 104 hospitalizations
2005	Hemel Hempstead, England	3 explosions in an oil storage facility (Buncefield depot)	▪ 43 injuries reported ▪ 2,000 persons evacuated
2006	Abidjan, Côte d'Ivoire	Dumping of toxic waste in the city of Abidjan	▪ 10 deaths ▪ Thousands made ill
2006	Panama	Diethylene glycol in a cough syrup	▪ At least 100 deaths
2007	Angola	Sodium bromide confused with tablet salt	▪ At least 460 people ill, most of them children
2008	Senegal	Lead from informal battery recycling	▪ People exposed, with many children showing symptoms of lead intoxication

Reproduced from World Health Organization. Examples of Chemical Incidents Worldwide. *Manual for the Public Health Management of Chemical Incidents*. 2009;WA 670:4. Available at: http://www.who.int/environmental_health_emergencies/publications/FINAL-PHM-Chemical-Incidents_web.pdf. Accessed April 2017.

BOX 2-3 Assassination by Ricin

In 1978, a Bulgarian exile named Georgi Markov was waiting for a bus in London. A man poked him with the tip of an umbrella, apologized, and got into a taxi. Four days later, Markov was dead.

Ten days prior to this incident, another Bulgarian exile, Vladimir Kostov, was stabbed in the back in Paris, and when he turned around, he witnessed someone running away with an umbrella. This particular umbrella had been adapted and rebuilt into a makeshift gun that fired ricin pellets from its tip. After learning of Markov's death, Kostov sought medical attention immediately. A doctor removed the pellet that had lodged in his back. Fortunately, the ricin that was contained within the pellet had not fully expelled into his blood stream. The doctor successfully removed it, confirmed the presence of ricin, and Kostov survived the incident.

One of the reasons ricin was such an effective assassination tool was that it was virtually impossible to detect what was killing Markov, and there was little authorities could have done even if it was identified. Ricin, a poison extracted from castor beans, prevents cells in the body from making proteins, and without proteins, cells die, which can eventually lead to death. Once exposed, it can take up to 6–8 hours for symptoms to occur, depending on the route of exposure, and death can occur rapidly within 36–72 hours. The symptoms of ricin exposure include respiratory distress if inhaled, vomiting and diarrhea if ingested, and redness and pain of skin and eyes if absorbed through skin. There is no available antidote at present, and the only treatment is supportive medical care.

Data from Centers for Disease Control and Prevention. Facts about Ricin. *Emergency Preparedness and Response*. Available at: https://emergency.cdc.gov/agent/ricin/facts.asp. March 5, 2008. Accessed April 2017.

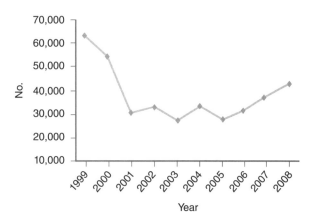

FIGURE 2-2 Number of persons evacuated for chemical incidents, by year in nine states (Colorado, Iowa, Minnesota, New York, North Carolina, Oregon, Texas, Washington, and Wisconsin) in the United States between 1999 and 2008

Reproduced from Melnikova N, Wu J, Orr MF. Number of Persons Evacuated for Chemical Incidents, by Year. Public Health Response to Acute Chemical Incidents—Hazardous Substances Emergency Events Surveillance, Nine States, 1999–2008. *MMWR*. 2015; 64(2): 28. Available at: https://www.cdc.gov/mmwr/pdf/ss/ss6402.pdf. Accessed April 2017.

adulterated with industrial rapeseed oil and distributed throughout southern Europe. Over 15,000 people became sick and 203 died after consuming the contaminated oil.[21]

In some instances, the release of chemical agents may not have been entirely accidental, but one assumes that the public health consequences were unintentional. In 2006, a Panamanian-flag, Greek-owned, Swiss oil company chartered tanker, the *Probo Koala*, avoiding European disposal fees, carried over 500 tons of petrochemical waste to Côte d'Ivoire, which was then dumped by a local contractor in more than 12 different sites around Abidjan. Fifteen people died as a result of exposure to this toxic waste, 69 were hospitalized, and over 100,000 sought medical treatment, easily overwhelming the existing public health and medical infrastructures.[22–24]

Unfortunately, these types of exposures to chemical agents are not infrequent. On May 29, 2010, a worker at a scrap yard in Nigeria tried to cut a gas cylinder into pieces, resulting in an explosion that released a cloud of chlorine gas into the air, sickening 300 people who eventually required medical treatment.[25]

The largest chemical agent accidental exposure took place on December 3, 1984, in Bhopal, India. A Union Carbide pesticide plant released 40 tons of methyl isocyanate (MIC) gas into the air in the middle of the night. Nearly 4,000 people died instantly, and the total number of deaths is estimated to be between 15,000 and 22,000; 500,000 people were exposed; and as many as 120,000 continue to suffer detrimental health effects.[26]

Accidents that expose populations to chemical agents can occur anywhere, including the United States. For example, a community in Graniteville, South Carolina, was left with 9 dead and 250 injured after a train carrying toxic chemicals, including chlorine gas, crashed.[27] Accidents such as these remind us that all public health communities, regardless of location, must have a level of awareness regarding preparedness for a variety of potential public health emergencies, including the need to know how to respond to an emergency.

▶ Nuclear and Radiological Threats

Nuclear Weapons

A nuclear weapon that involves fission (the splitting of atoms)—like the bomb that the United States detonated in Hiroshima, Japan, during World War II, or the devastating weapons created and stockpiled by a small number of nations since—leaves a limited role for the public health community. Such weapons, if released, would instantly destroy people, buildings, and anything else in the vicinity. There would be no need for a public health response, because the chances of survival would be minimal. The explosion, however, would leave behind large amounts of radioactivity. We discuss the challenge of radioactivity next in the "Radiological Threats" section.

Radiological Threats

A radiologic event is an explosion or other release of radioactivity. Such an event might be caused by any of the following: a simple, nonexplosive radiological device; an improvised nuclear device designed to release large amounts of radiation with a large blast radius (such as a "suitcase bomb"); a dispersal device that combines explosive materials and radioactive material (such as a "dirty bomb"); or damage to a nuclear reactor that results in the release of radiation.[28]

Even a small dose of radiation can cause some detectable changes in blood. Large doses of radiation can lead to acute radiation syndrome (ARS). First signs of ARS are typically nausea, vomiting, headache, diarrhea, and some loss of white blood cells. These signs are followed by hair loss, damage to nerve cells and cells that line the digestive tract, and severe loss of white blood cells. The higher the dose of radiation, the less likely the person will survive. Those who survive may take several weeks to 2 years to recover, and survivors may suffer from leukemia or other cancers.[29]

The public health implications of radiologic exposure can be significant. In addition to all other functions, the public health community will be responsible for the following:

- Participating in shelter-in-place or evacuation decisions
- Identifying exposed populations through surveillance activities
- Conducting or assisting with environmental decontamination
- Determining safety requirements for working in or near the site of the incident
- Conducting near and long-term follow up with exposed populations[30]

In recent years, we have seen radiation used as an assassination tool. In 2006, Alexander Litvinenko, a former agent of the Federal Security Service (FSS) in Russia who was living in the United Kingdom under political asylum, was poisoned with polonium-210 in his tea, resulting in ARS. Over the course of a month, officials in the United Kingdom had identified additional individuals who had been exposed to the material. The poisoning and the subsequent investigation created a series of challenges for the public health community, including deciding who to screen for exposure, how to screen for exposure, who to treat for radiation exposure, and how to treat.[31] All of these decisions had to be made in an environment of uncertainty, with a public that was rightfully concerned and confused about the risk, and with an undercurrent of international diplomatic tension between the United Kingdom and Russia.

To date, most radiologic exposure has occurred via accidents. An often-cited event occurred in Goiânia, Brazil, in 1987. Two men were rummaging through an abandoned hospital and found an old nuclear medicine source—a radioactive cesium-137 teletherapy head. They took it home, partially dismantled it, and eventually sold it to a scrap yard. The owner of the scrap yard discovered that the cesium capsule omitted a blue light; many came to see it and children rubbed the material on their bodies to glow in the dark. Four people, including a young child, died from the exposure. Another 249 individuals suffered serious health consequences.[32]

The most serious radiation accidents have been associated with nuclear power plants. Sixty-three accidents have occurred at nuclear power plants, with the most serious occurring in Chernobyl, Ukraine. On April 26, 1986, at 1:23 A.M., Reactor 4 of the Chernobyl Nuclear Power Plant exploded, instantly killing three and sending a plume of radioactive fallout into the air, which eventually drifted over parts of the Soviet Union, eastern Europe, western Europe, northern Europe, and eastern North America. Approximately 350,000 individuals had to be evacuated and resettled. Fifty-six people died as a direct result of the accident. Another 4000 have died from cancers linked to radiation exposure (**FIGURES 2-3** and **2-4**).[33]

The public health community's immediate and long-term responsibility in response to the Chernobyl disaster was significant, including assessing the safety of the environment for human habitation, addressing the psychological impact of the disaster on affected populations, monitoring the long-term health and well-being of exposed populations, and planning for the treatment of untold numbers of current and future cancer patients.[33,34]

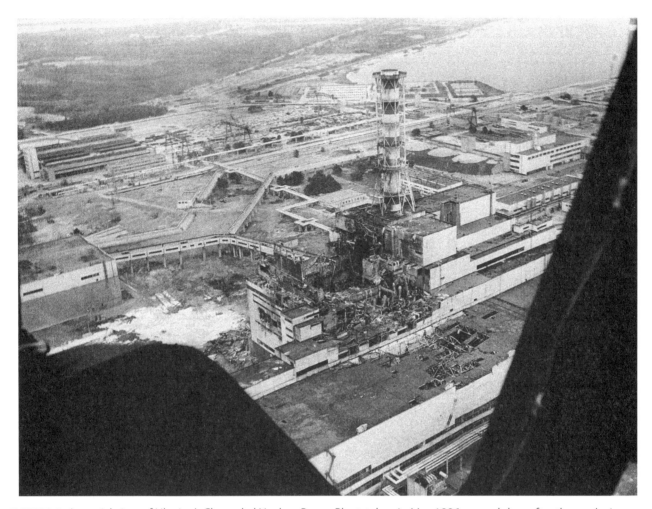

FIGURE 2-3 An aerial view of Ukraine's Chernobyl Nuclear Power Plant, taken in May 1986, several days after the explosion on April 26, 1986

© Associated Press.

In 2011, another major disaster occurred at a nuclear power plant. On March 11, 2011, following a massive earthquake and subsequent tsunami, three reactors at the Fukushima Daiichi power plant in Japan melted over the course of 3 days (after the tsunami led to the failure of the emergency generators needed to cool the reactors; **FIGURE 2-5**). While no direct deaths from the power plant accident occurred, over 100,000 people were evacuated from their homes (everyone within a 30-km radius), and radiation was tracked to have spread across the ocean. U.S. researchers also found that over 1000 people have died as a result of the evacuation.[35] Additionally, public health officials tracked radioactivity in vegetables, milk, and water near the reactor sites.

A 2013 report by the World Health Organization (WHO) found that the greatest impact to health from the Fukushima disaster was an increased risk of cancer for the exposed population. The lifetime risk of most cancers over baseline ranged from 4% to 7%, with the exception being an increase of 70% over baseline for the risk of developing thyroid cancer.[36]

In addition to the public health risk of accidental radiologic exposure, the global community continues to be concerned about the intentional use of a nuclear or radiologic device. In April 2010, President Barack Obama called the global community to a Nuclear Security Summit, where the nations of the world clearly acknowledged the threat of nuclear terrorism. President Obama delivered the following statement:

Two decades after the end of the Cold War, we face a cruel irony of history—the risk of a nuclear confrontation between nations has gone down, but the risk of nuclear attack has gone up.

Nuclear materials that could be sold or stolen and fashioned into a nuclear weapon exist in dozens of nations. Just the smallest amount of plutonium—about the size of an apple—could kill and injure hundreds of thousands

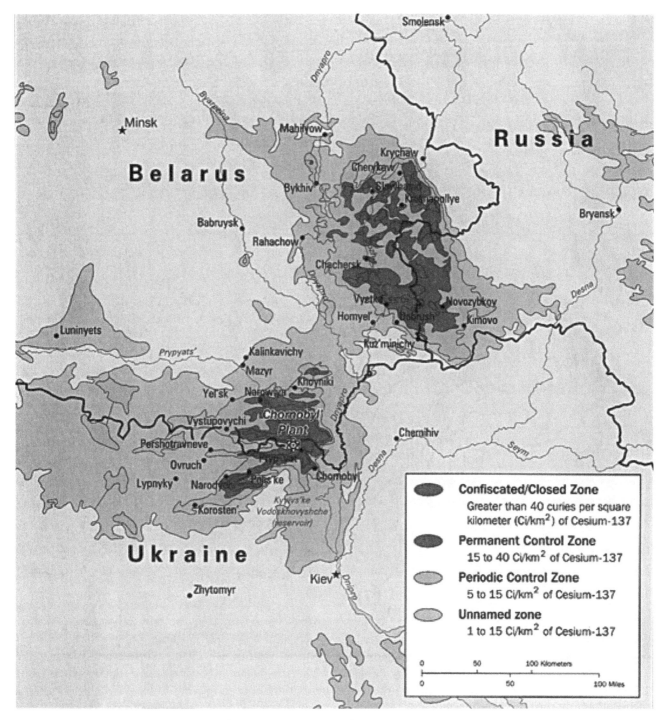

FIGURE 2-4 Radiation hot spots resulting from the Chernobyl Nuclear Power Plant accident

Reproduced from Central Intelligence Agency. Radiation Contamination after the Chernobyl Disaster. *Making the History of 1989*. Item #173. Available at: http://chnm.gmu.edu/1989/items/show/173. Accessed April 2017.

of innocent people. Terrorist networks such as al Qaeda have tried to acquire the material for a nuclear weapon, and if they ever succeeded, they would surely use it. Were they to do so, it would be a catastrophe for the world—causing extraordinary loss of life, and striking a major blow to global peace and stability.

In short, it is increasingly clear that the danger of nuclear terrorism is one of the greatest threats to global security—to our collective security.[37]

The International Atomic Energy Agency (IAEA) receives, on average, a report every 2–3 days on an incident of illicit trafficking of nuclear or radiological material.[38,39] Unfortunately, the nuclear and radiological threats are very real and it is essential that the public health community be prepared.

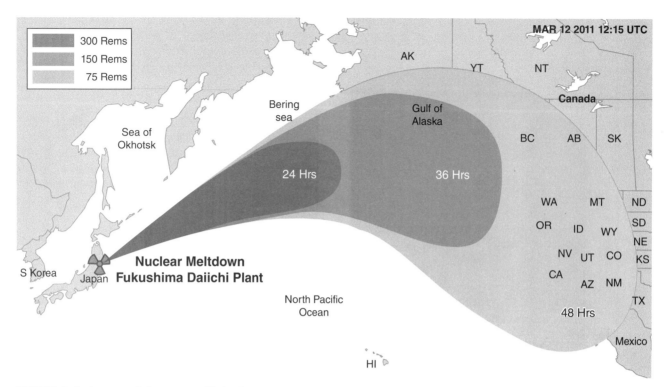

FIGURE 2-5 Radioactive fallout map of Fukushima, Japan

Data from NRC. Infinite Unknown. *Radioactive Fallout Map.* 2011. Available at: http://www.infiniteunknown.net/wp-content/uploads/2011/03/US-NRC-Japan-Fallout-Map-From-Destroyed-Fukushima-Daiichi-Nuclear-Plant.jpg. Accessed April 2017.

▶ Biological Threats

The biological threat can be thought of as along a continuum, to include everything from naturally occurring diseases to the intentional release of a biological agent. **FIGURE 2-6** shows how the impact of each type of threat can range from global to individual: how a deliberately caused event could have global consequences, while a naturally occurring outbreak of an only slightly contagious disease or a lab accident could be limited to a handful of individuals.

This text focuses on the threat from natural disease and emerging and pandemic threats in later chapters, as here we focus exclusively on the deliberate threat. Biological warfare (BW) is the military use of a biological agent to cause death or harm to humans, animals, or plants. In warfare, the targets of biological agents are typically governments, armed forces, or resources that might affect the ability of a nation to attack or defend itself. Similarly, bioterrorism (BT) is the threat or use of a biological agent to harm or kill humans, plants, or animals. Unlike BW though, the target of BT is typically the civilian population or resources that might affect the civilian economy. Agroterrorism refers to the knowing or malicious use of biological agents to affect the agricultural industry or food supply.[40]

As with chemical and radiological threats, there is a long history of the intentional use of biological agents. One example that is cited regularly comes from the 1346–1347 siege by Mongols of the city of Kaffa, now Feodosija, Ukraine. The Mongols reportedly catapulted corpses contaminated with plague over the walls of the city, causing an outbreak of *Yersinia pestis*.[41] Another historical example comes from 1767 when British troops under the direction of Sir William Amherst gave smallpox-infested blankets to Native Americans, causing a massive outbreak of smallpox among this previously unexposed population.

There was little use of biological weapons during World War I. In fact, the only reported use was by Germany, who used anthrax and glanders to infect Allied livestock.[42(p513)] After World War I, however, the Japanese began a robust offensive biological weapons program, housed in what was called "Unit 731." This unit was based in Harbin, Manchuria, and conducted extensive research and experiments, often using prisoners of war as subjects.

In 1940, the Japanese dropped rice and wheat mixed with plague-carrying fleas over China and Manchuria, leading to localized plague outbreaks. In 1942, the United States, with data from Unit 731, began its offensive biological weapons program (**BOX 2-4**).[43]

Several additional high-profile biological weapons events occurred starting in the late 1970s. In 1979, in the Siberian town of Sverdlovsk in the Soviet Union (now Yekaterinburg), at least 77 people became ill with anthrax, resulting in 66 fatalities. Originally, the Soviet Union claimed that the cause of the outbreak was

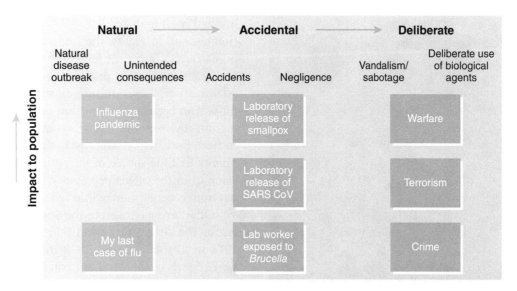

FIGURE 2-6 The biological threat spectrum

1942	The National Academies of Sciences Biological Warfare Committee recommends that the United States should develop an offensive and defensive biological weapons program. Secretary of War Henry L. Stimson recommends to the president that a civilian organization be set up to run the program, and the president approves. The War Research Service (WRS) is established and George Merck, president of Merck and Co., Inc., becomes the leader.
1943	A biological weapons research and development facility is constructed in Frederick, Maryland, at Camp Detrick, and becomes operational. Research begins on the offensive potential of botulinum toxin and anthrax.
1944	The BW program is transferred from the WRS to the War Department. The War Department divides the program between the Chemical Warfare Service (CWS) and the U.S. Army Surgeon General. CWS works mostly on offensive research and production, while the Surgeon General focuses more on defensive measures. The research and development program is housed at Camp Detrick. An existing industrial plant near Terre Haute, Indiana, is acquired for conversion to a biological weapons production plant. Research on biological agents is expanded to include brucellosis, psittacosis, tularemia, and glanders.
1946	The War Department publically acknowledges that the United States has developed an offensive biological weapons program.
1950	Several open-air/sea tests are conducted using simulants. Field testing is also conducted at Dugway Proving Ground, Utah. The construction of a production facility at Pine Bluff Arsenal, Arkansas, is authorized.
1950–1960	Research and production of at least seven biological agents continues. Airborne testing continues and the program is expanded.
1960–1970	Funding for the BW program starts to decline, but the army continues to work on antipersonnel, anti-plant, and anti-animal agents, and runs several open-air tests using simulants in populated areas. The program also works on developing vaccines for defensive purposes.
1969	President Nixon directs the National Security Council to review the chemical and biological weapons policy. The Senate Armed Services Committee votes to cease funding for the biological weapons program and prohibit additional open-air testing. On November 25, President Nixon renounces the development, production, stockpiling, and use of BW agents. The Department of Defense is ordered to destroy existing biological weapons and only engage in research for defensive purposes.
1971–1973	The United States destroys all BW agents and munitions.
1972	The United States signs the Biological and Toxin Weapons Convention.
1975	The Senate approves, and the president ratifies both the Biological and Toxin Weapons Convention and the Geneva Protocol of 1925.

Data from The Henry L. Stimson Center. *History of the US Offensive Biological Warfare Program (1941–1973)*. Biological and Chemical Weapons. Available at: http://www.stimson.org /cbw/?sn=cb2001121275. Accessed July 10, 2010; Smart JK. History of Chemical and Biological Warfare: An American Perspective. *Textbook of Military Medicine: Medical Aspects of Chemical and Biological Warfare*. Washington, DC: Office of the Surgeon General, US Department of the Army; 1989. Available at: http://www.au.af.mil/au/awc/awcgate/medaspec/cwbwfmelectrv699.pdf; Bernstein B. *Origins of the Biological Warfare Program*. 1990; MIT Press: 1–25. Available at: https://mitpress.mit.edu/sites/default/files/titles/content/9780262730969_sch_0001.pdf. Accessed April 2017.

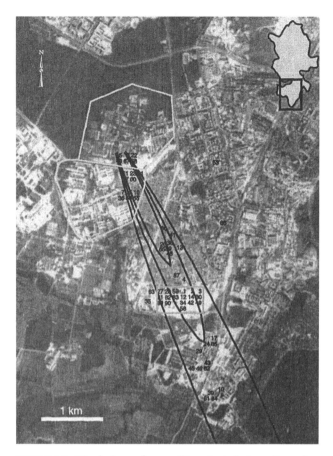

FIGURE 2-7 Wind plume from military installation allegedly producing anthrax in Sverdlovsk, Russia, and the location of anthrax cases in 1979

infected meat and that the route of infection was gastrointestinal. In reality, the cause of the outbreak was human error—someone forgetting to replace a filter—at a military installation that was producing anthrax for offensive purposes. Anthrax escaped into the air and those who became ill fell within the wind plume leading directly from the military compound (**FIGURE 2-7**). In 1992, Boris Yeltsin admitted to the international community that the source of the anthrax in this outbreak came from the offensive military production site, and not from consumption of infected meat.[44,45]

Other events linked to the Soviet Union occurred during the same time period. Starting in 1976 in Laos, 1978 in Cambodia, and 1979 in Afghanistan, there were reports of chemical or toxin weapons use against the Hmong, Khmer, and Mujuhadin, respectively. The alleged attacks were often said to begin with a helicopter or plane flying over a village or resistance group and release of a colored gas that would fall in a manner that often looked, felt, and sounded like rain. The most common color reported was yellow, and thus the collective name for these incidents became "Yellow Rain." The alleged causative agent was trichothecene mycotoxin (T2), and the alleged supplier of this toxin was the Soviet Union, who provided it to the Pathet Lao in Laos, to the Vietnamese for use against Khmer resistance groups in Cambodia, and for direct use by the Soviets in Afghanistan (**FIGURE 2-8**). High levels of morbidity and mortality were associated with the

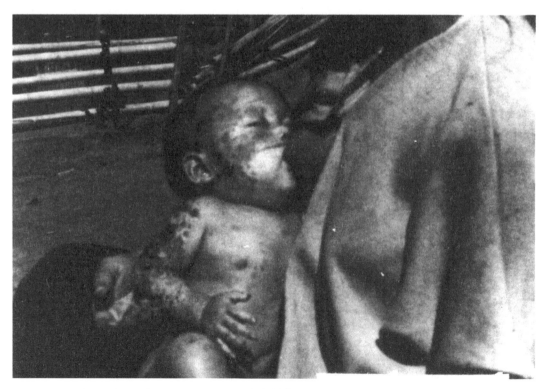

FIGURE 2-8 (A) A picture of Hmong woman and child from Laos

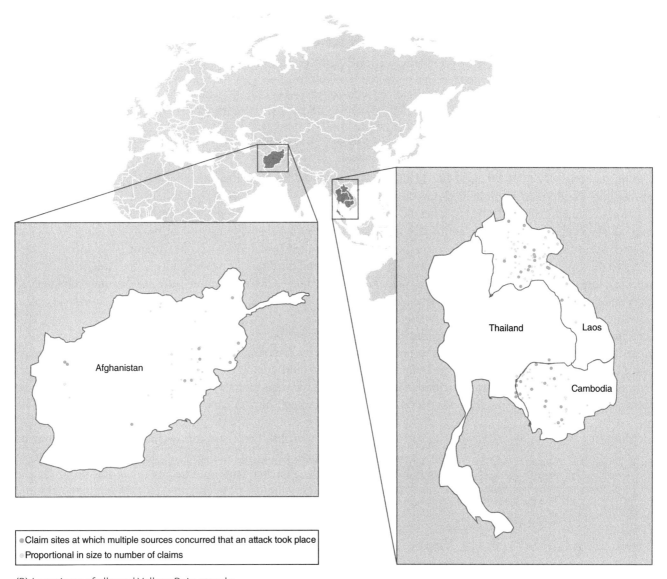

(B) Locations of alleged Yellow Rain attacks

Data from Katz R, Singer B. Can an attribution assessment be made for Yellow Rain? *Politics and the Life Sciences.* 2007;26(1):24–42. Accessed April 2017; © Hemera/Thinkstock/Getty.

alleged Yellow Rain attacks. In 1982, the United States estimated that over 10,700 people had been killed. Some estimated the loss of life to be much greater, particularly within the Hmong community. Some estimates go up to 20,000 and the Lao Human Rights Council puts the number as high as 40,000.[46,47]

The first large-scale BT event in the United States occurred in 1984 in The Dalles, Oregon. The Rajneeshee cult, living in the area at the time, wished to influence a local election. Their plan was to make people in the town too sick to show up to vote in the election, have all of the members of the cult vote, and thereby vote their candidate into office. As a trial run, cult members infected multiple salad bars in local restaurants with *Salmonella.* As a result, 751 people became ill and 45 were hospitalized. This case demonstrates how difficult it is to distinguish between a naturally occurring event and an intentional release of an agent, which enables plausible deniability on the part of the perpetrators. Members of the Epidemic Intelligence Service (EIS) from the CDC were called in to help with the investigation (**BOX 2-5**). While the EIS officers felt that something was not right with the outbreak, they were unable to definitively say that the cases were not of natural origin. It was not until a year after the event, when a member of the cult confessed to authorities, were the public health officials able to fully understand the nature of the outbreak.[48,49]

The most well-known BT event in the United States occurred in the fall of 2001, just weeks after the 9/11 attacks. The case, eventually named "Amerithrax" by the Federal Bureau of Investigation (FBI), involved finely milled anthrax sent through the mail, targeting senators and media outlets (**FIGURES 2-9** and **2-10**). In all, 22 people became ill and 5 died. Thousands of post office workers, congressional staff, and other potentially exposed individuals received prophylactic antibiotics and were offered a vaccine. Thousands more were potentially exposed during this incident, and many more who were worried about possible effects of exposure demanded antibiotics from their personal physicians. Vast sums of money were spent decontaminating post office facilities and Senate office buildings. In 2010, the FBI finally closed the Amerithrax case, claiming the perpetrator was a U.S. government researcher at Fort Detrick named Bruce Ivins. Dr Ivins committed suicide before being formally charged, and thus never stood trial.[50]

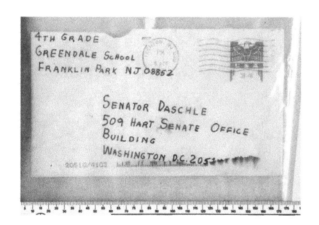

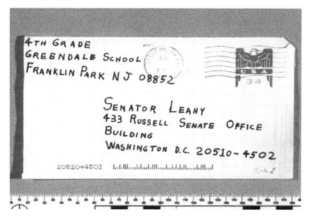

FIGURE 2-9 Anthrax letters sent to Senators Patrick Leahy and Tom Daschle

Reproduced from Federal Bureau of Investigation. *Photo Gallery Amerithrax Case*. Available at: https://archives.fbi.gov/archives/about-us/history/famous-cases/anthrax-amerithrax/the-envelopes. Accessed April 2017.

The total disruption caused by what was—in the end—the equivalent of about a sugar packet amount of anthrax demonstrates how destructive and disruptive biological weapons can be. In fact, they have been called "weapons of mass disruption." Vast infrastructure and funding came in response to the Amerithrax attack, which is discussed more fully in subsequent chapters.

Biological Agents

For a biological agent to be an effective weapon, it should ideally (from the perpetrator's perspective) have high toxicity; be fast acting; be predictable in its impact; have a capacity for survival outside the host for enough time to infect a victim; be relatively indestructible by air, water, or food purification; and be susceptible to medical countermeasures available to the attacker, but not the intended victim(s). Of the many biological agents that exist in nature (including parasites, fungi and yeasts, bacteria, *Rickettsia* and *Chlamydia*, viruses, prions, and toxins), most effort is directed at a small group of bacteria, viruses, and toxins as the primary source of potential biological weapons (**BOX 2-6**).

Classification of Biological Weapons

There have been a series of attempts to classify and characterize biological threat agents over the past 15 years. Here we present two of the major classifications and then the simple list of major biological threats.

This first classification was used primarily by policy planners at the federal level between 2005 and 2010. It looks at the spectrum of agents and defines them as follows:

- **Traditional:** These are naturally occurring microorganisms or toxins that have long been connected with BT or BW, either because they have been used in the past or they have been studied for use. There are a finite number of agents that are relatively well understood. The policy and public

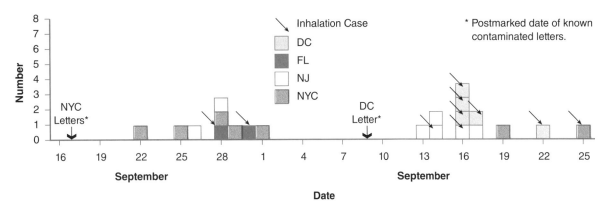

FIGURE 2-10 Number of bioterrorism-related anthrax cases, by date of onset and work location—District of Columbia (DC), Florida (FL), New Jersey (NJ), and New York City (NYC), September 16–October 25, 2001

Reproduced from Centers for Disease Control and Prevention. Number of bioterrorism-related anthrax cases, by date of onset and work location. Update: Investigation of Bioterrorism-Related Anthrax and Interim Guidelines for Clinical Evaluation of Persons with Possible Anthrax. *MMWR*. 2001;50(43): 941. Available at: https://www.cdc.gov/mmwr/PDF/wk/mm5043.pdf.

BOX 2-6 Biological Agents in Nature

Bacteria   Free-living unicellular organisms
Viruses   Core of DNA or RNA surrounded by a coat of protein, require host cell in order to replicate, and much smaller than bacteria
Toxins   Toxic substances produced by living organisms

---

health community has devised specific plans to address the potential use of these agents. Examples include smallpox and anthrax.

- **Enhanced:** Enhanced agents are traditional biological agents that have been altered to circumvent medical countermeasures. This group includes agents that are resistant to antibiotics.
- **Emerging:** This category includes any naturally occurring emerging organism or emerging infectious disease. Examples include severe acute respiratory syndrome (SARS), H5N1, and novel H1N1.
- **Advanced:** The final category on the spectrum of biological threats encompasses novel pathogens and other artificial agents that are engineered in laboratories. It is virtually impossible to plan for the specific threats posed by this category of agents, thus forcing policy makers to look at biological threats with a much broader strategic approach.[51]

The second classification method for biological threat agents is the Category A, B, and C list (**BOX 2-7**). This categorization originated with a 1999 CDC Strategic Planning Workgroup, which looked at the public health impacts of biological agents, the potential of those agents to be effective weapons, public perception, and fear and preparedness requirements. They also examined existing lists, including the Select Agent Rule list, the Australia Group list for export control, and the WHO list of biological weapons.[52]

The resulting list begins with Category A, which includes the highest priority pathogens and highest threat. They can cause large-scale morbidity and mortality, and often require specific preparedness plans on the part of the public health community. Category B includes the second highest threat group. Most of the agents in this category are waterborne or foodborne. These agents have often been used intentionally in the past, or were part of offensive research programs. The morbidity and mortality from these agents is not as significant as from Category A agents, but still considerable, and they often require the public health community to enhance surveillance and diagnostic capacity. The last group is Category C, which encompasses emerging pathogens or agents that have become resistant to medical countermeasures. These agents may cause high morbidity and mortality, and may be easily produced and transmitted.[53]

Biological weapons are unique from other potential WMD, in that the agents themselves are relatively available, as many occur naturally and may be endemic in some parts of the world. The technology to work with these agents has progressed to a point where knowledge is widespread and those with minimal formal education may possess the skills to work with and maliciously use certain agents. Compared to other WMD,

---

BOX 2-7 Major Biological Threat Agents

Anthrax (*Bacillus anthracis*)
Arenaviruses
Botulism (*Clostridium botulinum* toxin)
Brucellosis (*Brucella* species)
Burkholderia mallei (glanders)
Burkholderia pseudomallei (melioidosis)
Chlamydia psittaci (psittacosis)
Cholera (*Vibrio cholerae*)
E. coli O157:H7 (*Escherichia coli*)
Food safety threats (e.g., *Salmonella* species, *E. coli* O157:H7, and *Shigella*)
Q fever (*Coxiella burnetii*)
Ricin toxin
Rickettsia prowazekii (typhus fever)
Salmonella species (salmonellosis)
Shigella (shigellosis)
Smallpox (*Variola major*)
Staphylococcal enterotoxin B
Tularemia (*Francisella tularensis*)
Typhoid fever (*Salmonella typhi*)
Viral encephalitis (alphaviruses, e.g., Venezuelan equine encephalitis (VEE), Eastern equine encephalitis (EEE), and Western equine encephalitis (WEE))
Viral hemorrhagic fevers (filoviruses [e.g., Ebola and Marburg] and arenaviruses [e.g., Lassa and Machupo])
Water safety threats (e.g., *V. cholerae* and *Cryptosporidium parvum*)
Yersinia pestis (plague)
Emerging infectious diseases such as Zika, Nipah virus, and hantavirus.

Modified from Centers for Disease Control and Prevention. Bioterrorism Agents/Diseases—A to Z. *Emergency Preparedness and Response*. 2015. Available at: https://emergency.cdc.gov/agent/agentlist.asp. Accessed April 2017.

---

biological weapons are inexpensive. While it is extraordinarily complicated to distribute biological weapons through a missile or other munition, other means of dissemination are quite easy (e.g., spraying salad bars or self-infecting and passing to others). Intentional attacks may be very difficult to detect and differentiate from a naturally occurring event, thus allowing for plausible deniability on the part of the offender.

Finally, biological weapons can be extremely lethal. A 1993 study by the now defunct Congressional Office of Technology Assessment (OTA) concluded that a crop duster plane flying over Washington, DC, and disseminating 100 kg of anthrax powder had the potential to be more deadly than a 1-megaton hydrogen bomb (**FIGURE 2-11**). An earlier study by the WHO using a similar scenario of a line source dissemination of agent from an airplane also demonstrates the large-scale morbidity and mortality that can result from the intentional release of a biological weapon (**TABLE 2-2**).

The Biological Threat

In December 2008, the Commission on the Prevention of Weapons of Mass Destruction Proliferation and Terrorism released the *World at Risk* report, in which they concluded there will likely be a biological attack some place in the world within the next 5 years and biological weapons are to be considered a threat of primary importance to the United States.[54]

Obviously, there was no large scale biological attack between 2008 and 2013, but the fear of an event has not lessoned. In 2017, Bill Gates delivered a speech in Munich, Germany, warning,

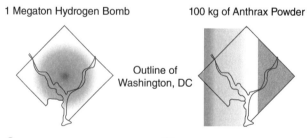

1 Megaton Hydrogen Bomb   100 kg of Anthrax Powder

Outline of
Washington, DC

570,000 – 1,900,00 Deaths   1,000,000 – 3,000,00 Deaths

FIGURE 2-11 Lethality of anthrax compared to a nuclear weapon. A 1993 study by the Congressional Office of Technology Assessment

Reproduced from U.S. Congress, Office of Technology Assessment. *Proliferation of Weapons of Mass Destruction: Assessing the Risk*. 1993. OTA-ISC-559. 53–54. Available at: http://www.au.af.mil/au/awc/awcgate/ota/9341.pdf. Accessed April 2017.

TABLE 2-2 WHO (1970) Analysis of Morbidity and Mortality that Would Result from an Airplane Release of 50 kg of Agent Along a 2-km Line Upwind of a Population Center of 500,000

Agent	Downwind Reach (km)	Casualties	Dead
Rift Valley fever	1	35,000	400
Tick-borne encephalitis	1	35,000	9,500
Typhus	5	85,000	19,000
Brucellosis	10	100,000	500
Q fever	>20	125,000	150
Tularemia	>20	125,000	30,000
Anthrax	>>20	125,000	95,000

Data from World Health Organization. Estimated Possible Primary Effects of Limited (Single Bomber). *Health Aspects of Chemical and Biological Weapons*. 1970. p 98. Available at: http://apps.who.int/iris/bitstream/10665/39444/1/24039.pdf. Accessed April 2017.

Whether it occurs by a quirk of nature or at the hand of a terrorist, epidemiologists say a fast-moving airborne pathogen could kill more than 30 million people in less than a year. And they say there is a reasonable probability the world will experience such an outbreak in the next 10–15 years.[55]

And a bipartisan working group, The Blue Ribbon Study Panel on Biodefense, wrote, "We have reached a critical mass of biological crises. Myriad biological threats, vulnerabilities, and consequences have collectively and dramatically increased the risk to the Nation."[56] So while the massive biological event predicted in 2008 has not materialized, it is clear that the threat has not diminished.

The threat of a biological weapons attack derives from multiple sources. An attack may be carried out by a lone actor, a terrorist group, an organization, or from a state-sponsored program. At one point in time, there were probably a dozen nations that sponsored offensive biological weapons programs. Fewer programs exist today,[57] but the agents created and knowledge gained from state-sponsored offensive programs have become a threat unto itself, as terrorist organizations lure scientists with financial and other incentives. For example, the former Soviet Union had an extensive offensive biological weapons program, spanning the military, the Komitet Gosudarstvennoy Bezopasnosti (KGB), and civilian sectors. In the civilian program, called Bioprepa-rat, there were up to 40,000 scientists and technicians, all working on biological weapons research and production.[58] This program was inherited by Russia after the fall of the Soviet Union, although in 1992, President Boris Yeltsin promised to terminate the program. While much effort and money has gone toward redirecting former weapons scientists into more peaceful lines of work, it is unclear whether all of the scientists involved in the program, or the material they worked with, are accounted for. Thus, the threat of knowledge and agents moving to other nations or terrorist organizations remains.

Terrorist organizations also present a significant threat that biological weapons will be used. As previously mentioned, the Rajneeshee cult successfully engaged in bioterrorism, as did Aum Shinrikyo. In addition to the sarin gas attack, Aum Shinrikyo had attempted to use biological weapons, but was unsuccessful in causing any injuries (they used a vaccine strain of the agent that would not cause disease and utilized inefficient dissemination mechanisms). When police raided their compound after the sarin attack, they found cultures of anthrax, botulism, and spray tanks.[59]

Al Qaeda has yet to use biological weapons, but expressed interest in this means of terrorism. The United States found a facility in Afghanistan that had been used by Al Qaeda, possibly to experiment with or eventually produce a biological weapon. At this location, called Tarnak Farms, several documents were found, including notes about where to acquire seed cultures, and analyses of the potential casualties from different agents. In addition to Al Qaeda, at least 11 other terrorist organizations have at least expressed interest in using biological weapons.[60] Current terrorist organizations, including the Islamic State, have expressed interest, but at the time of this writing, had not used biological weapons.[61]

Overall, the current threat posed by biological weapons has increased significantly in the past decade. The potential consequences of an attack would go beyond population morbidity and mortality and could include such disruptions as a slow down or shut down of international travel and trade, economic shocks, potential civil disorder, public panic or confusion, and national or regional instability.

This text examines the role of the public health community in addressing these threats and some of the challenges faced. Multiple sectors of society must work together to effectively prevent, prepare for, and manage the consequences of an attack, but the core of any effective detection and response capacity is public health. It is the public health community that can identify an event through population surveillance and clinical reporting. The public health community is central in mounting a response that treats those who are ill, protects those who may have been exposed, addresses immediate and long-term health consequences, and reconstitutes the infrastructure after the event has occurred.

Key Words

Accidental exposures
Biological weapons
Bioterrorism

Chemical weapons
Deliberate use
Intentional use

Radiological weapons
Toxins

Discussion Questions

1. Do you believe there will be a biological attack in the next 5 years? Why or why not?
2. What role would the public health community play if a radiological weapon was dispersed in a major metropolitan area?
3. Do you believe the public health community is prepared to address the threats from WMD? If not, what would you do to remedy the situation and what information do you think would be important for public health professionals to know?
4. How should public health professionals communicate with security officials to be kept aware of the latest threats? Is that an appropriate role for public health?

References

1. *Chemical Weapons Convention.* Available at: http://www.cwc.gov/cwc_treaty_full.html. Accessed June 26, 2010.
2. League of Nations. *Geneva Protocol: Protocol for the Prohibition of the Use of War of Asphyxiating, Poisonous or Other Gases, and of Bacteriological Methods of Warfare.* June 17, 1925. Available at: https://www.state.gov/t/isn/4784.htm. Accessed May 2017.
3. Nuclear Threat Initiative. Introduction to Chemical Weapons Nonproliferation. *Chemical Weapons Nonproliferation Tutorial.* 2004. Available at: http://tutorials.nti.org/chemical-weapons-nonproliferation/introduction/. Accessed April 2017.
4. Hu H, Fine J, Epstein P, et al. Tear Gas: Harassing Agent or Toxic Chemical Weapon? *JAMA.* August 1989;262(5):660–663. doi:10.1001/jama.1989.03430050076030.
5. Melnikova N, Wu J, Orr MF. Number of Persons Evacuated for Chemical Incidents, by Year. Public Health Response to Acute Chemical Incidents—Hazardous Substances Emergency Events Surveillance, Nine States, 1999–2008. *MMWR.* 2015;64(2):28. https://www.cdc.gov/mmwr/pdf/ss/ss6402.pdf. Accessed April 2017.
6. Fitzgerald GJ. Chemical Warfare and Medical Response During World War I. *American Journal of Public Health.* April 2008;98(4):611–625. doi:10.2105/AJPH.2007.11930.
7. Middlebury Institute of International Studies at Monteray, James Martin Center for Nonproliferation Studies. *Chronology of Major Events in the History of Biological and Chemical Weapons.* August 2008. Available at: http://cns.miis.edu/cbw/pastuse.htm. Accessed June 2017.
8. Kang HK, Dalager NA, Needham LL, et al. Health Status of Army Chemical Corps Vietnam Veterans Who Sprayed Defoliant in Vietnam. *American Journal of Industrial Medicine.* November 2006;49(11):875–884. doi:10.1002/ajim.20385.
9. Stellman JM, Stellman SD, Christian R, et al. The Extent and Patterns of Usage of Agent Orange and Other Herbicides in Vietnam. *Nature.* April 2003;22:681–687.
10. Federation of American Scientists. Chemical Weapons Program. October 2, 1999. Available at: http://www.fas.org/nuke/guide/egypt/cw/. Accessed April 2017.
11. Ali J. Chemical Weapons and the Iran–Iraq War: A Case Study in Noncompliance. *The Nonproliferation Review.* 2001;8(1):43–58. doi:10.1080/10736700108436837.
12. ProCon. Iraq Statements by Former US Department of Defense Secretary Donald Rumsfeld. 2009. Available at: http://usiraq.procon.org/view.additional-resource.php?resourceID=000687. Accessed April 2017.
13. BBC On This Day. 1988: Thousands Die in Halabja Gas Attack. *BBC.* March 16, 1988. Available at: http://news.bbc.co.uk/onthisday/hi/dates/stories/march/16/newsid_4304000/4304853.stm. Accessed April 2017.
14. Amos D. In Syria, Opposition Stages Massive Protests. *NPR.* July 15, 2011. Available at: http://n.pr/oKyu3R. Accessed June 7, 2013.
15. Mid-East Unrest: Syrian Protests in Damascus and Aleppo. *BBC.* March 15, 2011. Available at: http://bbc.in/18kMa1N. Accessed June 9, 2013.
16. UN Official Calls Syria Conflict 'civil war.' *Al Jazeera.* June 13, 2012. Available at: http://www.aljazeera.com/news/middleeast/2012/06/201261222721181345.html. Accessed June 7, 2013.
17. Joint Investigative Mechanism Presents Its Third Report to Security Council [Press Release]. New York: United Nations; August 30, 2016. Available at: https://www.un.org/press/en/2016/dc3651.doc.htm. Accessed April 2017.
18. Schmitt E. ISIS Used Chemical Arms at Least 52 Times in Syria and Iraq, Report Says. *The New York Times.* November 21, 2016. Available at: https://www.nytimes.com/2016/11/21/world/middleeast/isis-chemical-weapons-syria-iraq-mosul.html?_r=0. Accessed April 2017.

19. Vale A. What Lessons Can We Learn from the Japanese Sarin Attacks? *Przegl Lek.* 2005;62(6):528–532.
20. Mossiker F. *The affair of the poisons; Louis XIV, Madame de Montespan, and One of History's Great Unsolved Mysteries*, 1st ed. New York: Knopf; 1969.
21. World Health Organization. *The World Health Report 2007: A Safer Future—Global Public Health Security in the 21st Century.* 2007. p xi. Available at: http://www.who.int /whr/2007/whr07_en.pdf?ua=1. Accessed April 2017.
22. United Nations News Centre. *Toxic Wastes Caused Deaths, Illnesses in Côte d'Ivoire—UN Expert.* September 16, 2009. Available at: http://www.un.org/apps/news/story .asp?NewsID=32072. Accessed July 8, 2010.
23. Polgreen L, Simons M. Global Sludge Ends in Tragedy for Ivory Coast. *The New York Times.* October 2, 2006. Available at: http://www.nytimes.com/2006/10/02/world/africa/02ivory .html. Accessed July 8, 2010.
24. Feit C. Ivory Coast Pollute. Global Sludge Ends in Tragedy for Ivory Coast. *The New York Times.* 2006; Image number 05978613. Available at: http://archive.reduxpictures.com /id/05978613. Accessed April 2017.
25. Agence France-Presse. Poison Gas Sweeps Nigerian City, 300 Sickened. *Google News.* May 30, 2010. Accessed July 8, 2010. Available at: https://www.pressreader.com /canada/windsor-star/20100531/281809985131205
26. Sharma DC. Bhopal: 20 Years On. *The Lancet.* January 2005;365(9454):111–112. doi:10.1016/S0140-6736(05)17722-8.
27. Dunning AE, Oswalt JL. Train Wreck and Chlorine Spill in Graniteville, South Carolina Transportation Effects and Lessons in Small-Town Capacity for No-Notice Evacuation. Transportation Research Record. *Journal of the Transportation Research Board.* 2009:130–135. doi:10.3141/2009-17.
28. Durham B. The Background and History of Manmade Disasters. *Topics in Emergency Medicine.* June 2002;24(2):1–14.
29. Centers for Disease Control and Prevention. Acute Radiation Syndrome (ARS): A Fact Sheet for the Public. *Emergency Preparedness and Response.* May 10, 2006. Available at: https:// emergency.cdc.gov/radiation/ars.asp. Accessed July 8, 2010.
30. Centers for Disease Control and Prevention. Radiation Emergencies—Information for Public Health Professionals. *Emergency Preparedness and Response.* March 31, 2010. Available at: https://emergency.cdc.gov/radiation/publichealth.asp. Accessed July 8, 2010.
31. Nemhauser J. The Polonium-210 Public Health Assessment: The Need for Medical Toxicology Expertise in Radiation Terrorism Events. *Journal of Medical Toxicology.* 2010;6:355–359. doi:10.1007/s13181-010-0090-x.
32. International Atomic Energy Agency. *The Radiological Accident in Goiânia.* 1988. Available at: http://www-pub .iaea.org/MTCD/publications/PDF/Pub815_web.pdf. Accessed July 8, 2010.
33. The Chernobyl Forum: 2003–2005. *Chernobyl's Legacy: Health, Environmental and Socio-Economic Impacts and Recommendations to the Governments of Belarus, the Russian Federation and Ukraine.* International Atomic Energy Agency (IAEA). April 2006. Available at: https://www.iaea.org/sites /default/files/chernobyl.pdf. Accessed July 8, 2010.
34. Jargin SV. Overestimation of Thyroid Cancer Incidence after the Chernobyl Accident. *BMJ.* October 11, 2008. Available at: http: //www.bmj.com/rapid-response/2011/11/02/overestimation -thyroid-cancer-incidence-after-chernobyl-accident. Accessed July 8, 2010.
35. World Nuclear Association. Fukushima Accident. January 2017. Available at: http://www.world-nuclear.org/information -library/safety-and-security/safety-of-plants/fukushima -accident.aspx. Accessed April 2017.
36. WHO. *Health Risk Assessment from the Nuclear Accident after the 2011 Great East Japan Earthquake and Tsunami, Based on a Preliminary Dose Estimation.* 2013. Available at: http:// www.who.int/ionizing_radiation/pub_meet/fukushima _risk_assessment_2013/en/. Accessed April 2017.
37. The White House, Office of the Press Secretary. *Remarks by the President at the Opening Plenary Session of the Nuclear Security Summit.* April 13, 2010. Available at: https:// obamawhitehouse.archives.gov/the-press-office/2012/03/26 /remarks-president-obama-opening-plenary-session -nuclear-security-summit. Accessed June 2017.
38. IAEA. *IAEA Incident and Trafficking Database (ITDB): Incidents of Nuclear and Other Radioactive Material Out of Regulatory Control 2016 Fact Sheet.* 2016. Available at: https:// www-ns.iaea.org/downloads/security/itdb-fact-sheet.pdf. Accessed April 2017.
39. IAEA Director General Amano Y. Statement Presented at: Nuclear Security Summit. April 13, 2010; Washington, DC. Available at: http://www.iaea.org/NewsCenter/Statements/2010 /amsp2010n007.html. Accessed July 8, 2010.
40. Monke J. *CRS Report for Congress: Agroterrorism: Threats.* Federation of American Scientists. August 13, 2004. Available at: http://www.fas.org/irp/crs/RL32521.pdf. Accessed July 10, 2010.
41. Wheelis M. Biological Warfare at the 1346 Siege of Caffa. *Emerging Infectious Diseases.* September 2002;8(9):971–975.
42. Lesho ME, Dorsey MD, Bunner CD. Feces, Dead Horses, and Fleas: Evolution of the Hostile Use of Biological Agents. *Western Journal of Medicine.* June 1998;168(6):512–516.
43. Kristof N. Unmasking Horror—A special report; Japan Confronting Gruesome War Atrocity. *The New York Times.* March 17, 1995. Available at: http://www.nytimes .com/1995/03/17/world/unmasking-horror-a-special -report-japan-confronting-gruesome-war-atrocity .html?pagewanted=all. Accessed April 2017.
44. Meselson M, Guillemin J, Hugh-Jones M, et al. The Sverdlovsk Anthrax Outbreak of 1979. *Science.* November 1994;266(5188):1202–1208.
45. Guillemin J. *Anthrax: The Investigation of a Deadly Outbreak.* Berkeley, CA: University of California Press; 2001: p 163.
46. Katz R. *Yellow Rain Revisited: Lessons Learned for the Investigation of Chemical and Biological Weapons Allegations.* Dissertation ed. Princeton, NJ: Princeton University; 2005.
47. Katz R, Singer B. Can An Attribution Assessment be Made for Yellow Rain? *Politics and the Life Sciences.* 2007;26(1): 24–42.
48. Török TJ, Tauxe RV, Wise RP, et al. A Large Community Outbreak of Salmonellosis Caused by Intentional Contamination of Restaurant Salad Bars. *JAMA.* August 1997;278(5):389–385.
49. Carus WS. The Rajneeshees (1984). In: Tucker JB, ed. *Toxic Terror: Assessing Terrorist Use of Chemical and Biological Weapons.* Cambridge, MA: The MIT Press; 2000.
50. The United States Department of Justice. *Amerithrax Investigative Summary.* February 19, 2010. Available at: https:// www.justice.gov/archive/amerithrax/docs/amx-investigative -summary.pdf. Accessed April 2017.
51. The White House. *Homeland Security Presidential Directive/ HSPD—18.* January 31, 2007. Available at: https://fas.org /irp/offdocs/nspd/hspd-18.html. Accessed June 2017.

52. Elrod S. Category A–C Agents. In: Katz R, Zilinikas R, eds. *Encyclopedia of Bioterrorism Defense.* 2nd ed. Hoboken, NJ: Wiley & Sons; 2011.

53. Centers for Disease Control and Prevention. Bioterrorism Agents/Diseases—By Category. *Emergency Preparedness and Response.* Available at: https://emergency.cdc.gov/agent /agentlistchem-category.asp. Accessed July 10, 2010.

54. Graham B, Talent J, Allison G, et al. *World at Risk: The Report of the Commission on the Prevention of WMD Proliferation and Terrorism.* December 2008. Available at: http://www.preventwmd.gov/static/docs/report /worldatrisk_full.pdf. Accessed July 10, 2010.

55. Bill Gates. Speech Given at: 53rd Munich Security Conference; February 18, 2014; Munich, Germany. Available at: https:// www.securityconference.de/en/activities/munich-security -conference/msc-2017/speeches/speech-by-bill-gates/. Accessed April 2017.

56. Blue Ribbon Study Panel on Biodefense. *A National Blueprint for Biodefense: Leadership and Major Reform Needed to Optimize Efforts—Bipartisan Report of the Blue Ribbon Study Panel on Biodefense.* Washington, DC: Hudson Institute. October 2015. p viii. Available at: http://www.biodefensestudy .org/LiteratureRetrieve.aspx?ID=144258. Accessed April 2017.

57. U.S. Department of State. *2015 Report on Adherence to and Compliance with Arms Control, Nonproliferation, and Disarmament Agreements and Commitments.* June 5, 2015. Available at: https://www.state.gov/t/avc/rls/rpt/2015/243224 .htm. Accessed April 2017.

58. Alibek K. *Biohazard: The Chilling True Story of the Largest Covert Biological Weapons Program in the World—Told from Inside by the Man Who Ran It.* New York: Dell Publishing; 1999.

59. Clinehens MNA. *Aum Shinrikyo and Weapons of Mass Destruction: A Case Study.* Air Command and Staff College, Air University. April 2000. Available at: http://www.au.af.mil /au/awc/awcgate/acsc/00-040.pdf. Accessed July 10, 2010.

60. U.S. Department of State, Office of the Coordinator for Counterterrorism. *Country Reports on Terrorism 2009.* August 2010. Available at: http://www.state.gov/documents /organization/141114.pdf. Accessed November 19, 2010.

61. Doornbos H, Moussa J. Found: The Islamic State's Terror Laptop of Doom. *Foreign Policy.* August 28, 2014. Available at: http://foreignpolicy.com/2014/08/28/found-the-islamic -states-terror-laptop-of-doom/. Accessed April 2017.

CHAPTER 3

Threats from Naturally Occurring Disease and Natural Disaster

▶ Introduction

This chapter describes the links between disease and security, and explores how and why naturally occurring disease events can and sometimes do become national security threats. We look at the historical evolution of policy commitments to disease as a security threat, how health security is defined and embraced by different communities, and the burden of disease and emerging biological threats, including recent examples of disease outbreaks. We then examine how the foreign policy and security community are organizing to incorporate naturally occurring disease outbreaks into the security and preparedness context.

The term "health security" has evolved in recent years. During much of the George W. Bush administration, there was a debate around the "securitization

of health" and the "healthification of security," but by the end of the Obama administration, there was an emerging consensus not just about what health security means, but also about the importance of incorporating it into national security and foreign policy.[1]

The definition of health security in **BOX 3-1** is provided by the U.S. National Health Security Strategy (NHSS), which emphasizes a continual state of preparedness necessary to protect and respond to health threats. More specifically, the NHSS explains that a health emergency, such as a large outbreak of a naturally occurring infectious disease, can impact communities and be exacerbated by vulnerabilities from weak local networks to the ability of governments to provide appropriate medical countermeasures.[2(p3)]

The World Health Organization (WHO), on the other hand, defines health security as the activities that

National health security is a state in which the nation and its people are prepared for, protected from, and resilient in the face of incidents with health consequences. The threats and risks that communities face are diverse— they can be intentional or naturally occurring and can result from both persistent and emerging threats, including severe weather, infectious diseases, hazardous material exposures, and terrorist attacks. The impact of these incidents can be exacerbated by vulnerabilities that vary from community to community, such as a large number of at-risk individuals, weak social networks, unprotected critical infrastructure, a lack of training and exercising for health security, and a lack of available countermeasures for emerging infectious diseases.

Reproduced from U.S. Department of Health and Human Services. *National Health Security Strategy and Implementation Plan 2015–2018.* p 1. Available at: https://www.phe.gov/Preparedness/planning/authority/nhss/Documents/nhss-ip.pdf; http://www.astho.org/Preparedness/DPHP-Annual-Meeting/NHSSUpdate/. Accessed April 2017.

are necessary to "minimize vulnerability to acute public health events that endanger the collective health of populations."[3] The WHO also adds that health security can impact "economic or political stability, trade, tourism, access to goods and services, and . . . demographic stability."[3]

The health of a population, which can be affected by human behavior, disease, and natural and manmade threats, directly impacts the security of a nation. Thus, a multisectoral approach is needed to effectively address health security and build the capacities to prevent, detect, and respond to biological threats around the world.

▶ Evolution of Disease and Security Links

Massive disease outbreaks, such as the 1918 influenza pandemic that impacted every sector of society and killed millions around the world, clearly impacted the security and prosperity of populations.[4] Yet, the formal recognition of disease as security threat did not begin to take form until the 1990s. Fueled by the HIV/AIDS pandemic, emergence of Ebola, large-scale plague outbreak in India, the reemergence of cholera, introduction of new subtypes of dengue in the Americas, and the onset of drug-resistant tuberculosis (TB), the Clinton White House issued an assessment in 1996 called Addressing

the Threat of Emerging Infectious Diseases.[5] The Presidential Decision Directive called for strengthening the national infectious disease surveillance system, building a global surveillance and response system, and expanding the mandate of the Department of Defense to "better protect American citizens."[6]

The year 2000 initiated greater political recognition of the link between health and security. In January, the National Intelligence Council (a "think tank" for the U.S. Intelligence Community) released a report titled "The Global Infectious Disease Threat and Its Implications for the United States." This report responded to concerns by U.S. government officials that the spread of infectious diseases may affect health, economics, and national security. The report signaled the Intelligence Community's interest in considering disease as a nontraditional threat to national security.[7]

Also, in January 2000, the U.N. Security Council recognized the catastrophic impact of HIV/AIDS pandemic as a security issue.[8] This marked the first time the Security Council considered an infectious disease. Several months later, on April 29, 2000, the Clinton White House formally recognized infectious diseases as a threat to U.S. national security.[9] Together, these actions marked a paradigm shift in thinking about security threats and the relationship between disease and security. It would take, however, almost a decade to solidify health as a security threat and to attract the attention and resources of the security community.

The understanding and commitment to disease as a nontraditional security threat by senior security officials in the U.S. government continued to evolve. In 2002, President George W. Bush released the National Security Strategy (NSS) (**FIGURE 3-1**), which was heavily influenced by the 9/11 terrorist attacks and the anthrax letters immediately afterward. Public health and health promotion are mentioned several times but only as components of development assistance. HIV/AIDS is mentioned as a condition that, due to its devastation to sub-Saharan Africa, required direct assistance, and this call eventually led to the establishment of the President's Emergency Plan for AIDS Relief (PEPFAR). Medical preparedness for bioterrorism threats is mentioned briefly, in the sense that preparedness efforts will also benefit infectious disease and other mass casualty events.[10] Both public health preparedness and disease are addressed in the strategy, but no direct link is made between disease and security.

After the 2002 NSS was published, the global community was faced with the need to coordinate an international response to severe acute respiratory syndrome (SARS), followed by the emergency of highly

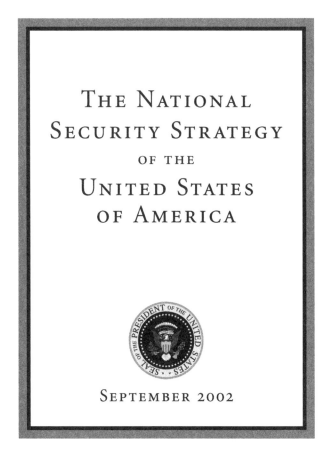

FIGURE 3-1 National Security Strategy 2002

Reproduced from The White House. *The National Security Strategy of the United States of America.* September 2002. Available at: https://www.state.gov/documents/organization/63562.pdf. Accessed April 2017.

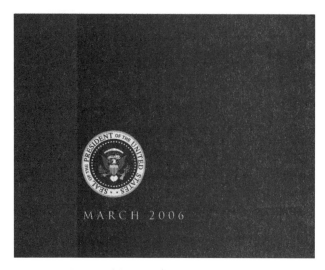

FIGURE 3-2 National Security Strategy 2006

Reproduced from The White House. *The National Security Strategy of the United States of America.* March 2006. Available at: https://www.state.gov/documents/organization/64884.pdf. Accessed April 2017.

pathogenic H5N1 avian influenza (AI) in East and Southeast Asia. The administration, worried about the potential spread of AI, developed pandemic preparedness plans as well as all-hazards U.S. policy frameworks. These efforts were paired with the launch of the International Partnership on Avian and Pandemic Influenza (IPAPI) in 2005, a U.S.-led effort to strengthen global surveillance and response and to mobilize resources. During this same period of time, the United States was engaged in international negotiations and the eventual adoption of a treaty focused on emerging infectious disease (EID), the International Health Regulations (addressed in detail in Chapter 5).

By 2006, President Bush released an updated NSS that included more language on the threat of both biological weapons and infectious diseases (**FIGURE 3-2**). The updated strategy explicitly mentioned the need to improve capacity to detect and respond to biological attacks, as well as the need to secure dangerous pathogens, strengthen global surveillance, develop medical countermeasures, and improve public health infrastructure—all in support of countering a biological attack. In regard to disease, the strategy declares that pandemics pose "a catastrophic challenge to national security with risks to social disorder."[11] At the time,

the country was preparing for a potential pandemic of H5N1 and had become well aware of the potential threat posed by this strain of influenza. In addition to declaring the need to prepare for the pandemic threat, the strategy also calls for transparent public health systems and emphasizes the need for governmental efforts to control and contain HIV/AIDS, TB, and malaria.

In 2009, Barack Obama became president and immediately had to face an evolving pandemic of influenza A H1N1 that emerged in North America, and issued a presidential directive on countering biological threats (to be discussed in later chapters). A year later, the Obama administration released the 2010 NSS, which more fully recognized the relationship between health and security, as well as the need to strengthen public health system in order to address biological threats.[12] To counter the biological threat, the strategy provided the following guidance:

> The effective dissemination of a lethal biological agent within a population center would endanger the lives of hundreds of thousands of people and have unprecedented economic, societal, and political consequences. We must continue to work at home with first responders and health officials to reduce the risk associated

with unintentional or deliberate outbreaks of infectious disease and to strengthen our resilience across the spectrum of high-consequence biological threats. We will work with domestic and international partners to protect against biological threats by promoting global health security and reinforcing norms of safe and responsible conduct; obtaining timely and accurate insight on current and emerging risks; taking reasonable steps to reduce the potential for exploitation; expanding our capability to prevent, attribute, and apprehend those who carry out attacks; communicating effectively with all stakeholders; and helping to transform the international dialogue on biological threats.[12(p24)]

In addition to addressing the biological threat, the 2010 strategy fully and explicitly defined the connections between pandemic and infectious diseases and security, and the need to build and maintain public health infrastructure to protect population health and national security (**BOX 3-2**).

Following the 2010 NSS, the Obama administration continued to release presidential directives, further develop global health activities and integrate health and security objectives. Also in 2010, Secretary of State Hillary Clinton described the objectives for U.S. global health engagement in terms of development, diplomacy, and the need to

> invest in global health to protect our nation's security. To cite one example, the threat posed by the spread of disease in our interconnected world in which thousands of people every day step on a plane in one continent and step off in another. We need a comprehensive, effective global system for tracking health data, monitoring threats, and coordinating responses.[13]

In September 2011, the political discourse of health security was raised to the highest levels when President Obama spoke about the importance of building capacity to prevent and respond to biological threats at the U.N. General Assembly (**BOX 3-3**).

Over the course of the next few years, the Obama administration worked to develop what would eventually become the Global Health Security Agenda, contributed to existing efforts, like the Global Health Security Initiative, invested in capacity building under the International Health Regulations, and eventually coordinated a multisectoral response to the West Africa Ebola Outbreak that started in 2014. In 2015, the Obama administration released its final NSS, which not only addressed health security, but also listed severe

---

BOX 3-2 May 2010 National Security Strategy: Section on Pandemic and Infectious Disease

The threat of contagious disease transcends political boundaries and the ability to prevent, quickly detect and contain outbreaks with pandemic potential has never been so important. An epidemic that begins in a single community can quickly evolve into a multinational health crisis that causes millions to suffer, as well as spark major disruptions to travel and trade. Addressing these transnational risks requires advance preparation, extensive collaboration with the global community, and the development of a resilient population at home.

Recognizing that the health of the world's population has never been more interdependent, we are improving our public health and medical capabilities on the front lines, including domestic and international disease surveillance, situational awareness, rapid and reliable development of medical countermeasures to respond to public health threats, preparedness education and training, and surge capacity of the domestic health care system to respond to an influx of patients due to a disaster or emergency. These capabilities include our ability to work with international partners to mitigate and contain disease when necessary.

We are enhancing international collaboration and strengthening multilateral institutions in order to improve global surveillance and early warning capabilities and quickly enact control and containment measures against the next pandemic threat. We continue to improve our understanding of emerging diseases and help develop environments that are less conducive to epidemic emergence. We depend on U.S. overseas laboratories, relationships with host nation governments, and the willingness of states to share health data with nongovernmental and international organizations. In this regard, we need to continue to work to overcome the lack of openness and a general reluctance to share health information. Finally, we seek to mitigate other problem areas, including limited global vaccine production capacity, and the threat of emergent and reemergent disease in poorly governed states.

Reproduced from The White House. Pandemic and Infectious Disease. *National Security Strategy.* May 2010; pp 48–49. Available at: https://obamawhitehouse.archives.gov/sites/default/files/rss_viewer/national_security_strategy.pdf. Accessed April 2017.

---

global infectious disease outbreaks as a top strategic risk to the United States (**BOX 3-4** and **FIGURE 3-3**). The 2015 NSS included specific language on Ebola, the spread of EIDs, antimicrobial resistance (AMR), and the need to build public health capacity around the world to prevent, detect, and respond to outbreaks.

To stop disease that spreads across borders, we much strengthen our system of public health. We will continue the fight against HIV/AIDS, TB, and malaria. We will focus on the health of mothers and of children. And we must come together to prevent, and detect, and fight every kind of biological danger—whether it's a pandemic like H1N1, or a terrorist threat, or a treatable disease.

Reproduced from President Barack Obama. Speech given at: United Nations General Assembly, New York, NY. Available at: https://obamawhitehouse.archives.gov/the-press-office/2011/09/21/remarks-president-obama-address-united-nations-general-assembly. Accessed April 2017.

The spread of infectious diseases constitute a growing risk. The Ebola epidemic in West Africa highlights the danger of a raging virus. The spread of new microbes or viruses, the rise and spread of drug resistance, and the deliberate release of pathogens all represent threats that are exacerbated by the globalization of travel, food production and supply, and medical products. Despite important scientific, technological, and organizational accomplishments, most countries have not yet achieved international core competencies for health security, and many lack sufficient capacity to prevent, detect, or respond to disease outbreaks.

America is the world leader in fighting pandemics, including HIV/AIDS, and in improving global health security.

At home, we are strengthening our ability to prevent outbreaks and ensure sufficient capacity to respond rapidly and manage biological incidents. As an exemplar of a modern and responsive public health system, we will accelerate our work with partners through the Global Health Security Agenda in pursuit of a world that is safer and more secure from infectious disease. We will save lives by strengthening regulatory frameworks for food safety and developing a global system to prevent avoidable epidemics, detect and report disease outbreaks in real time, and respond more rapidly and effectively. Finally, we will continue to lead efforts to combat the rise of antibiotic resistant bacteria.

Reproduced from The White House. *National Security Strategy*. February 2015; pp 13–14. Available at: https://obamawhitehouse.archives.gov/sites/default/files/docs/2015_national_security_strategy.pdf. Accessed April 2017.

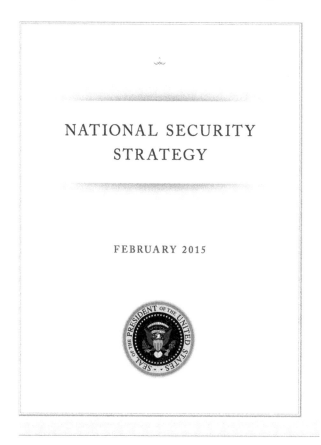

FIGURE 3-3 National Security Strategy 2015

Reproduced from The White House. *National Security Strategy*. February 2015; pp 13–14. Available at: https://obamawhitehouse.archives.gov/sites/default/files/docs/2015_national_security_strategy.pdf. Accessed April 2017.

▶ Defining the Link Between Disease and Security

We have traced the political evolution of health security in the United States, but how exactly does health impact national security? There are both direct and indirect links between health and national security (**BOX 3-5**).

The direct impact of disease on national security arises from the potential proliferation or use of a biological weapon, or the intentional spread of disease within specific populations. In addition, the impact of disease on the armed forces directly affects security because morbidity and mortality affects "readiness"—the ability of the nation to defend itself militarily and to engage in armed battles around the world. It is interesting to note that until World War II, more soldiers died from infectious diseases than from direct combat injuries.[14] Disease altered the outcomes of conflicts and affected the balance of power among states. Even today, troop exposure to diseases affects morbidity and mortality, which then impacts overall military readiness. Hospital admissions from disease continue to outnumber injuries and wounds during

This box, quoting text from the report, highlights the relationship between infectious diseases and national security.

> Human and animal health will increasingly be interconnected. Increasing global connectivity and changing environmental conditions will affect the geographic distribution of pathogens and their hosts, and, in turn, the emergence, transmission, and spread of many human and animal infectious diseases. Unaddressed deficiencies in national and global health systems for disease control will make infectious disease outbreaks more difficult to detect and manage, increasing the potential for epidemics to break out far beyond their points of origin.

Reproduced from NIC. *Trends Transforming the Global Landscape*. January 2017. Available at: https://www.dni.gov/index.php/global-trends/trends-transforming -the-global-landscape. Accessed June 2017.

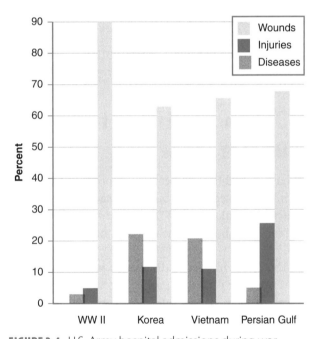

FIGURE 3-4 U.S. Army hospital admissions during war

Data from Noah D, Fidas G. *The global infectious disease and its implications for the United States*. Washington, DC, National Intelligence Council (NIC), 2000. NIE 99-17D. Available at: https://permanent.access.gpo.gov/websites/www.cia.gov /www.cia.gov/cia/reports/nie/report/372307.gif. Accessed April 2017.

U.S. military deployments (see **FIGURE 3-4**). As a result, the military has invested significant resources in infectious disease research, building diagnostic laboratory capacity around the world, disease surveillance infrastructure, and vaccine development.[15–18]

Indirectly, disease affects security because it can create large-scale morbidity and mortality, leading to massive loss of life and affecting all sectors of society. Such morbidity and mortality could result in economic loss and even long-term deterioration of economic viability. Fear of disease, in addition to disease itself, can lead to societal disruption, which can lead to civil disorder, political unrest, and, ultimately, destabilization. Also indirectly, chronic diseases—now the leading cause of morbidity and mortality around the world—can impact economies, government stability, and military readiness in strategic countries and regions.[19]

Globalization; movement of peoples, animals, and goods; rapid urbanization; and changing human behaviors and land use all create opportunities for the emergence of infectious diseases. These diseases emerge from every corner of the world and because of rapid transportation networks, can spread from international airports around the world in 24–48 hours. Pathogens with differing routes of exposure will spread at varying rates, but it has been estimated that a respiratory virus could spread globally and kill as many as 30 million people in a single year.[20]

While disease can emerge anywhere and spread everywhere, it tends to adversely affect regions and countries that are less able to address the threat.[3] Over the past four decades, there has been a fourfold increase in the number of EIDs and these diseases continue to emerge in all corners of the world.[21,22] Additionally, researchers have conducted "hot spot analysis" to identify conditions such as the presence of vectors, land use, and climate to identify where particular types of disease (like mosquito borne) are likely to occur.[23]

The regions where public health emergencies are most likely to emerge are the same regions experiencing critical shortages of healthcare personnel and tend to have the least developed healthcare infrastructure (**FIGURE 3-5**).[3,24] On top of this, many of the current and developing megacities (10 million people or more) can be found in these same regions as poor healthcare infrastructure, understaffed healthcare workforce, and the most public health emergencies.[24] This means that it is possible that a public health emergency will emerge in a place that is understaffed, under-resourced, and overpopulated—all conditions that may contribute to the spread of disease.

▶ Global Interconnectedness and the Threat of Emerging Infectious Diseases

There have been several examples in recent history that underscore just how connected the world is, and that people, animals, and pathogens travel the world with remarkable speed. Below are examples of EID or reemerging diseases, how they have spread around the world, and their impact on society.

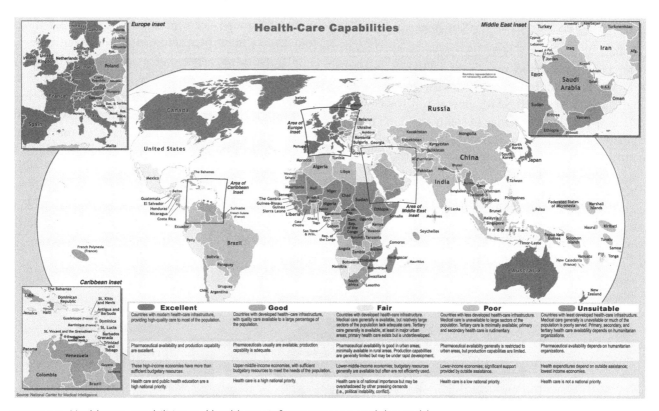

FIGURE 3-5 Healthcare capabilities and healthcare infrastructure around the world

Reproduced from Office of the Director of National Intelligence. *Health-care Capabilities*. Available at https://www.dni.gov/files/documents/Special%20Report_ICA%20Global%20Health%202008%20foldout.pdf. Accessed April 2017.

Monkeypox

In April 2003, a shipment of 800 small animals from Ghana arrived in Texas. Included in this shipment were Gambian rats, which were incidentally infected with monkeypox. The Gambian rats were kept in a location close enough to a group of prairie dogs to infect them with the disease. An Illinois animal vendor then sold these infected prairie dogs. Prairie dog owners—many of whom were children—were bitten by or touched either blood or rash on the infected animals (**FIGURE 3-6**). This resulted in 71 cases of monkeypox throughout the Midwest United States (**TABLE 3-1**).[25] Given that poxviruses, with the exception of chickenpox, are not commonly seen in the United States, the public health community was not prepared to treat the almost 80 cases and address public fear associated with the outbreak. In one instance, a 10-year-old girl struggled to find a doctor who would treat her. When she did find medical care, she was relegated to a small medical staff who were willing to interact with her.[26]

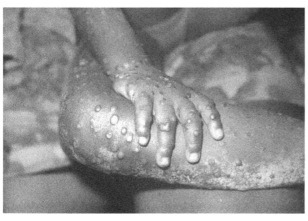

FIGURE 3-6 Close-up of monkeypox lesions on the arm and leg of a female child in Liberia

Reproduced from CDC Public Health Image Library. *Close-up of monkeypox lesions on the arm and leg of a female child*. Available at: https://phil.cdc.gov/phil_images/20021115/32/PHIL_2329.tif. Accessed April 2017.

TABLE 3-1 Location and Number of Confirmed and Suspected Monkeypox Cases Resulting from 2003 Shipment of Infected Gambian Rats to the United States

State	Number of Cases
Illinois	12
Indiana	16
Kansas	1
Missouri	2
Ohio	1
Wisconsin	39
Total	**71**

Data from Centers for Disease Control and Prevention. Update: Multistate Outbreak of Monkeypox—Illinois, Indiana, Kansas, Missouri, Ohio, and Wisconsin, 2003. *MMWR.* July 2003;52(27):643. Available at: https://www.cdc.gov/mmwr/PDF/wk /mm5227.pdf.

Severe Acute Respiratory Syndrome

The best example of global interdependence, speed of air travel, and rapid movement of people comes from the SARS outbreak in 2003. The first case of what came to be called SARS emerged in November 2002 in Guangdong Province in southern China from exposure, slaughter, and consumption of small wild mammals. The outbreak grew over the course of several months, but the causative agent was not correctly identified, and little was done to contain the spread of disease. By early February 2003, there were almost 300 cases in Guangdong Province and 5 deaths.[27(p6)] China, however, did not report this EID to the outside world. The WHO queried China after receiving news of an outbreak through electronic reporting systems, but was told it was a nonurgent acute respiratory syndrome.[27]

The worldwide spread of SARS began on February 21, 2003 (**FIGURE 3-7**). An infected physician traveled to Hong Kong and stayed at the Metropole Hotel, where he infected 12 other people at the hotel, who then left Hong Kong and brought the disease to the United States, Canada, Singapore, Vietnam, and Ireland.[28] In each instance, except for Ireland, these infected travelers then spread the disease in the next country. In at least one documented instance, SARS was spread on a transnational flight.[29] By September 2003, there had been 8098 cases and 774 deaths reported in 29 countries.

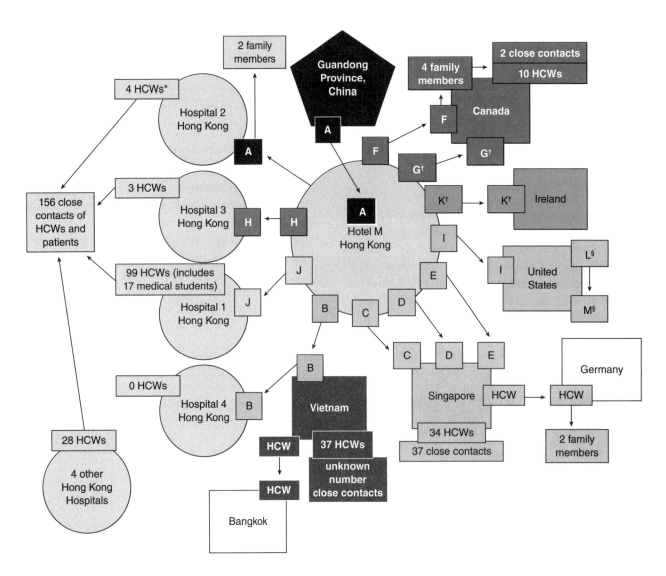

* Healthcare workers.
† All guests except G and K stayed on the 9th floor of the hotel. Guest G stayed on the 14th floor, and Guest K stayed on the 11th floor.
§ Guests L and M (spouses) were not at the Hotel M during the same time as index Guest A but were at the hotel during the same times as Guests G, H, and I, who were ill during this period.

FIGURE 3-7 How SARS spread around the world: chain of transmission among guests at a hotel in Hong Kong in 2003.

The global experience with SARS and the actions taken to try to contain the disease as it spread throughout the world highlight our interconnectedness, as well as the challenges of global health governance. The WHO advised airlines to screen passengers and advised travelers to avoid all but essential travel to certain areas, resulting in significant economic consequences. Thailand saw a 55% decline in tourism, and SARS cut gross domestic product growth in Vietnam by 1.1% in 2003. The full economic cost of the outbreak has been estimated to be approximately $30 billion, hitting Southeast Asia and Canada hardest.[27(pp91–136)] The epidemic led to discrimination, unnecessary isolation and quarantine, and political upheavals.[27(pp91–136),30] SARS was a naturally occurring disease that caused morbidity and mortality, invoked fear, affected travel, led to population discrimination, created an economic burden on certain nations, and affected security.

Almost a decade later, another coronavirus emerged; this time in the Middle East. Middle East Respiratory Syndrome (MERS) first emerged in 2012, identified in an outbreak in Jordan, and has now spread to over two dozen countries. Between 2012 and April 2017, there have been over 1900 cases, with the majority of cases occurring in Saudi Arabia.[31] Over 30% of cases result in death and it appears that camels are the major reservoir for the disease, although human-to-human transmission is possible and has been documented around the world through close contact (**FIGURE 3-8**).[32]

In the summer of 2015, a traveler from the Middle East arrived in South Korea. The traveler sought health care in multiple clinical settings, eventually transmitting the disease before it was identified. This single case resulted in over 180 MERS cases in South Korea, and a response that involved large-scale quarantines at a significant societal cost.

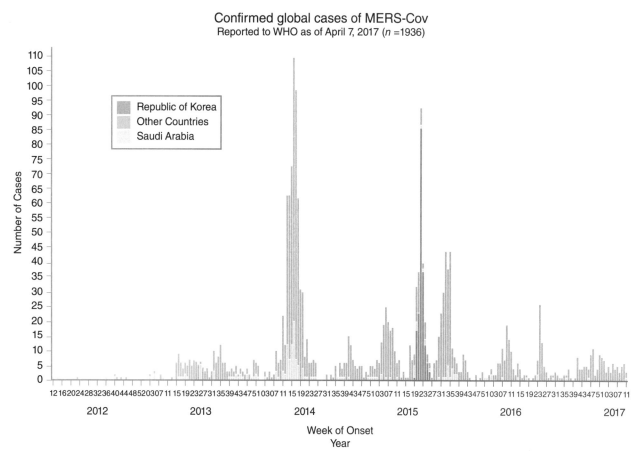

Other countries: Algeria, Austria, Bahrain, China, Egypt, France, Germany, Greece, Iran, Italy, Jordan, Kuwait, Lebanon, Malaysia, Netherlands, Oman, Philippines, Qatar, Thailand, Tunisia, Turkey, United Arab Emirates, United Kingdom, United States of America, Yemen

Please note that the underlying data is subject to change as the investigations around cases are ongoing. Onset date estimated if not available.

FIGURE 3-8 Confirmed global cases of Middle East Respiratory Syndrome Coronavirus, which was reported to the WHO as of April 7, 2017 (*n* = 1936)

HIV/AIDS

The HIV/AIDS pandemic provides the most illustrative example to date of the ways in which a disease with high levels of morbidity and mortality can affect the security and viability of nations. HIV/AIDS has already caused approximately 35 million deaths worldwide. There were an estimated 36.7 million people living with HIV in 2015.[33] The disease tends to affect the working-age population and has dramatically reduced life expectancy in some nations. The disease has impacted all sectors of society, from education to agriculture. The labor force in some countries has shrunk dramatically and the number of orphans from HIV/AIDS has grown—there are now nearly 17 million HIV/AIDS orphans, with 90% of these children living in sub-Saharan Africa.[34] Without enough workers to sustain an economically viable society, too few teachers, and a growing number of orphans and children who cannot be provided for, nations without global support become almost destined for civil unrest and government instability.

One of the most direct ways HIV/AIDS has affected national security is through the effect of the disease on militaries. Initial research suggested that armed conflict increased the spread and severity of HIV/AIDS in society. These claims, however, have not been proven through empirical analysis; more recent concern focuses on how disease may spread at the end of conflict.[35] The absolute numbers of HIV-positive individuals in militaries, however, remains of great concern. Nations need to be capable of fielding healthy armed forces and when the prevalence of disease amongst military age citizens is high, this can be a challenge. For example, the prevalence of HIV has risen dramatically among Russian military recruits, posing unique challenges to both the civilian and military sectors to address the problem.[36] As HIV/AIDS incidence and prevalence rise in countries such as China and India, and retains its foothold in sub-Saharan Africa and Russia, the security implications of the disease cannot be underestimated. Aside from direct military security concerns, approximately 1.7 million of the 314 million people affected by emergencies were living with HIV, complicating the lives of already vulnerable people trying to survive in insecure environments.[37]

Ebola in West Africa

In late December 2013, a small boy who had interacted with bats became sick with what would eventually be identified as Ebola. The boy spread the disease to his family in his rural village in Guinea, and it rapidly spread from there into the urban environment.[38] By March 2014, authorities had identified the outbreak as Ebola, but international resources to aid in the response were slow in coming; it wasn't until August 2014 that the outbreak was declared a public health emergency by the WHO and international aid began to flow in earnest.[39] The disease spread rapidly between Guinea, Sierra Leone, and Liberia: a region that had emerged from civil wars only a bit over a decade earlier and where the population of the three countries transverse over national boundaries with regularity. Disease spread to other parts of the world as well, with limited examples of both ill West Africans leaving the region and infected healthcare workers and first responders going back to their country of origin. In all, there were 28,616 cases and 11,310 deaths (**FIGURE 3-9**).[40]

Zika

Zika virus was first discovered in 1947 in Uganda, but little attention was paid to the virus until the spring of 2015, when Brazil and other nations in the Americas starting reporting significant numbers of Zika infections.[41,42] While it wasn't entirely clear at the time,

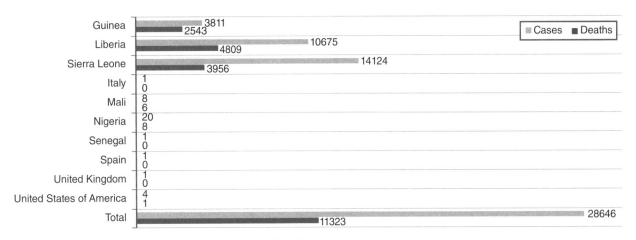

FIGURE 3-9 Ebola cases and deaths data up to March 27, 2016

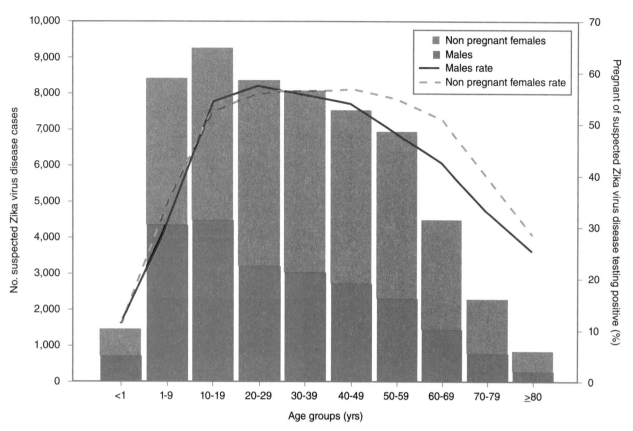

* Sex was not reported for 33 cases; age or date of birth was not reported for 251 cases.

FIGURE 3-10 Number of suspected Zika virus disease cases among males and nonpregnant females reported, and percent that tested positive for Zika virus by age group and sex (*n* = 57,727)—including Puerto Rico, November 1, 2015–October 20, 2016

Reproduced from Lozier M, Adams L, Febo M.F, et al. Incidence of Zika Virus Disease by Age and Sex—Puerto Rico, November 1, 2015–October 20, 2016. *MMWR*. November 11, 2016;65(44): 1221. Available at: http://apps.who.int/iris/bitstream/10665/204714/1 /ebolasitrep_30mar2016_eng.pdf?ua=1. Accessed April 2017.

public health officials suspected that the Zika virus was linked to unusually high numbers of infants born with microcephaly. The virus, spread via mosquito as well as through sexual transmission, evoked significant fear for people of childbearing age. From South America, the virus has spread north, leading to large numbers of cases in the Caribbean, including Puerto Rico, and documented cases in the United States (**FIGURE 3-10**).

▶ Antimicrobial Resistance

While it is virtually impossible to predict what the next naturally occurring disease outbreak will be or where it will emerge, we know for certain that AMR threatens public health around the world. AMR is what happens when organisms develop resistance to drugs commonly used to treat disease and improve population health. It can complicate treatment of particular diseases. For example, 480,000 people develop multidrug-resistant TB every year.[43] Some classes of drugs, like chloroquine for malaria, are now ineffective, as chloroquine resistance has spread to almost all parts of the world.[44]

AMR will continue to threaten public health around the world and could make even the most

common surgeries and treatments impossible (**FIGURE 3-11**). New approaches, from animal practices to economic models, are currently being considered by governments in an attempt to address this threat.

▶ Response

To date, the response to the health security nexus has been to try to establish stronger public health infrastructure and to direct assistance to address, contain, and mitigate natural disease threats. This has been accomplished by trying to strengthen global disease surveillance (see later chapters) and through disease and development assistance, primarily in the United States through U.S. Agency for International Development, PEPFAR, the Global Fund, Centers for Disease Control and Prevention, and the Department of Defense (**BOX 3-6**).

Domestic efforts have focused on improving surveillance, research, countermeasures and diagnostics, surge capacity for catastrophic events, and community resilience. These topics are all addressed throughout the course of this text.

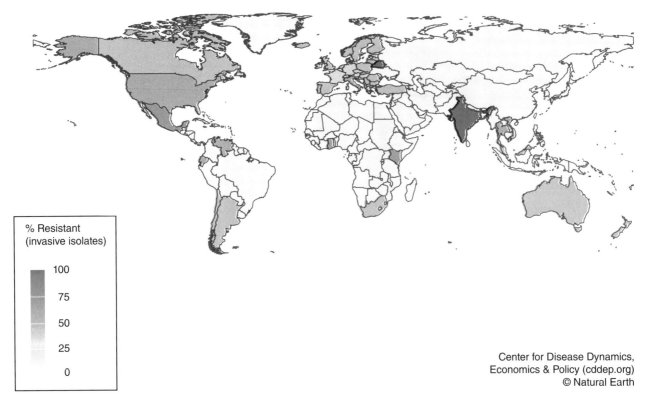

FIGURE 3-11 Resistance of *Escherichia coli* to fluoroquinolones

Reproduced from The Center for Disease Dynamics, Economics and Policy. *Resistance of Escherichia coli to Fluoroquinolones.* Available at: https://resistancemap.cddep.org/AntibioticResistance.php. Accessed April 2017.

BOX 3-6 Disease, Security, Foreign Policy, and Diplomacy

In 1978, Peter Bourne, the then special assistant to President Carter for health issues, completed a study on international health policy and called for a diplomatic strategy to both improve global health and utilize health efforts to affect foreign policy. In recent years, this concept of health and its relationship to foreign policy and opportunities for diplomacy has been reinvigorated. There is still much debate over exactly how and when global health efforts impact foreign policy and whether the health concern also needs to be a security concern in order to raise its importance in policy circles. But there is a growing recognition of the opportunities presented by health diplomacy and the importance of significantly contributing to efforts to detect, control, and treat diseases around the world.

Data from Bourne PG. A Partnership for International Health Care. *Public Health Reports.* March–April 1978;93(2):114–123; Feldbaum H, Michaud J. Health Diplomacy and the Enduring Relevance of Foreign Policy Interests. *PLoS Medicine.* April 2010;7(4); Fidler DP. Eastphalia Emerging?: Asia, International Law, and Global Governance. *Indiana Journal of Global Legal Studies.* Winter 2010;17(1):1–12.

Key Words

Antimicrobial resistance	HIV/AIDS	SARS
Ebola	MERS	Zika
Health security	Monkeypox	

Discussion Questions

1. What is health security?
2. Why and when is a natural infectious disease a security threat? To whom?
3. How does urbanization in one part of the world become a security interest to others?
4. Is it necessary to securitize a health issue in order to gain political support to direct resources to the global community?
5. Can you think of an example of "health diplomacy"?
6. Should health be used as a diplomatic tool?
7. Are there any detriments to making disease a security issue?

References

1. Weber AC (Assistant to the Secretary of Defense for Nuclear and Chemical and Biological Defense Programs). *Second Annual Richard and Janet South by Distinguished Lectureship in Comparative Health Policy.* The George Washington University School of Public Health and Health Services; Washington, DC; April 6, 2010.

2. U.S. Department of Health and Human Services. *National Health Security Strategy of the United States of America.* December 2009. p 3. Available at: http://www.phe.gov/Preparedness/planning/authority/nhss/strategy/Documents/nhss-final.pdf. Accessed July 25, 2010.

3. World Health Organization. *The World Health Report 2007: A Safer Future—Global Public Health Security in the 21st Century.* 2007. Available at: http://www.who.int/whr/2007/overview/en/. Accessed April 2017.

4. Barry JM. *The Great Influenza: The Epic Story of the Deadliest Plague in History.* New York, NY: Penguin Books; 2005.

5. Clinton WJ. *Presidential Decision Directive NSTC-7.* Federation of American Scientists. 1996. Available at: http://www.fas.org/irp/offdocs/pdd/pdd-nstc-7.pdf. Accessed June 2017.

6. The White House, Office of the Vice President. *Vice President Announces Policy on Infectious Diseases.* Federation of American Scientists. June 12, 1996. Available at: http://www.fas.org/irp/offdocs/pdd_ntsc7.htm. Accessed June 2017.

7. National Intelligence Council. *The Global Infectious Disease Threat and Its Implications for the United States.* NIE 99-17D. January 2000. Available at: https://www.dni.gov/files/documents/infectiousdiseases_2000.pdf. Accessed June 2017.

8. United Nations Security Council. *Security Council Resolution 1308: On the Responsibility of the Security Council in the Maintenance of International Peace and Security: HIV/AIDS and International Peacekeeping Operations.* July 17, 2000. Available at: http://www.unaids.org/sites/default/files/sub_landing/files/20000717_un_scresolution_1308_en.pdf. Accessed June 2017.

9. Gellman B. AIDS Is Declared Threat to Security. *The Washington Post.* April 2000. A01. Available at: https://www.washingtonpost.com/archive/politics/2000/04/30/aids-is-declared-threat-to-security/c5e976e4-3fe8-411b-9734-ca44f3130b41/?utm_term=.b3f2ca0b7a5a.

10. The White House. *The National Security Strategy of the United States of America.* September 2002. Available at: https://www.state.gov/documents/organization/63562.pdf. Accessed April 2017.

11. The White House. *The National Security Strategy of the United States of America.* March 2006. Available at: https://www.state.gov/documents/organization/64884.pdf. Accessed April 2017.

12. The White House. *National Security Strategy.* May 2010. Available at: https://obamawhitehouse.archives.gov/sites/default/files/rss_viewer/national_security_strategy.pdf. Accessed April 2017.

13. Clinton HR. Global Health Initiative: The Next Phase of American Leadership in Health around the World. Speech Presented at: Paul H. Nitze School of Advanced International Studies; August 16, 2010; Washington, DC. Available at: https://geneva.usmission.gov/2010/08/17/ghi-next-phase/. Accessed April 25, 2017.

14. Institute of Medicine (IOM), Medical Follow-Up Agency (MFUA). Introduction and History—Naturally Occurring Infectious Diseases in the U.S. Military. In: Lemon SM, Thaul S, Fisseha S, O'Maon HC, eds. *Protecting Our Forces: Improving Vaccine Acquisition and Availability in the U.S. Military.* Washington, DC: The National Academies Press; 2002; Available at: http://www.nap.edu/openbook.php?record_id=10483&page=9.

15. Murry CK, Hinkle MK, Yun HC. History of Infections Associated With Combat-Related Injuries. *The Journal of Trauma: Injury, Infection, & Critical Care.* March 2008;64(3):S221–S231; Available at: http://www.afids.org/Prevention%20and%20Management%20of%20CRI%20(4)%20-%20History.pdf.

16. Writer JV, DeFraites RF, Keep LW. Non-battle injury casualties during the Persian Gulf War and other deployments. *American Journal of Preventive Medicine.* April 2000;18 (3, Suppl 1):64–70.

17. Military Health System. Global Emerging Infections Surveillance and Response System. Available at: https://www.health.mil/Military-Health-Topics/Health-Readiness/Armed-Forces-Health-Surveillance-Branch/Global-Emerging-Infections-Surveillance-and-Response. Accessed September 2017.

18. Walter Reed Army Institute of Research. U.S. Army Medical Research and Materiel Command. Available at: http://mrmc.amedd.army.mil . Accessed September 2017.

19. U.S. Department of State. Infectious and Chronic Disease. Available at: https://2001-2009.state.gov/g/oes/id/. Accessed August 1, 2010.

20. Gates B. Speech Given at: 53rd Munich Security Conference; February 18, 2014; Munich, Germany. Available at: https://www.securityconference.de/en/activities/munich-security-conference/msc-2017/speeches/speech-by-bill-gates/. Accessed April 2017.

21. Doucleff M, Greenhalgh J. Why Killer Viruses Are on the Rise. *NPR.* February 14, 2017. Available at: http://www.npr.org/sections/goatsandsoda/2017/02/14/511227050/why-killer-viruses-are-on-the-rise. Accessed May 2017.

22. Fauci A. *Pandemic Preparedness in the Next Administration: A View from the National Institutes of Health.* Speech Given at: Georgetown University/Harvard University symposium on Pandemic Preparedness; January 10, 2017; Washington, DC. Available at: https://www.youtube.com/watch?v=wB7j_7vgZvY, Accessed March 16, 2010.

23. Jones K, Patel NG, Levy M, et al. Global Trends in Emerging Infectious Diseases. *Nature.* 2008;451:993. doi:10.1038/nature06536.

24. National Intelligence Council. *Strategic Implications of Global Health.* December 2008. ICA 2008-10D. Available at: https://www.dni.gov/files/documents/Special%20Report_ICA%20Global%20Health%202008.pdf. Accessed June 2017.

25. Centers for Disease Control and Prevention. Update: Multistate Outbreak of Monkeypox—Illinois, Indiana, Kansas, Missouri, Ohio, and Wisconsin, 2003. *MMWR.* July 2003;52(27):642–646.

26. Reynolds G. *Why Were Doctors Afraid to Treat Rebecca McLester?* [So they called-in doctors Michael and Stephanie Anderson who both stepped-up.] Children's Pediatric Center—East Main. April 18, 2004. Available at: http://www.childrenspediatrics.com/monkey_pox.htm. Accessed August 1, 2010.

27. Institute of Medicine. *Learning from SARS: Preparing for the Next Disease Outbreak.* Washington, DC: The National

Academies Press; 2004; Available at: http://www.nap.edu /catalog.php?record_id=10915.

28. Centers for Disease Control and Prevention. Update: Outbreak of Severe Acute Respiratory Syndrome—Worldwide, 2003. *MMWR*. March 2003;52(12):241–248.

29. Olsen SJ, Chang HL, Cheung TYY, et al. Transmission of the Severe Acute Respiratory Syndrome on Aircraft. *The New England Journal of Medicine*. December 2003;349(25):2416–2422.

30. National Intelligence Council. *SARS: Down but Still a Threat*. National Intelligence Council. August 2003. Available at: https://fas.org/irp/nic/sars.pdf. Accessed April 2017.

31. WHO. Middle East Respiratory Syndrome Coronavirus (MERs-CoV). 2017. Available at: http://www.who.int /emergencies/mers-cov/en/. Accessed April 2017.

32. WHO Media Centre. Middle East Respiratory Syndrome Coronavirus (MERs-CoV). *Fact Sheet*. June 2015. Available at: http://www.who.int/mediacentre/factsheets/mers-cov/en/. Accessed April 2017.

33. UNAIDS. Global HIV Statistics. *Fact Sheet*. November 2016. Available at: http://www.unaids.org/sites/default /files/media_asset/UNAIDS_FactSheet_en.pdf. Accessed April 2017.

34. USAID. Orphans and Vulnerable Children affected by HIV and AIDS. February 23, 2016. Available at: https:// www.usaid.gov/what-we-do/global-health/hiv-and-aids /technical-areas/orphans-and-vulnerable-children-affected-hiv. Accessed April 2017.

35. Waal Ad. HIV/AIDS and the Challenges of Security and Conflict. *The Lancet*. January 2010; 375(9708):22–23.

36. Holachek J. *Russia's Shrinking Population and the Russian Military's HIV/AIDS Problem*. The Atlantic Council. September 2006. Available at: https://www.files.ethz.ch /isn/32369/2006_09_Russia%27s_Shrinking_Population_.pdf. Accessed May 2017.

37. UNAIDS. HIV and Security: Past, Present and Future. June 7, 2016. Available at: http://www.unaids.org/en/resources /presscentre/featurestories/2016/june/20160607_hivandsecurity. Accessed April 2017.

38. WHO. *Emergencies Preparedness, Response: Origins of the 2014 Ebola Epidemic*. January 2015. Available at: http:// who.int/csr/disease/ebola/one-year-report/virus-origin/en/. Accessed April 2017.

39. WHO Media Centre. Statement on the 1st Meeting of the IHR Emergency Committee on the 2014 Ebola Outbreak in West Africa [News Release]. August 8, 2014. Available at: http:// www.who.int/mediacentre/news/statements/2014/ebola -20140808/en/. Accessed April 2017.

40. WHO Media Centre. Final Trial Results Confirm Ebola Vaccine Provides High Protection against Disease [News Release]. December 23, 2016. Available at http://www.who .int/mediacentre/news/releases/2016/ebola-vaccine-results /en/. Accessed April 2017.

41. WHO. *Emergencies: The History of Zika Virus*. 2017. Available at: http://www.who.int/emergencies/zika-virus/timeline/en/. Accessed April 2017.

42. WHO. Zika Virus Outbreaks in the Americas. *Weekly Epidemiological Record*. 2015;90(45): 609–616, Available at: http://www.who.int/wer/2015/wer9045.pdf?ua=1. Accessed April 2017.

43. WHO Media Centre. Antimicrobial Resistance. *Fact Sheet*. September 2016. Available at: http://www.who.int/mediacentre /factsheets/fs194/en/. Accessed April 2017.

44. CDC. Drug Resistance in the Malaria-Endemic World. 2015. Available at: https://www.cdc.gov/malaria/malaria_worldwide /reduction/drug_resistance.html. Accessed April 2017.

PART III
Infrastructure

© f00sion/E+/Getty

CHAPTER 4

9/11 and Its Aftermath

▶ Introduction

The public health community does not operate in a vacuum, and public health preparedness, in particular, functions within a large, relatively new, and often shifting infrastructure of organizations and policies. In this chapter, we review the federal government's role in preparedness and response to biological threats in the United States, how it has developed over time, and the shifts that occurred after the September 11, 2001 (9/11) terrorist disaster. We also look at the offices, organizations, and policies that have emerged in the past two decades that relate directly to public health preparedness. Finally, this chapter introduces readers to the Intelligence Community (IC). In the past, the public health community had minimal interaction with the IC. While most local and state public health professionals still do not interface with this community, many federal public health professionals working on preparedness have begun to coordinate with their IC colleagues. This community, though, is foreign to most public health professionals, therefore this chapter provides an overview of the organizations within the community and some of the basic concepts associated with intelligence.

In the wake of 9/11, the U.S. government stepped up efforts to develop, exercise, and solidify plans to address all types of emergencies that might threaten the population. We follow the path for the development of these plans and delve deeper into the emergency preparedness plans that have been created, tested, and retested since 2001. We focus primarily on the federal level plans, but also look at state and local preparedness planning efforts, and some of the efforts that have emerged to track state and local preparedness. We examine international preparedness activities in later chapters of this book.

▶ Constitutional Framework and History of Federal Assistance for Preparedness and Disaster Response

Under the U.S. Constitution, powers are delegated to both the federal and state governments. Under this arrangement, state and local governments are responsible for public health and safety from domestic threats (including natural threats).[1(amend. 10)] The federal government is responsible for protection from external threats or internal rebellion.[1(Art. I §§ 8–10, Art. II § 2, Art. IV § 4)] Note that the U.S. Constitution contains no provision ensuring federal assistance during a disaster. Although the federal government may assist, the 10th Amendment does reserve to the states those powers are not specifically enumerated. By this delineation, the federal government when it was established had only a supportive role in disaster response, with the states and local governments responsible for preparedness and response. According to George M. Foster, there were both practical and philosophical reasons for the limited federal role. The practical reasons were that prior to the Civil War, the federal government was very small, with almost all of its workforce located in Washington, D.C. The government had limited infrastructure to support the logistics involved in sending relief and supplies to an affected region.[2,3(p4)] The philosophical rationale for a limited federal role in disaster response was based on the prevailing concept of self-help, and if need be, assistance from private organizations, as opposed to government aid.

In 1803, Congress passed the first law related to domestic disaster assistance (BOX 4-1). This act came after Portsmouth, New Hampshire, experienced massive fires in late December 1802. The assistance was in the form of long-term financial aid to rebuild

---

BOX 4-1 Text of the 1803 Federal Domestic Disaster Aid Bill from January 14, 1803

A Bill for the Relief of Sufferers by Fire, in the town of Portsmouth

Be it enacted, by the Senate and House of Representatives of the United States of America, in Congress assembled, That the Secretary of the Treasury be, and he hereby is authorized and directed to cause to be suspended for months, the collection of bonds due to the United States by merchants of Portsmouth, in New Hampshire, who have suffered by the late conflagration of that town.

Reproduced from *A Bill for the relief of the sufferers by fire, in the town of Portsmouth*, H.R. 7th Cong. (January 14, 1803).

---

and recover, as opposed to immediate assistance.[2] Congress acted similarly in response to subsequent disasters, and there was no attempt to create a comprehensive policy for federal disaster assistance. Between 1803 and 1950, Congress passed legislation to provide relief in 128 separate natural disaster instances. Over time, the assistance shifted from financial aid (relief from bond payments) to in-kind assistance.[4]

After the Civil War, there was a shift in how the federal government perceived its responsibilities toward disaster relief, as well as a greater willingness—and need—on the part of individuals to ask for assistance. In March 1865, Congress created the Bureau of Refugees, Freedmen and Abandoned Lands, known as the Freedmen's Bureau, located administratively within the War Department. The purpose of the organization, which only existed for 7 years, was to aid former slaves. It took on multiple projects, though, including land reform, labor practices, and the development of social institutions.[5] It also provided relief in the form of shelter and supplies to refugees and newly freed men.[6] Through the Freedmen's Bureau, the U.S. Army became the federal entity tasked with providing disaster relief.

Federal disaster assistance had become not only popular but also expected; and in the 1930s, the Reconstruction Finance Corporation (RFC) became responsible for providing loans for disaster recovery. RFC was only quasi-governmental; it was owned by the federal government but staffed by nongovernment employees.[7] Other federal agencies were given more authority to assist in both disaster response and preparedness. This was done on a piecemeal basis and not as part of a comprehensive approach to preparedness or response.[8] In 1953, President Harry S. Truman issued Executive Order 10427, which emphasized that federal assistance was only to supplement—not supplant—state, local, and private organization's resources in response to disasters. This was restated and supported by President Richard Nixon in 1973.[9] By the late 1970s, there were over 100 federal agencies involved in some aspect of disaster preparedness and response. Yet, the policy firmly stated that the federal government was only to assist state and local entities, who were in charge of response. The National Governor's Association asked President Jimmy Carter to centralize federal government functions, and Carter responded in 1979 with Executive Order 12127, which created the Federal Emergency Management Agency (FEMA).[8,10]

In 1974, Congress passed the Disaster Relief Act, which created a process for Presidential Disaster Declarations, as a requirement to trigger financial and physical assistance from FEMA for any domestic disaster.[11] In 1988, the Stafford Disaster Relief and Emergency Assistance Act (Stafford Act) amended the Disaster Relief Act, and became the principal document for federal

BOX 4-2 Robert T. Stafford Disaster Relief and Emergency Assistance Act, Public Law 93-288, as Amended, 42 U.S.C. 5121–5207, and Related Authorities

TITLE I—FINDINGS, DECLARATIONS AND DEFINITIONS

SEC. 101. CONGRESSIONAL FINDINGS AND DECLARATIONS (42 U.S.C. 5121)

It is the intent of the Congress, by this Act, to provide an orderly and continuing means of assistance by the Federal Government to State and local governments in carrying out their responsibilities to alleviate the suffering and damage which result from such disasters by—

1. revising and broadening the scope of existing disaster relief programs;
2. encouraging the development of comprehensive disaster preparedness and assistance plans, programs, capabilities, and organizations by the States and by local governments;
3. achieving greater coordination and responsiveness of disaster preparedness and relief programs;
4. encouraging individuals, States, and local governments to protect themselves by obtaining insurance coverage to supplement or replace governmental assistance;
5. encouraging hazard mitigation measures to reduce losses from disasters, including development of land use and construction regulations; and
6. providing Federal assistance programs for both public and private losses sustained in disasters.

Reproduced from Robert T. Stafford Disaster Relief and Emergency Assistance Act (Stafford Act), Public Law No. 100-707

authority and funds for assisting state and local governments in responding to any type of disaster (**BOX 4-2**).[12] This act mandates that the governor of a state make a formal request to the president to declare either a major disaster or an emergency. Once the declaration is made, FEMA is then responsible for coordinating relief efforts across 28 federal agencies and nongovernmental organizations, including the American Red Cross (**FIGURE 4-1**). The Stafford Act has been amended several times, including in 2000 with passage of the Disaster Mitigation Act and in 2006 with the Pets Evacuation and Transportation Standards (PETS) Act (**BOX 4-3**).[13,14] It was amended again in 2013 through the Sandy Recovery Improvement Act to improve how public assistance is delivered to state, local, and tribal governments.[15]

The 1995 Presidential Decision Directive 39 (PDD-39), "United States Policy on Counterterrorism," was the last major policy guidance that addressed disaster preparedness and response prior to 2001. This directive reaffirmed that FEMA would be in charge of consequence management during an emergency—including any terrorist event—while the Federal Bureau of Investigation (FBI) would handle crisis management for threats or acts of terrorism within the United States (**FIGURE 4-2**). All other federal agencies would provide support where appropriate, under coordination by the National Security Council (NSC).

▶ Immediate Response to 9/11

Prior to 2001, plans and policies were in place for federal response efforts, primarily designed for natural disasters. The federal government had historically taken a position of assisting state and local agencies,

not running a disaster response. On September 9, 2001, the United States experienced a terrorist event resulting in over 3000 deaths, which forced a paradigm shift in thinking about federal responsibilities. 9/11 was a major national emergency, not caused by a natural disaster. This was a disaster related to national security, in an arena where the federal government is responsible for "providing for the common defense." Many were forced to rethink how they conceive of disasters, federal roles, national security, and a new term that entered the vocabulary—homeland security.

In November 2002, the National Commission on Terrorist Attacks upon the United States was convened to review the events leading up to the 9/11 attacks and to make recommendations for moving forward. The commission's final report was released in July 2004, and is known as the "9/11 Commission Report." The commission found "the 9/11 attacks revealed four kinds of failures: in imagination, policy, capabilities, and management."[16(p339)] On imagination, many in government and across the country did not give adequate consideration to the possibility of a foreign terrorist attack on U.S. soil. On policy, terrorism was not a major priority for either the Clinton or Bush administration. It was considered and there were expertise devoted to it, but not nearly enough given the true nature of the threat. On capabilities, the United States operated in a Cold War mind-set, focusing on past threats instead of thinking about future conflicts. Military and intelligence organizations were not concentrating on a terrorist threat. There was very little link between local FBI agents and national priorities. The Federal Aviation Administration (FAA) was not strong enough. On management, the commission found an inability on the part of the federal government to manage new problems. Not enough information was shared

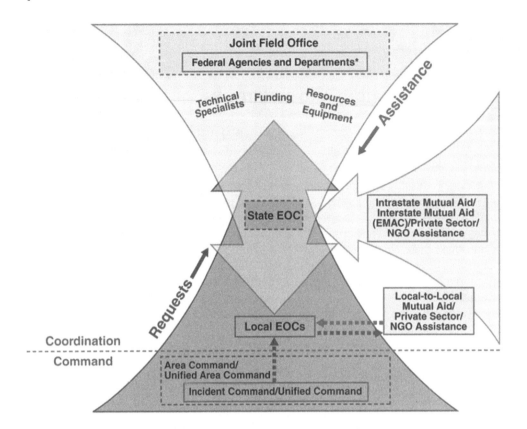

*Some Federal agencies (U.S. Coast Guard, Environmental Protection Agency, etc.) have statutory responsibility for response and may coordinate and/or integrate directly with affected jurisdictions.

FIGURE 4-1 Flow of requests and assistance when an incident occurs

Reproduced from Department of Homeland Security. *National Incident Management System*. December 2008. p. 36. Available at: https://www.fema.gov/pdf/emergency/nims/NIMS_core.pdf. Accessed May 2017.

BOX 4-3 Pets Evacuation and Transportation Standards Act

In 2006, Congress passed the PETS Act to ensure that household pets and service animals are provided for during an emergency. The development and passage of this act came about in the wake of Hurricane Katrina, when disaster response professionals became acutely aware that people would not evacuate or go to a shelter if there were no accommodations for their animals.

Data from AVMA. PETS Act FAQ. Available at: www.avma.org/KB/Resources/Reference /disaster/Pages/PETS-Act-FAQ.aspx. Accessed May 2017.

between agencies, duties were not clearly assigned, and there was limited management of how top leaders set priorities and allocated resources, particularly within the IC.

A main finding of the 9/11 Commission Report was that the U.S. federal government did not have a fully integrated, communicative, functional homeland security infrastructure, including emergency preparedness, which includes everything from first responders to public health infrastructure (**BOX 4-4**).

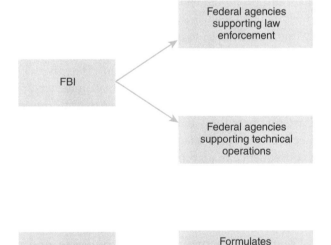

FIGURE 4-2 Presidential Decision Directive 39 from 1995: Relationship among federal agencies for crises and consequence management in response to terrorist acts

Data from FEMA. Figure 2-Relationship Among Federation Agencies Under PDD-39. *Federal Response Plan, Notice of Change*. February 7, 1997. Available at: https://www.fas.org/irp/offdocs/pdd39_frp.htm. Accessed May 2017.

▶ Post 9/11

Almost immediately after 9/11, and in the wake of the anthrax letters that followed, the United States began to make a series of changes, resulting in the most massive reorganization of the federal government since World War II. The following are some of the initial changes:

- Executive Order 13228, October 8, 2001: Established the Office of Homeland Security and the Homeland Security Council. Executive Order 13228 was the first effort by President George W. Bush following the 9/11 attacks. This established an Office of Homeland Security within the White House, and directed that the assistant to the president for homeland security should be the individual primarily responsible for coordinating the domestic response efforts of all departments and agencies in the event of an imminent terrorist threat and immediately following an attack. Tom Ridge, the former governor of Pennsylvania, was appointed to fill this position.
- National Security Presidential Directive 8 (NSPD 8), 2001: With the establishment of the Office and Council of Homeland Security, also came the creation of a deputy national security advisor for combating terrorism, tasked with operational coordination of combating transnational terrorist activities.
- Homeland Security Act of 2002, passed in 2003. This act created the Department of Homeland Security (DHS), reorganizing multiple existing agencies under a single department, as well as creating new responsibilities for security and preparedness.
- A series of Homeland Security Presidential Directives (HSPD) aimed at national preparedness and response policies and guidance documents (**BOX 4-5**). (More on these later in the book.)

In July 2002, the Bush administration released the National Strategy for Homeland Security, which identified six critical mission areas: intelligence and warning, border and transportation security, domestic counterterrorism, protecting critical infrastructure and key assets, defending against catastrophic events, and emergency preparedness and response. While the public health community was not directly referenced in this strategy (although emergency medical providers are identified as America's first line of defense in the aftermath of an attack), public health contributes to at least three of the

---

BOX 4-4 9/11 Commission Report Findings: The U.S. Government Challenges and Failures Leading up to 9/11

Unsuccessful Diplomacy

- As early as February 1997, the U.S. government attempted to use diplomatic pressure to convince different states to cease support to al-Qaeda and Osama bin Laden, including the Taliban Regime in Afghanistan, Pakistan, and the United Arab Emirates. These attempts included incentives, sanctions, and even warnings of retribution, but the United States could not find the right balance between these approaches and diplomatic attempts were largely fruitless.

Lack of Military Options

- In the summer of 1998, policymakers requested the military prepare options for conducting an attack on bin Laden and al-Qaeda. A great emphasis was placed on the need for actionable intelligence before launching any strike. The lack of such intelligence tied the hands of the military and frustrated policymakers, as they could not risk the possibility of inflicting serious collateral damage and could not afford to have any attack fail, because either scenario would make bin Laden appear strong and the United States appear weak.

Problems Within the Intelligence Community

- Due to competing priorities, budget constraints, an inefficient structure, and typical bureaucratic rivalries, the IC's effort to combat transnational terrorism was inadequate. Not only was there a lack of any comprehensive review of what the Central Intelligence Agency knew or did not know on the matter, it was also limited to using proxies in its efforts to disrupt terrorist activities by capturing Bin Laden or his lieutenants, which produced a frustrating lack of results.

Problems Within the FBI

- Following the first terrorist attack on the World Trade Center in 1993, the FBI became increasingly involved in the counterterrorism effort. However, its resources were primarily devoted to investigating and prosecuting terrorists after attacks, not preventing them from happening in the first place. Efforts to change this policy were fairly unsuccessful, mostly due to the FBI's bureaucratically limited capacity or wish to share information.

Permeable Borders and Immigration Controls

- Intelligence and law enforcement officials were both presented with opportunities to prevent al-Qaeda's attacks by exploiting their travel vulnerabilities, as the 9/11 participants included known al-Qaeda operatives who both behaved

(continues)

suspiciously and presented suspicious paperwork. Prior to the 9/11 attacks, however, protecting national borders was not a priority and the Immigration and Naturalization Service was not considered a partner in the counterterrorism effort.

Permeable Aviation Security

■ The hijackers in the 9/11 attack only needed to get past the security checkpoint process to carry out their attack, an obstacle easily overcome by simply studying publicly available materials on the subject. After some of the hijackers were selected for extra screening, the only action taken was a more highly scrutinized examination of their checked baggage.

Financing

■ The 9/11 attacks cost between $400,000 and $500,000 to execute, making them an extremely economical means of attack. The operatives' transactions were not suspicious and were effectively invisible amidst the billions of daily purchases in the United States.

An Improvised Homeland Defense

■ Both the FAA and North American Aerospace Defense Command (NORAD) were unprepared for the type of attack launched against the United States on 9/11. Both implemented the best course of action possible given the information at hand, but communication at more senior levels was poor. The military and the FAA had little to no communication with each other, and senior officials of the president's staff such as the secretary of defense were not brought into the chain of command until the key events of the morning had already occurred.

Reproduced from Zelikow P, Jenkins BD, May ER; National Commission on Terrorist Attacks upon the United States. *The 9/11 Commission Report*. Available at: https://www.9-11commission.gov/report/911Report.pdf. Accessed May 2017.

BOX 4-5 Overview of Presidential Directives

The president uses several instruments to establish, continue, or cease federal policies. Here are some of the most common directives, including those referenced in this text:

■ **Executive Order (EO)**: A presidential directive with the authority of a law that directs and governs action by executive officials and agencies.
■ **Homeland Security Presidential Directives**: Following 9/11, the George W. Bush administration created the Homeland Security Council, which then released a series of directives to record and communicate presidential decisions and policies related to homeland security in the United States.
■ **National Security Council Directives:** Different administrations have had their own names for national security directives use for decision and review of national security policies and strategies. These are a type of EO, but done with the advice and consent of the National Security Council. Like EO's, they have the effect of law. Typically, Republican presidents select a name that begins with "N," while Democrats select a name that begins with "P." Nomenclatures used by different administrations include the following:

  – National Security Decision Directive (NSDD)—Reagan
  – National Security Directive (NSD)—Bush
  – Presidential Decision Directive (PDD)—Clinton
  – National Security Presidential Directive (NSPD)—Bush
  – Presidential Policy Directive (PPD)—Obama
  – National Security Presidential Memorandum (NSPM)—Trump

Data from Relyea H. Presidential Directives: Background and Overview. CRS Report for Congress. November 26, 2008. Available at: https://fas.org/sgp/crs/misc/98–611.pdf. Accessed May 2017; Bellinger J. National Security Memorandum 2 - President Trump's NSC and HSC. *Lawfare*. January 28, 2017. Available at: https://www.lawfareblog.com/national-security-presidential -memorandum-2—president-trumps-nsc-and-hsc. Accessed May 2017.

---

six critical mission areas.[17(p41)] The three critical mission areas are, specifically, intelligence (disease surveillance and development of medical intelligence), defending against catastrophic events (improving sensor and decontamination techniques, developing vaccines and medical countermeasures, harnessing scientific knowledge and tools to counter terrorism, and controlling access to dangerous agents), and emergency preparedness and response (preparing the healthcare community for catastrophic terrorism, augmenting medical countermeasure supplies, preparing for decontamination needs, building volunteer systems, enhancing victim support systems, preparing hospitals for surge capacity, training and deploying disaster medical assistance teams, and preparing first responders to work safely in areas where dangerous weapons have been used).

▸ Offices and Organizations—The Federal Preparedness Infrastructure

In addition to the creation of the DHS in the wake of 9/11, many existing organizations established new offices, expanded existing ones, and redirected resources toward preparedness and homeland security. Here are the offices and organizations most directly linked to public health preparedness in the United States.

Department of Homeland Security
Office of Health Affairs

The main office within DHS that addresses public health preparedness is the Office of Health Affairs. This office has several divisions: the Health Threats Resilience Division and the Workforce Health and Medical Support Division. Workforce Health and Medical Support Division works to strengthen national medical emergency response capacity. The division encompasses a suite of programs, including Behavioral Health, Medical Countermeasures, Medical First Responder Coordination, Medical Quality Management, and a medical liaison program to place senior clinicians within DHS. The Health Threats Resilience Division is primarily focused on preparedness and response to chemical and biological incidents. Programs include Biowatch, which tries to provide early detection of biological events (**FIGURE 4-3**); the National Biosurveillance Integration Center (NBIC); the Chemical Defense Program; Food, Agriculture and Veterinary Defense programs; Integrated Consortium of Laboratory Networks; State and Local Initiatives; and radiological health experts.[18,19]

Federal Emergency Management Administration

FEMA is also located within DHS. The role of FEMA is discussed in detail in subsequent chapters, particularly their coordination role for responding to emergencies.

Department of Health and Human Services
Office of the Assistant Secretary for Preparedness and Response

The Office of the Assistant Secretary for Preparedness and Response (ASPR) was created by the Pandemic and All-Hazards Preparedness Act of 2006, and replaced the office previously known as the Office of Public Health Emergency Preparedness. ASPR is composed of multiple components, including the Biomedical Advanced Research and Development Authority (BARDA), the Office of Emergency Management, and Policy and Planning.[20] ASPR is responsible for "preventing, preparing for, and responding to adverse health effects of public health emergencies and disasters."[21] In addition to policy development, the office supports state and local capacity during emergencies by providing federal support. This includes deployment of clinicians through the National Disaster Medical System. ASPR also hosts a series of preparedness programs, including the Hospital Preparedness Program (**FIGURE 4-4**).[22]

Centers for Disease Control and Prevention

The Centers for Disease Control and Prevention (CDC) has a vast array of offices and subject matter expertise that would be utilized during a public health emergency. Many of the preparedness and response activities are consolidated in the Office of Public Health Preparedness and Response (OPHPR). This office coordinates and responds to public health threats through a multitude of programs, including an emergency operations division that constantly maintains situational awareness of potential threats; a division dedicated to supporting preparedness at the states, local, tribal, and territorial levels through cooperative agreements providing approximate funding to state and local entities for preparedness for all-hazard threats; a division that hosts and manages the strategic national stockpile of medical countermeasures and supplies necessary to address a large-scale public health emergency; and a division devoted to regulating the federal select agent program.[23]

National Institutes of Health

The National Institutes of Health (NIH) is engaged in public health preparedness through a variety of offices. The two primary locations are the Office of Science Policy, which houses the National Science Advisory Board for Biosecurity (NSABB). Additionally, the National Institute of Allergy and Infectious Diseases (NIAID) hosts a robust research agenda, both intramural and in support of extramural programs, that supports the research and development of medical countermeasures against radiological, nuclear, and chemical threats, and that supports biodefense activities.[24,25] Additionally, divisions across NIH support research programs that might focus on special population or clinical outcomes from public health emergencies, like mental health, children's health, or disease mapping for preparedness.

The Food and Drug Administration

The Food and Drug Administration (FDA) has multiple offices that focus on emergency preparedness and response. These offices focus on regulatory oversight, monitoring infrastructure, and facilitating the delivery

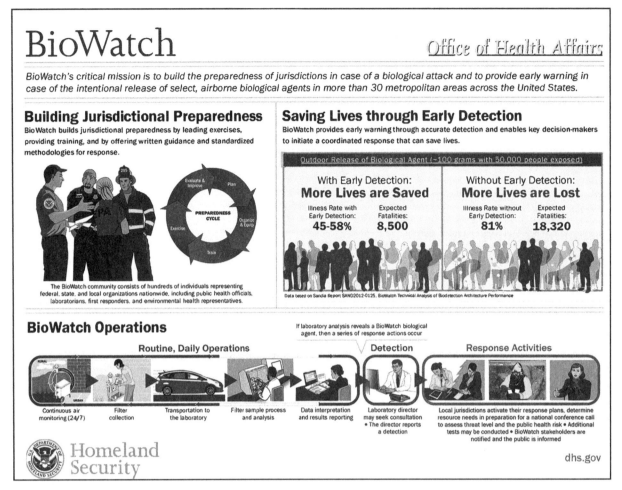

FIGURE 4-3 Biowatch

Reproduced from Office of Health Affairs. *The Biowatch Program Infographic*. August 2016. Available at: www.dhs.gov/sites/default/files/publications/BioWatch%20Infographic_0.pdf. Accessed May 2017.

of appropriate countermeasures. Specifically, the Office of Crises Management coordinates emergency and crises response, as related to FDA regulated products. The Center for Biologics and Evaluation Research oversees safety and effectiveness of biologic products, including chemical, biological, radiological, and nuclear (CBRN) medical countermeasures. The Office of Counterterrorism and Emerging Threats works on policies, strategies, and interagency communication around counterterrorism. It also coordinates activities around Emergency Use Authorization for medical countermeasures.[26]

U.S. Department of Agriculture

The Animal and Plant Health Inspection Service (APHIS) at U.S. Department of Agriculture (USDA) has a broad mission to protect and promote U.S. agricultural health. APHIS also works with DHS and FEMA to provide assistance and coordination during emergencies. This assistance ranges from disease containment in poultry (such as in cases of avian influenza) to protecting health of livestock and crops from foreign disease.[27] The Agricultural Research Service (ARS) provides research support that may be essential during an emergency.[28]

Department of Justice, Federal Bureau of Investigation

The FBI created a new Weapons of Mass Destruction (WMD) Directorate in 2006. This directorate works in several areas, including countermeasures and preparedness, investigations and operations, and intelligence analysis. The investigative component directs the WMD threat credibility assessments and manages all WMD criminal investigations. On preparedness, the FBI works with field components as well as with other agencies. In particular, the FBI works closely with CDC on "Crim-Epi," the cooperation between law enforcement and epidemiologists in the investigation of potential WMD events in a way that enables the FBI not only to collect information that will lead to a prosecution, but that also enables epidemiologists to investigate, treat, and minimize morbidity and mortality.[29]

Department of Defense

The Department of Defense (DoD) has a massive infrastructure designed to address threats of any nature,

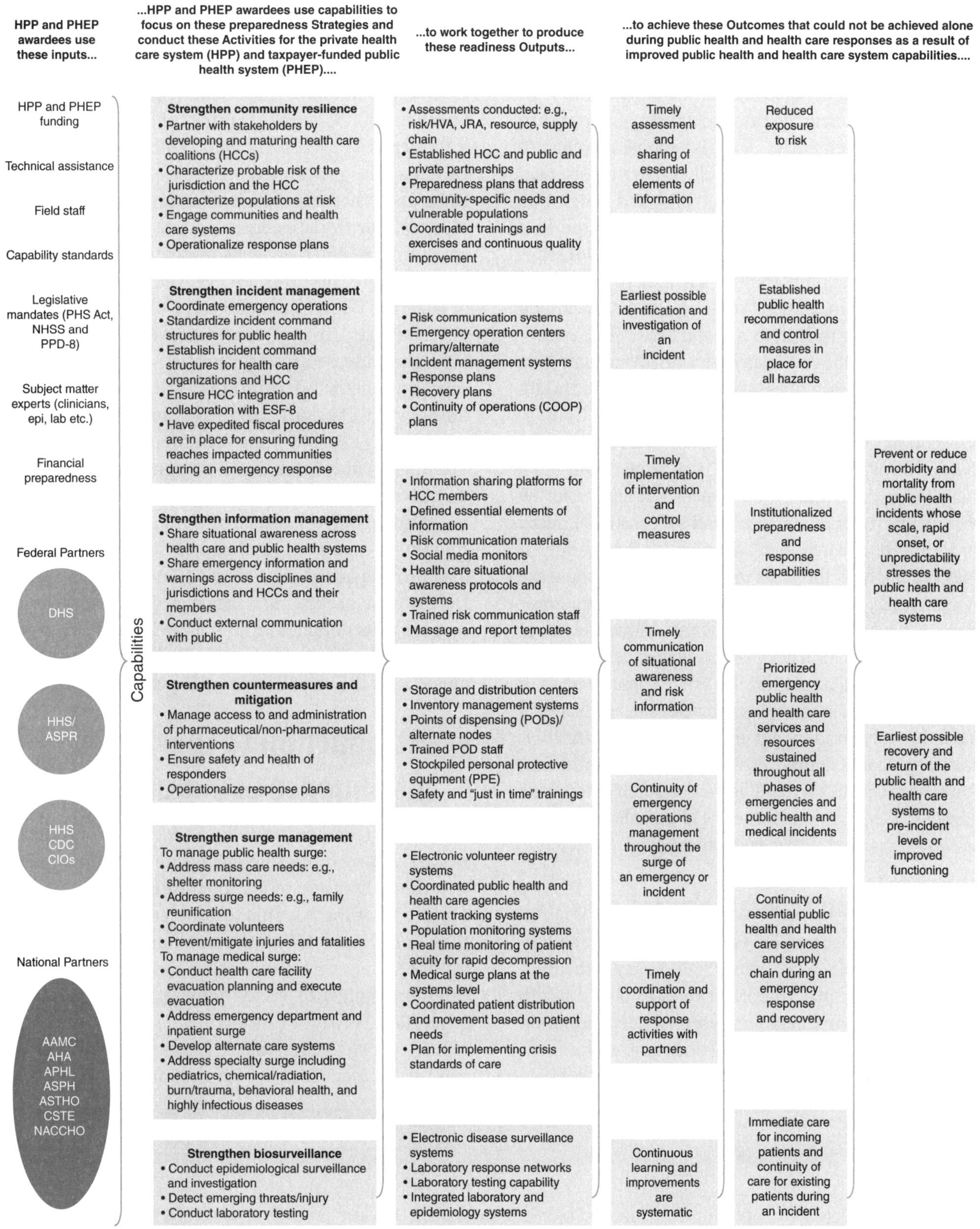

HPP and PHEP awardees use these inputs...
- HPP and PHEP funding
- Technical assistance
- Field staff
- Capability standards
- Legislative mandates (PHS Act, NHSS and PPD-8)
- Subject matter experts (clinicians, epi, lab etc.)
- Financial preparedness

Federal Partners
- DHS
- HHS/ASPR
- HHS CDC CIOs

National Partners
- AAMC
- AHA
- APHL
- ASPH
- ASTHO
- CSTE
- NACCHO

Capabilities

...HPP and PHEP awardees use capabilities to focus on these preparedness Strategies and conduct these Activities for the private health care system (HPP) and taxpayer-funded public health system (PHEP)....

Strengthen community resilience
- Partner with stakeholders by developing and maturing health care coalitions (HCCs)
- Characterize probable risk of the jurisdiction and the HCC
- Characterize populations at risk
- Engage communities and health care systems
- Operationalize response plans

Strengthen incident management
- Coordinate emergency operations
- Standardize incident command structures for public health
- Establish incident command structures for health care organizations and HCC
- Ensure HCC integration and collaboration with ESF-8
- Have expedited fiscal procedures are in place for ensuring funding reaches impacted communities during an emergency response

Strengthen information management
- Share situational awareness across health care and public health systems
- Share emergency information and warnings across disciplines and jurisdictions and HCCs and their members
- Conduct external communication with public

Strengthen countermeasures and mitigation
- Manage access to and administration of pharmaceutical/non-pharmaceutical interventions
- Ensure safety and health of responders
- Operationalize response plans

Strengthen surge management
To manage public health surge:
- Address mass care needs: e.g., shelter monitoring
- Address surge needs: e.g., family reunification
- Coordinate volunteers
- Prevent/mitigate injuries and fatalities
To manage medical surge:
- Conduct health care facility evacuation planning and execute evacuation
- Address emergency department and inpatient surge
- Develop alternate care systems
- Address specialty surge including pediatrics, chemical/radiation, burn/trauma, behavioral health, and highly infectious diseases

Strengthen biosurveillance
- Conduct epidemiological surveillance and investigation
- Detect emerging threats/injury
- Conduct laboratory testing

...to work together to produce these readiness Outputs...

- Assessments conducted: e.g., risk/HVA, JRA, resource, supply chain
- Established HCC and public and private partnerships
- Preparedness plans that address community-specific needs and vulnerable populations
- Coordinated trainings and exercises and continuous quality improvement

- Risk communication systems
- Emergency operation centers primary/alternate
- Incident management systems
- Response plans
- Recovery plans
- Continuity of operations (COOP) plans

- Information sharing platforms for HCC members
- Defined essential elements of information
- Risk communication materials
- Social media monitors
- Health care situational awareness protocols and systems
- Trained risk communication staff
- Massage and report templates

- Storage and distribution centers
- Inventory management systems
- Points of dispensing (PODs)/alternate nodes
- Trained POD staff
- Stockpiled personal protective equipment (PPE)
- Safety and "just in time" trainings

- Electronic volunteer registry systems
- Coordinated public health and health care agencies
- Patient tracking systems
- Population monitoring systems
- Real time monitoring of patient acuity for rapid decompression
- Medical surge plans at the systems level
- Coordinated patient distribution and movement based on patient needs
- Plan for implementing crisis standards of care

- Electronic disease surveillance systems
- Laboratory response networks
- Laboratory testing capability
- Integrated laboratory and epidemiology systems

...to achieve these Outcomes that could not be achieved alone during public health and health care responses as a result of improved public health and health care system capabilities....

- Timely assessment and sharing of essential elements of information
- Earliest possible identification and investigation of an incident
- Timely implementation of intervention and control measures
- Timely communication of situational awareness and risk information
- Continuity of emergency operations management throughout the surge of an emergency or incident
- Timely coordination and support of response activities with partners
- Continuous learning and improvements are systematic

- Reduced exposure to risk
- Established public health recommendations and control measures in place for all hazards
- Institutionalized preparedness and response capabilities
- Prioritized emergency public health and health care services and resources sustained throughout all phases of emergencies and public health and medical incidents
- Continuity of essential public health and health care services and supply chain during an emergency response and recovery
- Immediate care for incoming patients and continuity of care for existing patients during an incident

- Prevent or reduce morbidity and mortality from public health incidents whose scale, rapid onset, or unpredictability stresses the public health and health care systems
- Earliest possible recovery and return of the public health and health care systems to pre-incident levels or improved functioning

FIGURE 4-4 Hospital Preparedness Program: Logic model for Public Health Emergency Preparedness cooperative agreements

Reproduced from ASPR. *2017–2022 HPP Performance Measures Implementation Guidance.* p 80. Available at: www.phe.gov/Preparedness/planning/hpp/reports/Documents/hpp-pmi-guidance-2017.pdf. Accessed May 2017.

including public health emergencies. The military is trained in emergency response and preparedness as critical components of an effective armed forces. While most DoD programs focus on protecting the war fighter, several also have implications for the broader civilian population. There is an active chemical and biological defense program that involves research, development, and testing defense systems and equipment, including medical countermeasures. The Cooperative Threat Reduction (CTR) programs work to reduce the threat of

WMD around the world, while building global capacity for detection and response to biological threats. There is a large-scale laboratory network both in the United States and abroad engaged in basic scientific research for infectious diseases, as well as epidemiologic response to public health emergencies. There is a robust surveillance and response program for naturally occurring diseases. For emergency response within the United States, U.S. Northern Command (USNORTHCOM) has the lead within DoD and is charged with coordinating DoD support to civilian authorities (**BOX 4-6**). There are several consequence management response teams, including those specifically trained to respond to WMD events.[30]

While the DoD has many assets that can contribute to emergency preparedness and response to public health events, it must act within the limits of the Posse Comitatus Act (**BOX 4-7**). The act is an 1878 federal law intended to limit the ability of the federal government to use the military for civilian law enforcement.[31] It applies to the army, navy, marines, air force, and state national guard forces, but only when they are called for federal duty. It does not apply to the coast guard. In 2006, in the wake of Hurricane Katrina and under pressure from President Bush, Congress passed a law that allows the use of the armed forces in major public emergencies, to restore public order and enforce laws.[32(Sec. 1076)] These changes to Posse Comitatus, however, were repealed by the National Defense Authorization Act for FY 2008; and in 2011, President Obama signed the National Defense Authorization Act for FY 2012, extending the definition of someone subject to detention under the law to include an individual who supported al-Qaeda or other belligerent actors.[33]

Other Relevant Federal Agencies

In addition to Department of Health and Human Services (HHS), DHS, CDC, and USDA, several other federal entities may play important roles in public health emergency preparedness and response, depending on the type of event (**FIGURE 4-5**). For example, the Environmental Protection Agency (EPA) will assist HHS in developing and implementing sampling strategies and decontamination efforts. They also might assist in identifying water supplies for critical healthcare facilities in an emergency. The Department of Energy (DoE) may be called upon to monitor and decontaminate radiological emergency events. The National Laboratories under DoE may also provide expertise on biodefense, surveillance, and other technological factors. The Department of Labor may work to ensure the safety of first responders during an emergency. Department of Interior may be essential for outbreaks or events that impact wildlife or fisheries. Department of State (DoS) may coordinate international activities related to WMD or naturally occurring disease crossing borders. National Oceanic and Atmospheric Administration (NOAA) may provide transport, dispersion, and predictions of atmospheric releases of radioactive and hazardous. Department of Commerce may coordinate response activities with the private sector. Department of Transportation may be called upon to assist in the transport of response equipment and personnel across state lines. The IC may provide actionable information for response. The Department of Veteran's Affairs will provide clinical support to its population, as will the Indian Health Service. And the White House NSC will most likely coordinate all of the activities across the executive branch.

▶ Introduction to the Intelligence Community

A primary recommendation of the 9/11 Commission Report was to unify intelligence and knowledge and to create a Director of National Intelligence (DNI) to oversee all of the IC. This recommendation led to just that—a DNI, along with the creation of multiple intelligence entities within other agencies, including a DoD Counterintelligence Field Activity, the Joint Intelligence Task Force for Combating Terrorism, the Office of Intelligence Analysis at the Department of Treasury, and the National Security Services at the FBI.

BOX 4-6 2008 Plan for DoD USNORTHCOM Support for Civil Authorities During an Emergency

1. *Purpose.* Natural or man-made disasters and special events can be so demanding that local, tribal, state and non-military federal responders are temporarily overwhelmed by the situation. The Department of Defense (DoD) has a long history of supporting civil authorities in the wake of catastrophic events. When directed by the President or Secretary of Defense (SecDef), U.S. Northern Command (USNORTHCOM) will respond quickly and effectively to the requests of civil authorities to save lives, prevent human suffering, and mitigate great property damage. The Joint Strategic Capabilities Plan 2008 (JSCP) directs CDRUSNORTHCOM to prepare a plan to support the employment of Title 10 DoD forces providing DSCA in accordance with (IAW) the National Response Framework (NRF), applicable federal law, DoD Directives, and other policy guidance including those hazards defined by the national planning scenarios that are not addressed by other JSCP tasked plans. DSCA is a subset of DoD civil support that is performed within the parameters of the NERF.

Reproduced from United States Northern Command. CDRUSNORTHCOM CONPLAN 3501–08. DSCA. May 16, 2008. p v. Available at: www.northcom.mil/Portals/28/Documents/FOIA/Con%20 Plan%203501-08%20DSCA.pdf. Accessed May 2017.

BOX 4-7 Posse Comitatus Act

18 U.S.C. § 1385. *Use of Army and Air Force as posse comitatus*
  Whoever, except in cases and under circumstances
expressly authorized by the Constitution or Act of
Congress, willfully uses any part of the Army or the Air
Force as a posse comitatus or otherwise to execute the
laws shall be fined under this title or imprisoned not more
than two years, or both.

Reproduced from Use of Army and Air Force as posse comitatus, 18 U.S.C. § 1385, August 10,
1959. Available at http://www.law.cornell.edu/uscode/text/18/1385. Accessed May 2017.

The IC supports policymakers, but does not make policy or advocate for one policy choice over another. The community is an executive function of the federal government, composed of multiple agencies and offices from across the executive branch. The legislative branch provides oversight committees.

Organizationally, the IC reports to the NSC. The NSC is chaired by the president, with regular participants including the vice president; secretaries of state, treasury, and defense; the assistant to the president for National Security Affairs, the chairman of the Joint Chiefs of Staff, and the DNI.

The NSC oversees the DNI, and the DNI oversees the rest of the IC, including the Central Intelligence Agency (CIA). Within the DNI, there are several areas of focus. These include the following:

- National Counterterrorism Center (NCTC)
- National Counterproliferation Center (NCPC)
- Deputy Director of National Intelligence for Intelligence Integration (DDII)
- National Intelligence Council (NIC)
- National Counterintelligence and Security Center (NCSC)
- Cyber Threat Intelligence Integration Center (CTICC)[34]

Under the DNI, there are 16 additional members that make up the rest of the IC (**BOX 4-8**). The only independent agency in this community is the CIA. The other 15 elements are offices, bureaus, or agencies situated within executive branch departments.[35]

Each member of the IC tailors its work to the specific needs of its customers, specifically the priorities of the home agency. The entire IC, however, uses the same set of terminology. There are eight major types of intelligence utilized by the IC, with some members of the community focusing more on some types than others:

1. *Human Intelligence (HUMINT):* HUMINT uses people to gain information. It is the oldest form of information collection.

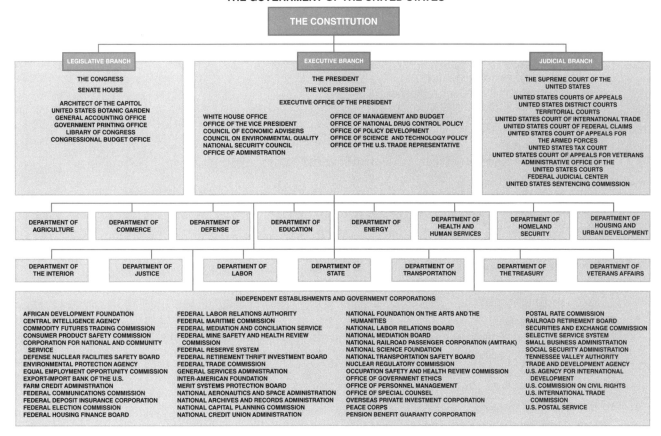

FIGURE 4-5 Government organization chart

Office of the Federal Register, National Archives and Records Administration. *The United States Government Manual 2003/2004.* June 15, 2003. Available at: www.gpo.gov/fdsys/pkg/GOVMAN-2003-06-15/pdf/GOVMAN-2003-06-15.pdf. Accessed May 2017.

2. *Geographic Intelligence (GEOINT)*: GEOINT comes from imagery and geospacial information, including photography, sensors, electro-optics, and radar. This type of intelligence can come from land, sea, air, or space platforms.

3. *Signals Intelligence (SIGINT)*: SIGINT includes foreign communications intercepts (COMINT), Electronic Intelligence (ELINT), and Foreign Instrumentation Signals Intelligence (FISINT).

4. *Measurement and Signature Intelligence (MASINT)*: MASINT is the quantitative and qualitative analysis of data coming from technical sensors.

5. *Open Source Intelligence (OSINT)*: OSINT is the exploitation of news media and public sources for uses by the IC.

6. *Technical Intelligence (TECHINT)*: TECHINT is the exploitation of foreign material.

7. *Cyber Intelligence (CYBINT)*: CYBINT is information collected through cyberspace or anything connected to the Internet.

8. *Financial Intelligence (FININT)*: FININT is intelligence on financial transactions.

Each member of the IC produces products (papers, briefings, etc.) for their respective agency and that information may be shared and coordinated with the DNI, and even reported up to the president, depending on the need for the intelligence information to inform policy development. The community also produces National Intelligence Estimates, under the purview of the National Intelligence Council within the DNI. These are the IC's most authoritative written judgments on specific national security issues, with input from the entire community.[36]

▶ The National Response Framework—Public Health and Medical Response

On February 28, 2003, the Bush administration released Homeland Security Presidential Directive 5 (HSPD 5): Management of Domestic Incidents. The purpose of this document was to establish a single,

---

BOX 4-8 Intelligence Community Members

- Independent Agency
  - Central Intelligence Agency
- Department of Defense
  - Agencies/Offices
    - Defense Intelligence Agency (DIA)
    - National Geospatial-Intelligence Agency (NGA)
    - National Reconnaissance Office (NRO)
    - National Security Agency (NSA)
  - Service Components
    - Air Force Intelligence, Surveillance and Reconnaissance Agency
    - Army Military Intelligence
    - Marine Corps Intelligence Activity
    - Office of Naval Intelligence
- Department of Energy
  - Office of Intelligence and Counterintelligence
- Department of Homeland Security
  - Office of Intelligence and Analysis (IA)
  - Coast Guard Intelligence
- Department of Justice
  - Drug Enforcement Administration (DEA), Office of National Security Intelligence
  - FBI, Directorate of Intelligence
- Department of State
  - Bureau of Intelligence and Research (INR)
- Department of the Treasury
  - Office of Intelligence and Analysis

comprehensive National Incident Management System (NIMS), ensuring that all agencies and levels of government could work together to best respond to an emergency event. HSPD 5 called for the creation of both a National Response Plan (NRP) and an NIMS, and clarified that the initial responsibility for managing an incident lies at the state and local levels. The federal government response is designed to be used only when state and local resources are overwhelmed, as assessed by the state and local authorities themselves.[37]

In December 2003, Homeland Security Presidential Directive 8 (HSPD 8): National Preparedness was released, building on the concepts addressed in HSPD 5. HSPD 8 called for the development of a National Preparedness Goal that would provide effective and efficient aid from the federal government, support first responders, and establish measurable priorities and targets (**BOX 4-9**).[38] It also called for an "all-hazards approach" to preparedness planning. An all-hazards approach refers to preparedness planning that is relevant to multiple types of disasters, including terrorist events, natural disasters, and any other large-scale emergency.

In September 2007, the government released the National Preparedness Guidelines, defining what it means for the nation to be prepared for all hazards. The purpose of the document was to strengthen and organize national preparedness efforts, guide investment, and inform the planning process. The guidelines contained four key elements:

1. *National preparedness vision*—The national preparedness vision stated: "A nation prepared with coordinated capabilities to prevent, protect against, respond to, and recover from all hazards in a way that balances risk resources and need."[39(p1)]
2. *15 National planning scenarios*—These were 15 scenarios that represent a broad range of natural and man-made threats that are designed to focus national planning, training, investments, and exercises.

3. *Universal task list*—The universal task list (UTL) is a menu of approximately 1600 tasks that were required to "prevent, protect against, respond to, and recover" from the events listed in the national planning scenarios.[39(p1)]
4. *Target capabilities list*—The target capabilities list (TCL) was 37 specific capabilities that organizations and individuals at all levels of government and the private sector should collectively develop and possess to respond to emergencies.

The National Preparedness System has been updated and revised in the past decade, yet continues to include many of the same core components. The current National Preparedness System starts with the National Preparedness Goal and then organizes capabilities into five discrete mission areas: prevention, protection, mitigation, response, and recovery (**TABLE 4-1**). The goal now has 32 core capabilities associated with preparedness (see **FIGURES 4-6** and **4-7**). The process for achieving this goal is through what is now called the National Preparedness System, which is composed of six major areas: identification and assessment of risk, estimating capability requirements using the core capabilities list, building and sustaining those capabilities, preparedness planning to deliver the capabilities, validating the capabilities through exercises and other activities, and engaging in constant review and updating of plans and capabilities (see **FIGURE 4-8**).[40]

Additional components of the National Preparedness System include a series of guidance plans, including the Threat and Hazard Identification and Risk Assessment (THIRA) guidance (more information on THIRA is provided in Chapter 11); a Comprehensive Preparedness Guide for assistance in rating operational plans; the National Planning Frameworks for unified guidance for strategic, operational, and tactical plans, including the National Prevention Framework, the National Protection Framework, the National Mitigation Framework, the National Response Framework (discussed further in this chapter), and the National Disaster Recovery Framework; and the NIMS (more information later in this chapter). Additionally, the DHS releases a National Preparedness Report to show annual progress toward building preparedness capacity in the United States.

To test preparedness and readiness, the DHS, through FEMA, runs an Exercise and Evaluation Program (formally, the Homeland Security Exercise and Evaluation Program (HSEEP)). The program standardizes exercises, attempts to establish common

---

BOX 4-9   National Preparedness Goal

A secure and resilient nation with the capabilities required across the whole community to prevent, protect against, mitigate, respond to, and recover from the threats and hazards that pose the greatest risk

Department of Homeland Security. FEMA. *National Preparedness Goal, Second Edition—What's New.* Available at: https://www.fema.gov/media-library-data/1443703117389-27c542ca395218d3154e5c1dfa8bfcb6/National_Preparedness_Goal_Whats_New_2015.pdf. Accessed May 2017.

TABLE 4-1 National Planning Scenarios				
Prevention	**Protection**	**Mitigation**	**Response**	**Recovery**
Planning				
Public Information and Warning				
Operational Coordination				
Intelligence and information sharing Interdiction and disruption Screening, search, and detection Forensics and attribution	Access control and identity verification Cybersecurity Physical protective measures Risk management for protection programs and activities Supply chain integrity and security	Community resilience Long-term vulnerability reduction Risk and disaster resilience assessment Threats and hazards identification	Infrastructure systems Critical transportation Environmental response/health and safety Fatality management services Fire management and suppression Logistics and supply chain management Mass care services Mass search and rescue operations On-scene security, protection, and law enforcement Operational communications Public health, healthcare, and emergency medical services Situational assessment	Economic recovery Health and social services Housing Natural and cultural resources

Reproduced from Department of Homeland Security. *National Preparedness Goal*, Second Edition. September 2015. p 3. Available at: https://www.fema.gov/media-library-data/1443799615171-2aae90be55041740f97e8532fc680d40/National_Preparedness_Goal_2nd_Edition.pdf. Accessed May 2017.

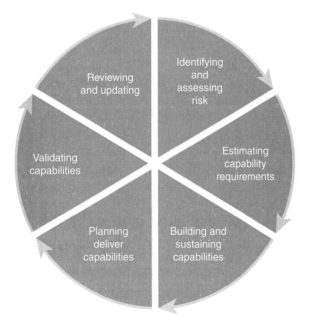

FIGURE 4-6 National Preparedness System components

Reproduced from Department of Homeland Security. *National Preparedness System*. November 2011. p 1. Available at: www.fema.gov/media-library-data/20130726-1855-25045-8110/national_preparedness_system_final.pdf. Accessed May 2017.

concepts, and synchronizes all exercises across the country. Importantly, this program supports state and local jurisdictions through direct funding, training, and exercises assistance. Ideally, these exercises enable jurisdictions to assess preparedness levels and take corrective action when necessary to improve capacities to respond to emergencies.[41]

▶ National Incident Management System

One of the directives in HSPD 5 was the need for the DHS to develop and administer an NIMS (**FIGURE 4-9**). What was developed, and subsequently revised, was a document that provides for standardized incident management protocols that can be used by those responding to any type of emergency at all levels of government. The document itself evolved out of a need for a common language, as well as a common

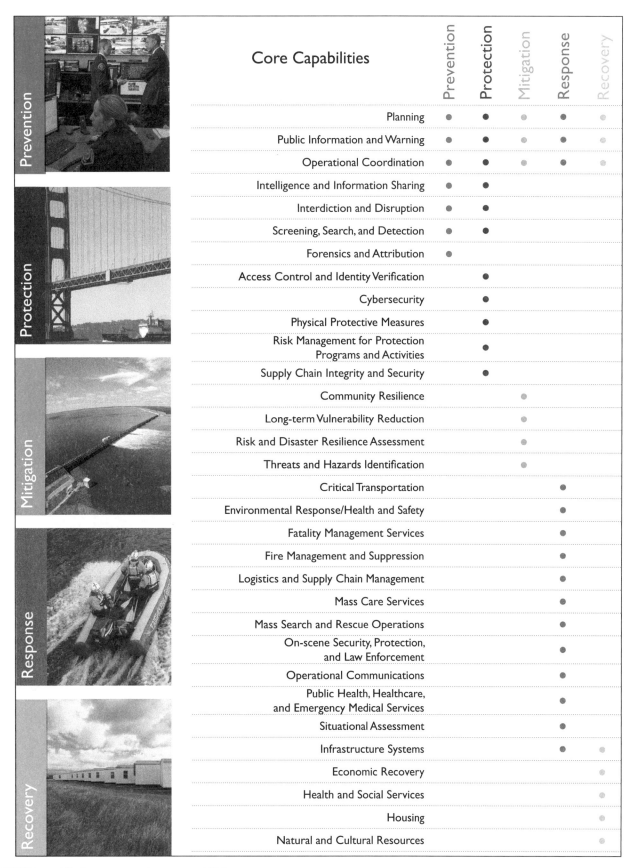

Core Capabilities	Prevention	Protection	Mitigation	Response	Recovery
Planning	●	●	●	●	●
Public Information and Warning	●	●	●	●	●
Operational Coordination	●	●	●	●	●
Intelligence and Information Sharing	●	●			
Interdiction and Disruption	●	●			
Screening, Search, and Detection	●	●			
Forensics and Attribution	●				
Access Control and Identity Verification		●			
Cybersecurity		●			
Physical Protective Measures		●			
Risk Management for Protection Programs and Activities		●			
Supply Chain Integrity and Security		●			
Community Resilience			●		
Long-term Vulnerability Reduction			●		
Risk and Disaster Resilience Assessment			●		
Threats and Hazards Identification			●		
Critical Transportation				●	
Environmental Response/Health and Safety				●	
Fatality Management Services				●	
Fire Management and Suppression				●	
Logistics and Supply Chain Management				●	
Mass Care Services				●	
Mass Search and Rescue Operations				●	
On-scene Security, Protection, and Law Enforcement				●	
Operational Communications				●	
Public Health, Healthcare, and Emergency Medical Services				●	
Situational Assessment				●	
Infrastructure Systems				●	●
Economic Recovery					●
Health and Social Services					●
Housing					●
Natural and Cultural Resources					●

FIGURE 4-7 Mission areas and core capabilities

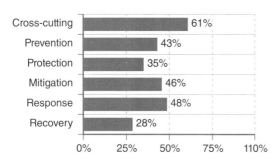

Cross-cutting — 61%
Prevention — 43%
Protection — 35%
Mitigation — 46%
Response — 48%
Recovery — 28%

0%   25%   50%   75%   110%

Percentage of state/territory responses indicating proficiency

FIGURE 4-8 U.S. preparedness capability in 2015: Percentage of state and territories indicating proficiency in the preparedness mission areas

Reproduced from Department of Homeland Security. 2015 State and Territory Self-Assessment of Preparedness Capability Based on State Preparedness Report Results. *National Preparedness Report.* March 30, 2016. p 21. Available at: www.fema.gov/media -library-data/1476817353589-987d6a58e2eb124ac6b19ef1f7c9a77d/2016NPR_508c_052716_1600_alla.pdf. Accessed 2017.

framework, for managing emergencies. In the past, most jurisdictions had plans in place for responding to an emergency, but many of these plans were not consistent with the plans of other localities, which had implications for coordination and management of large-scale events that involved multiple jurisdictions and multiple levels of government.

NIMS, as published in 2008, has five major components:

- *Preparedness:* Establishment of guidelines and standards for planning, training, and qualifications for responders
- *Communications and Information Management:* Requirements for an interoperable communications and information process
- *Resource Management:* Mutual-aid agreements, resource mobilization protocols, and the ability of all jurisdictional levels to access necessary resources to address an emergency
- *Command and Management:* Standards for an incident command system, a multiagency coordination system, and a public information system
- *Ongoing Management and Maintenance:* Through the National Integration Center and the NIMS standards development, maintenance of compliance, standards, and training[42]

Importantly, NIMS was developed as a comprehensive, systematic approach to manage an emergency, which can be used at all levels of government, in every jurisdiction. It provides a common set of principles and language, and standards that can be scaled to all levels of incidents. NIMS, however, is not a specific response plan.

▶ National Response Framework

NIMS was designed to be used in conjunction with a specific response plan, developed as the NRF (**FIGURE 4-10**). Originally, it was built upon the Federal

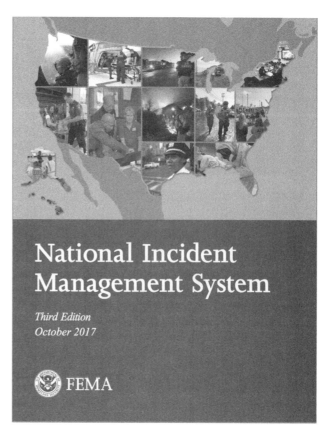

FIGURE 4-9 National Incident Management System

Reproduced from Department of Homeland Security. *National Incident Management System.* October 2017. Available at: www.fema.gov /media-library-data/1508151197225-ced8c60378c3936adb92c1a3ee6f6564/FINAL_NIMS_2017.pdf. Accessed October 2017.

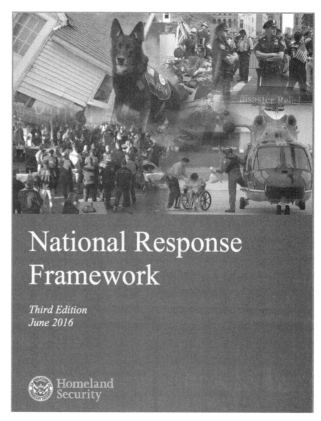

FIGURE 4-10 National Response Framework

Department of Homeland Security. *National Response Framework,* Third Edition. June 2016. Available at: https://www.fema .gov/media-library-data/1466014682982-9bcf8245ba4c60c120aa915abe74e15d/National_Response_Framework3rd.pdf. Accessed May 2017.

ESF #1: Transportation
ESF #2: Communications
ESF #3: Public Works and Engineering
ESF #4: Firefighting
ESF #5: Information and Planning
ESF #6: Mass Care, Emergency Assistance, Temporary Housing, and Human Services
ESF #7: Logistics
ESF #8: Public Health and Medical Services
ESF #9: Search and Rescue
ESF #10: Oil and Hazardous Materials Response
ESF #11: Agriculture and Natural Resources
ESF #12: Energy
ESF #13: Public Safety and Security
ESF #14 [Superseded by National Disaster Recovery Framework]
ESF #15: External Affairs

Data from Department of Homeland Security. *National Response Framework*. Third Edition. June 2016. p 34–37. Available at: www.fema.gov/media-library -data/1466014682982-9bcf8245ba4c60c120aa915abe74e15d/National_Response _Framework3rd.pdf. Accessed May 2017.

Response Plan from the early 1990s, revised into the National Response Plan in 2004, revised and renamed in 2007 as the NRF, and subsequently revised with the last update in 2016, reflecting lessons learned from past emergencies (**BOX 4-10**). The NRF is a broad national plan that tries to describe the "who, what, and how" of preparedness and response for disasters and emergencies. It was designed to address five basic principles of response: engaged partnership, tiered response, scalable and flexible capabilities, unity of effort, and readiness to act.[43]

The NRF is organized as a core document that contains doctrines, roles and responsibilities, and planning requirements. The core document is followed by Emergency Support Function (ESF) Annexes and Support Annexes. Of particular importance to the public health community is ESF #8 (**BOX 4-11**). Incident Annexes are now published in the Response Federal Interagency Operational Plan, including operational coordination for public health, health care, and emergency medical services. (See **FIGURE 4-11** for Coordination plan for ESF 8.)[44]

▶ Emergency Support Function #8

ESF #8 is devoted entirely to public health and medical services. This guidance document puts the secretary of HHS in charge of public health emergencies to coordinate preparedness, response, and recovery. The purpose of ESF#8 is to provide for coordinated federal assistance for public health and medical disasters. This document addresses a number of core functional areas:

BOX 4-11 Emergency Support Function #8 of the National Response Framework—Public Health and Medical Services Annex

ESF Coordinator	Support Team
Department of Health and Human Services	Department of Agriculture
Primary Agency	Department of Commerce
Department of Health and Human Services	Department of Energy
	Department of Homeland Security
	Department of the Interior
	Department of Justice
	Department of Labor
	Department of State
	Department of Transportation
	Department of Veteran Affairs
	Environmental Protection Agency
	General Services Administration
	U.S. Agency for International Development
	U.S. Postal Service
	American Red Cross

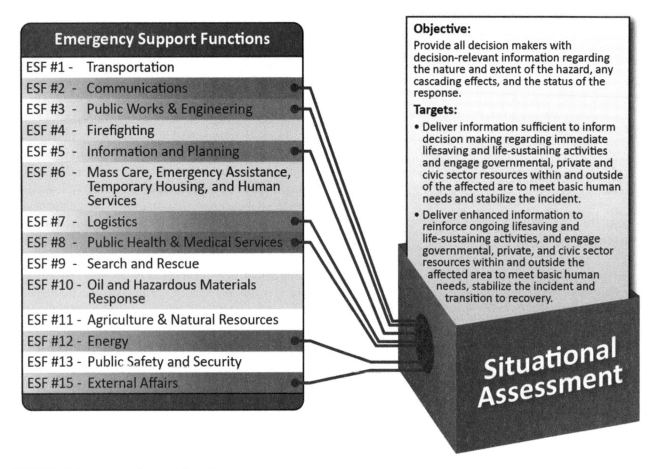

FIGURE 4-11 Emergency Support Functions

Reproduced from Department of Homeland Security. *Response Federal Interagency Operational Plan*, Second Edition. August 2016. p B.2–10. Available at: https://www.fema.gov/media-library-data/1471452095112-507e23ad4d85449ff131c2b025743101/Response_FIOP_2nd.pdf. Accessed May 2017.

- Assessment of public health and medical needs
- Health surveillance
- Medical surge
- Health, medical, and veterinary equipment and supplies
- Patient movement
- Patient care
- Safety and security of drugs, biologics, and devices
- Blood and tissues
- Food safety and defense
- Agriculture safety and security
- All-hazards public health and medical consultation, technical assistance, and support
- Behavioral health care
- Public health and medical information
- Vector control
- Guidance on potable water and solid waste disposal
- Fatality management, victim identification, and mitigation of health hazards from contaminated remains
- Veterinary medical support

One of the most challenging questions posed by these guidance documents is, "Who is in Charge?" If a public health emergency turns out to be caused by an intentional event, then not only does the public health community need to respond, but the law enforcement community becomes in charge of all legal and investigatory aspects. Because there may be both intelligence and foreign affairs equities at stake, those communities are brought into the fold as well. And the DHS remains tasked with coordinating communication with the public.

In all, NIMS and the NRF are designed to work together to better coordinate and prepare all entities that may be involved in responding to emergencies. NIMS is the "template for the management of incidents,"[19] while the NRF focuses on the mechanisms for policy and operational direction at the federal level.

▶ Who Does What

The National Preparedness System aims to improve the entire nation's ability to prepare, respond, and recover from emergencies. Response and recovery from a national emergency, however, requires appropriate funding and activations. Appropriate planning and financing, however, necessitates an understanding of the responsibilities of different levels of government. The entire national system is beyond the scope of this text, but in **TABLE 4-2**, we attempt to highlight the main areas of responsibility for response and recovery to a public health or medical disaster, divided by local, state, and federal levels.

TABLE 4-2 Local, State, and Federal Steps in Response and Recovery

	Municipal/Local Level	State/Tribal Level	Federal Level
Response	■ Activate the local Emergency Management Agency (EMA) ■ Coordinate with the local health officer ■ Develop and exercise local public health all-hazard plan ■ Monitor situation ■ Education, information, and communication activities for residents ■ Maintain essential public health functions ■ Notify the State Emergency Management Agency of the situation by regularly submitting Situation Reports (SITREP) ■ Contact state EMA when local capacity is exceeded	■ Review and evaluate situation reports ■ Activate the state EMA and Emergency Operations Center (EOC) ■ Coordinate emergency response ■ Provide technical assistance ■ Request assistance from neighboring states through Emergency Management Assistance Compact (EMAC) Act ■ If state capacity exceeded, proclaim a state of emergency and activate the State Disaster Preparedness Plan ■ Request federal assistance: a request for "emergency" or "major disaster declaration" under the Robert T Stafford Disaster Relief and Emergency Assistance Act or Public Health Emergency Declaration under the Public Health Service Act	■ Conduct joint Preliminary Damage Assessments (PDA) with state and local governments to identify damages ■ Approving or denying requests for federal assistance: • Stafford Act Declaration (emergency or major disaster) • Collaboration between state coordinating officer and federal coordinating officer • Identify Emergency Support Functions (ESF) to respond • HHS' Secretary Public Health Service Act (public health emergency) ■ Presidential declaration of national emergency ■ Presidential request for supplemental emergency funding to Congress
Recovery	■ If federal assistance is denied, the cost of recovery is the responsibility of the state and local governments. ■ Activate Disaster Recovery Centers (DRCs) ■ Prospective applicants fill out a Request for Public Assistance (to federal government).	■ If federal assistance is denied, the cost of recovery is the responsibility of the state and local governments. ■ Activate DRCs ■ FEMA and the state work with the applicant on hazard mitigation and insurance requirements.	■ If the president declares an emergency or a major disaster, all of the recovery provisions pursuant to the Stafford Act. ■ Activate DRCs ■ FEMA and the state work with the applicant on hazard mitigation and insurance requirements.

Data from FEMA. *Unit 3: Disaster Sequence of Events*. State Disaster Management Course—IS 208. Available at: https://www.training.fema.gov/emiweb/downloads/is208sdmunit3.pdf. Accessed May 2017.

Recognizing the importance of building local and state public health preparedness, the CDC has been investing in local and state health departments for over a decade to assist in capacity building, focusing on community resilience, incident management, information management, medical countermeasures and mitigation, surge management, and biosurveillance (**FIGURE 4-12**). A 2017 report assessed improvements in state and local public health emergency preparedness since 2001 (**TABLE 4-3**) and found that through targeted investments, there are now capacities in place to mobilize during an emergency, manage and collaborate with partners, and distribute medical countermeasures.

Independent analyses, however, show that while there have been significant improvements in public health preparedness at the state and local levels, it is

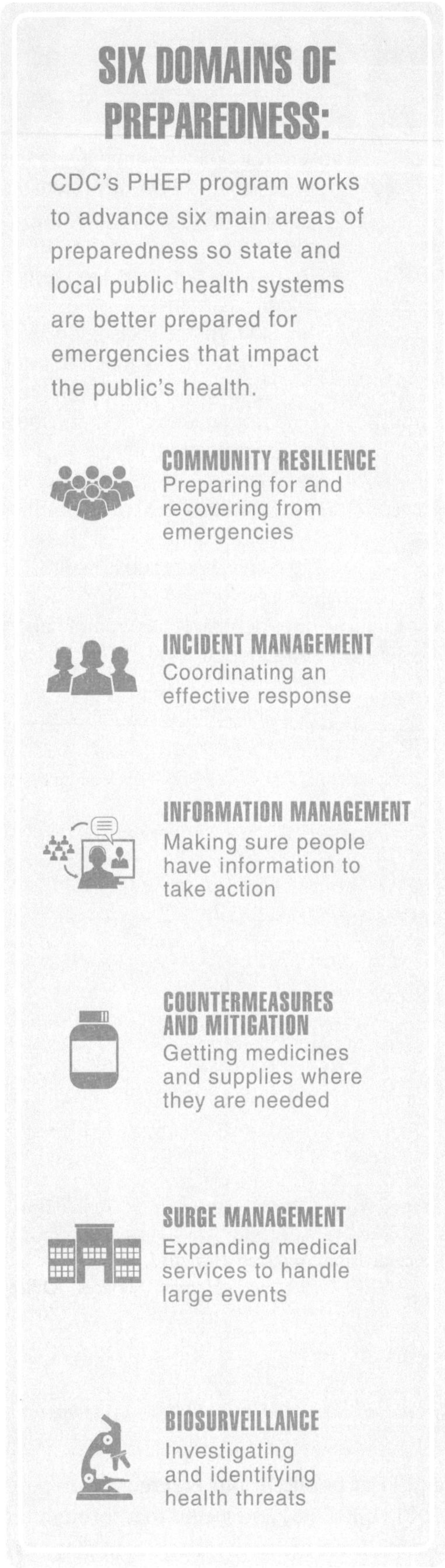

SIX DOMAINS OF PREPAREDNESS:

CDC's PHEP program works to advance six main areas of preparedness so state and local public health systems are better prepared for emergencies that impact the public's health.

COMMUNITY RESILIENCE
Preparing for and recovering from emergencies

INCIDENT MANAGEMENT
Coordinating an effective response

INFORMATION MANAGEMENT
Making sure people have information to take action

COUNTERMEASURES AND MITIGATION
Getting medicines and supplies where they are needed

SURGE MANAGEMENT
Expanding medical services to handle large events

BIOSURVEILLANCE
Investigating and identifying health threats

FIGURE 4-12 Six domains of preparedness

Reproduced from Six Domains of Preparedness. *CDC's Public Health Emergency Preparedness Program: Every Response is Local.* February 2017. Available at: https://www.cdc.gov/phpr/readiness/issuebrief.htm. Accessed May 2017.

TABLE 4-3 Improvements in Public Health Emergency Preparedness Since 9/11

Jurisdictions Who Can:	Then (%)	Now (%)
Can mobilize staff during an emergency	20	98
Have an incident command system with pre-assigned roles in place	5	100
Include collaboration with healthcare agencies in their preparedness plans	8	92
Have sufficient storage and distribution capacity for critical medicines and supplies	0	98

Reproduced from Improvements in Public Health Emergency Preparedness since 9/11. *CDC's Public Health Emergency Preparedness Program: Every Response is Local.* February 2017.

uneven and there is still much work to do. One study found that it will take 9 more years for the less prepared states to meet the same level of preparedness as more developed states, and 20 years to be fully prepared.[45] Another assessment found that there is still a lack of a near real-time biosurveillance system, not enough support for research and development, and the healthcare system is ill equipped to handle a mass casualty event.[46]

▶ Discussion

This entire chapter begs the following questions: Are we prepared? Is everyone ready for the next emergency? Will there be appropriate coordination of activities during the next emergency? The most honest answer probably is, "We don't know." Planning and preparedness is a difficult balancing act. Funding is often associated with the previous disaster, in that monies are appropriated so we can better respond to the exact type of emergency that happened last time. Yet, seldom does the next emergency mirror the last. Scenario-based planning is useful, but only as long as planners and responders are flexible enough to view these scenarios as illustrative of the potential set of capabilities that should be developed. A locality should not think it is fully prepared if it can check the box that it is ready for disasters A, B, and C. Because the next disaster will most certainly not match the planning scenarios. This means that the best we can do as a nation is to be as forward thinking as possible regarding potential emergencies so that we can enable a flexible and coordinated response, with appropriate resources, using best possible risk communication methods.

Key Words

9/11 Commission Report
    Disaster assistance
Exercise and Evaluation Program
    Intelligence Community

National Response
    Framework
National Incident Management
    System

Preparedness
    planning
Presidential directives
Stafford Act

Discussion Questions

1. Describe the events that led to the redesign of the national preparedness infrastructure.

2. Given the findings from the 9/11 Commission Report, which do you think are most important for future planning and policy development? Which most directly impact the public health community?

3. Do you think the IC works well together? Does it work well with outside entities? How do you think the public health community should engage the IC?

4. Try to create an organizational chart linking all of the federal agencies associated with preparedness activities.

5. Describe current U.S. government policies regarding management of domestic emergencies.

6. What is the division between federal, state, and local entities in an emergency?

7. What documents answer the questions: "Who is in charge"?

8. How is NIMS different from NRF? How do they work together?

9. How would you organize preparedness planning for federal, state, and local entities to best prepare for the next emergency?

References

1. Constitution of the United States of America.
2. Suburban Emergency Management Project. *History of Federal Domestic Disaster Aid before the Civil War.* July 24, 2006. Available at: http://www.semp.us/publications/biot_reader.php?BiotID=379. Accessed August 23, 2010.
3. Foster GM. *The Demands of Humanity: Army Medical Disaster Relief.* U.S. Army Medical Department, Office of Medical History. 1983. Available at: http://history.amedd.army.mil/booksdocs/misc/disaster/default.html. Accessed August 23, 2010.
4. Hoover M. Rowboat federalism: The politics of U.S. disaster relief. *MRZine.* November 28, 2005. Available at: http://mrzine.monthlyreview.org/2005/hoover281105.html. Accessed June 2017.
5. Du Bois WEB. The Freedmen's Bureau. *The Atlantic.* March 1901. Available at: https://www.theatlantic.com/magazine/archive/1901/03/the-freedmens-bureau/308772/. Accessed May 2017.
6. Dauber ML. The Sympathetic State. *Law and History Review.* 2005;23(2):387–442.
7. Federal Reserve. Banking Acts of 1932. History. February 1932. Available at: https://www.federalreservehistory.org/essays/banking_acts_of_1932. Accessed June 2017.
8. U.S. Department of Homeland Security, FEMA. FEMA History. August 11, 2010. Available at: https://www.fema.gov/about-agency. Accessed June 2017.
9. The White House. *The Federal Response to Hurricane Katrina Lessons Learned.* February 2006. Available at: http://library.stmarytx.edu/acadlib/edocs/katrinawh.pdf. Accessed September 2017.
10. Federation of American Scientists. Executive Order 12127—Federal Emergency Management Agency. March 31, 1979. Available at: http://www.fas.org/irp/offdocs/eo/eo-12127.htm. Accessed September 2017.
11. Disaster Relief Act of 1974; Public Law No. 93-288.
12. Robert T. Stafford Disaster Relief and Emergency Assistance Act (Stafford Act); Public Law No. 100-707.
13. Disaster Mitigation Act of 2000; Public Law No. 106-390.
14. Pets Evacuation and Transportation Standards Act, Public Law No. 109-308.
15. Homeland Security Watch. Stafford at Twenty-Six. November 26, 2014. Available at: http://www.hlswatch.com/2014/11/26/stafford-at-twenty-six/. Accessed May 2017.
16. Zelikow P, Jenkins BD, May ER; National Commission on Terrorist Attacks upon the United States. *The 9/11 Commission Report.* Available at: https://www.9-11commission.gov/report/911Report.pdf. Accessed May 2017.
17. Office of Homeland Security. *National Strategy for Homeland Security.* July 2002. Available at: https://www.dhs.gov/sites/default/files/publications/nat-strat-hls-2002.pdf. Accessed May 2017.
18. Department of Homeland Security. *Office of Health Affairs.* Available at: https://www.dhs.gov/office-health-affairs. Accessed May 2017.
19. Department of Homeland Security. *Health Threats Resilience Division.* Available at: https://www.dhs.gov/health-threats-resilience-division. Accessed May 2017.
20. Department of Health and Human Services. Office of the Assistant Secretary for Preparedness and Response Organization Chart. 2014. Available at: https://www.hhs.gov/about/agencies/orgchart/aspr/index.html. Accessed May 2017.
21. U.S. Department of Health and Human Services. Office of the Assistant Secretary for Preparedness and Response (ASPR). Public Health Emergency. April 27, 2017. Available at: http://www.phe.gov/about/aspr/pages/default.aspx. Accessed August 23, 2010.
22. U.S. Department of Health and Human Services. Hospital Preparedness Program. Public Health Emergency. April 14, 2017. Available at: https://www.phe.gov/preparedness/planning/hpp/pages/default.aspx. Accessed May 2017.
23. CDC, Office of Public Health Preparedness and Response. Divisions of Office of Public Health Preparedness and

Response. August 18, 2016. Available at: https://www.cdc.gov /phpr/whoweare/divisions.htm. Accessed May 2017.

24. NIH, Office of Science Policy. *Biosecurity.* Available at: http:// osp.od.nih.gov/office-biotechnology-activities/biosecurity /nsabb. Accessed May 2017.

25. NIH. National Institute of Allergy and Infectious Diseases. Available at: https://www.niaid.nih.gov. Accessed May 2017.

26. FDA. *Counterterrorism and Emerging Threats.* December 14, 2016. Available at: https://www.fda.gov/emergencypreparedness /counterterrorism /default.htm. Accessed May 2017.

27. U.S. Department of Agriculture. *Animal and Plant Health Inspection Service.* August 23, 2010. Available at: http://www .aphis.usda.gov/. Accessed June 2017.

28. USDA. *Agricultural Research Service.* February 7, 2017. Available at: https://www.ars.usda.gov/about-ars/. Accessed May 2017.

29. U.S. Department of Justice. *Federal Bureau of Investigation.* Available at: http://www.fbi.gov/homepage.htm. Accessed August 23, 2010.

30. Sandor K. Department of Defense. In: Katz R, Zilinikas R, eds. *Encyclopedia of Bioterrorism Defense,* 2nd ed. Wiley and Sons; forthcoming 2011.

31. Use of Army and Air Force as posse comitatus, 18 U.S.C. § 1385.

32. John Warner National Defense Authorization Act for Fiscal Year 2007, Public Law No. 109-364.

33. National Defense Authorization Act for Fiscal Year 2012, P.L. 112-81 (December 31, 2011).

34. Office of the Director of National Intelligence Organization. Available at: https://www.dni.gov/index.php/who-we-are /organizations. Accessed May 2017.

35. Agrawal N. There's more than the CIA and FBI: The 17 agencies that make up the U.S. intelligence community. *The LA Times.* January 17, 2017. Available at: http://www.latimes .com/nation/la-na-17-intelligence-agencies-20170112-story .html. Accessed May 2017.

36. Gruszczak A. *Intelligence Security in the European Union: Building a Strategic Intelligence Community.* London: MacMillen Publishers; 2016. https:// books.google.com/books?id=tM7MDAAAQBAJ &pg=PA75&lpg=PA75&dq=cyb erint+intelligence+gat hering&source=bl&ots=-ZlXNM28gP&sig=ZI777JoJafo uwsAZ1fg1Xd_1QlM&hl=en&sa=X&ved=0ahUKEwjl2 4WLqMfTAhWISiYKHVxNCW44ChDoAQgsMAI#v=

onepage&q=cyberint%20intellig ence%20gathering&f=false. Accessed May 2017.

37. Department of Homeland Security. *Homeland Security Presidential Directive-5.* February 28, 2003. Available at: https://www.dhs.gov/sites/default/files/publications /Homeland%20Security%20Presidential%20Directive%205 .pdf. Accessed May 2017.

38. Department of Homeland Security. *Homeland Security Presidential Directive/HSPD 8.* FAS. December 17, 2003. Available at: https://fas.org/irp/offdocs/nspd/hspd-8.html. Accessed May 2017.

39. Department of Homeland Security. *National Preparedness Guidelines.* September 2007. Available at: https://www.hsdl .org/?view&did=478815. Accessed May 2017.

40. Department of Homeland Security, FEMA. *National Preparedness System.* December 20, 2016. Available at: https://www.fema.gov/national-preparedness-system. Accessed 2017.

41. Department of Homeland Security. *Homeland Security Exercise and Evaluation Program (HSEEP).* April 2013. Available at: https://preptoolkit.fema.gov/documents /1269813/1269861 /HSEEP_Revision_Apr13_Fin al.pdf/65bc7843-1d10-47b7 -bc0d-45118a4d21da. Accessed May 2017.

42. Department of Homeland Security. *National Incident Management System.* December 2008. Available at: https:// www.fema.gov/pdf/emergency/nims/NIMS_core.pdf. Accessed May 2017.

43. Department of Homeland Security. *National Response Framework,* 3rd ed. June 2016. Available at: https:// www.fema.gov/media-library-data/1466014682982 -9bcf8245ba4c60c120aa915abe74e15d/National_Response _Framework3rd.pdf. Accessed May 2017.

44. Department of Homeland Security. *Response Federal Interagency Operational Plan,* 2nd ed. August 2016. Available at: https://www.fema.gov/media-library- data/1471452095112 -507e23ad4d85449ff131c2b025743101/Response_FIOP_2nd .pdf. Accessed May 2017.

45. Prepare: National. *2017 Preparedness Index Key Findings.* Available at: http://nhspi.org/tools-resources/2017-nhspi-key- findings/2017-nhspi-key-findings-2/. Accessed May 2017.

46. Trust for America's Health. *Ready or Not? Protecting the Public from Diseases, Disasters and Bioterrorism.* December 2016. Available at: http://healthyamericans.org/reports/readyornot 2016/. Accessed May 2017.

CHAPTER 5

Legislation, Regulations, and Policy Guidance

LEARNING OBJECTIVES

By the end of this chapter, the reader will be able to:

- Identify legislation, regulations, and policies that frame public health preparedness
- Describe current policy positions on preparedness, particularly as they relate to biological threats
- Understand the debate between security and civil liberties that arise as states look to update their legal and regulatory basis for response
- Introduce treaties and other multilateral agreements that impact public health preparedness
- Explore how one important piece of legislation was drafted through a case study

▶ Introduction

Legislation, regulations, and policy guidance documents form the foundation of public health preparedness.[1] In other disciplines, these documents might be considered the "theory" that underlies the study. In this always-evolving, operations-based field, it is the legal and regulatory framework that creates the baseline for which all policy, planning, and action is taken. As this is a relatively new discipline, the legislation, regulation, and policy guidance are also relatively new, changing to meet an evolving threat, incorporating lessons from previous experiences, and adapting to feedback from those directly affected by these documents. This chapter looks at a variety of public laws, regulations, and presidential directives that have shaped the field over the past decade and a half and currently guide preparedness efforts. Legislation and executive orders related to select agents are addressed in the next chapter.

Previous chapters looked at guidance documents that support emergency and disaster response. This included a review of the Stafford Act, which gives the president the power to issue major disaster declarations in response to emergencies that overwhelm state and local authorities. This chapter examines a series of laws and policy guidance that support preparedness efforts. We first look chronologically at a series of legislation, and then explore presidential national and homeland security directives. We then discuss a model piece of legislation and the debate it raises over the balance between individual rights and the powers needed to respond effectively to an emergency.

This chapter also explores the international legal regime that exists to guide public health emergency preparedness (PHEP) and global health security. While there are a multitude of international agreements related to public health (over 50 multilateral agreements and several hundred bilateral agreements between the United States and other nations), this chapter highlights the handful that directly relate to emergency preparedness for public health threats.[2]

▶ Public Health Emergency Preparedness Legislation in the United States (Starting in 2000)

Public Health Improvement Act of 2000 (Public Law 106-505)

The Public Health Improvement Act of 2000 has 10 titles (or sections), 9 of which address traditional public health interests, such as sexually transmitted diseases, Alzheimer's research, organ donation, clinical research, and laboratory infrastructure. Title 1, however, addresses emerging threats to public health. This section authorizes the secretary of Department of Health and Human Services (HHS) to take appropriate response actions during a public health emergency, including investigations, treatment, and prevention. The act established the Public Health Emergency Fund to support activities in response to such public health emergencies. The act also authorized 10 years of appropriations to the Centers for Disease Control and Prevention (CDC) to defend and combat public health threats. Of note, the act directs the secretary of HHS to establish a working group to focus on the medical and public health effects of a bioterrorist attack.

Uniting and Strengthening America by Providing Appropriate Tools Required to Intercept and Obstruct Terrorism Act of 2001 (Public Law 107-56)

The Uniting and Strengthening America by Providing Appropriate Tools Required to Intercept and Obstruct Terrorism (USA PATRIOT) Act was passed by Congress and signed into law in October 2001, immediately following the 9/11 attacks and during the height of the anthrax-letters scare. This law includes a multitude of terrorism-related policies. Among them are provisions related to acquiring, handling, and transporting particularly dangerous pathogens; assistance to first responders; and funding for substantial new investments in bioterrorism preparedness and response.[3]

Public Health Security and Bioterrorism Preparedness and Response Act of 2002 (Public Law 107-188)

Signed into law in June 2002, the Bioterrorism Act (as it is known) was the first major piece of legislation dedicated entirely to public health preparedness. The act has five titles:

1. *National Preparedness for Bioterrorism and Other Public Health Emergencies*: It addresses national preparedness and response planning by calling for the development and maintenance of medical countermeasures, creating a National Disaster Medical System (NDMS), supporting communications and surveillance among all levels of public health officials, creating a core academic curriculum concerning bioweapons and other public health emergencies, improving hospital preparedness, and addressing workforce shortages for public health emergencics. It also codifies what had already been established—a Strategic National Stockpile of medical countermeasures.[4]
2. *Enhancing Controls on Dangerous Biological Agents and Toxins*: It addresses the control over select agents.
3. *Protecting Safety and Security of Food and Drug Supply:* It addresses bioterrorist threats to the food supply and what the Food and Drug Administration (FDA) is permitted to do to address this threat. It also touches on the importance of ensuring the safety of drugs imported into the United States.
4. *Drinking Water Security and Safety*: It directs communities to do a full assessment of the vulnerabilities of the water supply to terrorist attacks.
5. *Additional Provisions:* This final section of the law includes miscellaneous provisions for prescription drug user fees, digital televisions, and Medicare plans.

Smallpox Emergency Personnel Protection Act of 2003 (Public Law 108-20)

In December 2002, the Bush administration announced a program to vaccinate both military personnel and civilian emergency health workers against smallpox (**BOX 5-1**). The vaccine program for the military was obligatory, while the civilian vaccination program was voluntary. The Smallpox Emergency Personnel Protection Act (SEPA), which became

On December 13, 2002, President George W. Bush announced a plan to vaccinate military and select civilian personnel against smallpox, citing national security concerns. These concerns were based on general fears of a bioterrorism attack against the United States using smallpox, a disease that has been eradicated and for which the general population had little to no immunity. The United States ceased routine vaccination of smallpox in 1972, and even for those who had been vaccinated prior, immunity had diminished significantly.

The administration's plan was to vaccinate 500,000 military personnel against smallpox as fast as possible, and then vaccinate 500,000 civilians, focusing first on healthcare workers and first responders. Initially, the debate amongst the civilian community was around who would be eligible, with multiple entities pushing for inclusion. When the time came to be vaccinated, however, far fewer civilians than expected participated. By January 2004, 578,286 military personnel were vaccinated, but only 34,213 civilians received the vaccine.

Many of the civilian health workers refused the vaccine, often citing the potential for adverse reactions, as the vaccine is a live virus that has the potential to cause severe side effects. In fact, two civilians and one military vaccine recipient (all in their 50s) died within days of receiving the smallpox vaccine from ischemic cardiac events (heart attacks). Approximately 20 additional vaccine recipients suffered nonfatal cardiac events.

The National Academies of Science (NAS) found this smallpox vaccination program to have several major flaws contributing to its overall failure within the civilian population. It found that the rational for the smallpox vaccination program was never clearly explained to key constituencies, the program assumptions were never reviewed, and CDC was constrained in its ability to communicate effectively to state and local public health officials. There were significant barriers to program implementation, such as lack of compensation at the start of the program, logistical and practical constraints, and confusion over program structure and goals. Additionally, the program did not explicitly link to preparedness, leaving stakeholders with questions about the utility of the program. NAS recommended that future preparedness programs better integrate public health and scientific reason, engage stakeholders, and establish strong communication lines to the public about preparedness efforts.

Data from Richards EP, Rathbun KC, Gold J. The Smallpox Vaccination Campaign of 2003: Why Did It Fail and What Are the Lessons for Bioterrorism Preparedness? *Louisiana Law Review.* 2004;64:851–904; Available at: http://biotech.law.lsu.edu/articles/smallpox.pdf; Centers for Disease Control and Prevention. Cardiac Deaths After a Mass Smallpox Vaccination Campaign—New York City, 1947. *Morbidity and Mortality Weekly.* October 2003;52(39):933–936.; Centers for Disease Control and Prevention. Update: Cardiac-Related Events during the Civilian Smallpox Vaccination Program—United States, 2003. *Morbidity and Mortality Weekly.* May 2003;52(21):492–496.; Committee on Smallpox Vaccination Program Implementation, Board on Health Promotion and Disease Prevention, Institute of Medicine. *The Smallpox Vaccination Program, Public Health in an Age of Terrorism.* Washington, DC: The National Academies Press; 2005.

law nearly 3 months after the vaccination program started, focuses on compensation related to medical care, lost income, or death resulting from receipt of the smallpox vaccine.

The Project Bioshield Act of 2004 (Public Law 108-276)

While the Bioterrorism Act of 2002 codified the Strategic National Stockpile, there remained a problem. Because of the vast costs involved with producing medical countermeasures and no guaranteed market in which to sell chemical, biological, radiological, and nuclear (CBRN) drugs and vaccines, pharmaceutical companies were reluctant to develop and bring to market these countermeasures. As a result, the Strategic National Stockpile remained under-resourced. The act aimed to create a guaranteed government-funded market for these countermeasures and included funding to purchase the products while they are still in the final stages of development. It also allowed HHS to expedite spending to procure products, hire experts, and award research grants pertaining to CBRN, and to allow for emergency use of countermeasures, even

if they lacked final FDA approval. However, most of the funds were used to target only three pathogens—anthrax, smallpox, and botulism—which led some to criticize the Obama administration for diverting funds that could have been used to develop therapeutics against other biological agents, such as the Ebola virus.

Public Readiness and Emergency Preparedness Act of 2005 (Division C of the Department of Defense Emergency Supplemental Appropriations, Public Law 109-148)

Because the Project Bioshield Act allowed the secretary of HHS to force the use of medical countermeasures for emergency purposes without final FDA approval, manufacturers, distributors, program administrators, prescribers, and dispensers expressed concern to policymakers that they could be held liable for any negative consequences associated with the use of unapproved countermeasures. In response, Congress and the Bush administration passed the Public Readiness and Emergency Preparedness (PREP) Act, which limits liability associated with public health countermeasures used on an emergency basis. The exception is in the event of "willful misconduct."

Pandemic and All-Hazards Preparedness Act of 2006 (Public Law 109-417)

The Pandemic and All-Hazards Preparedness Act, known as PAHPA, reauthorized the Bioterrorism Act of 2002 and added broad provisions aimed at preparing for and responding to public health and medical emergencies, regardless of origin. It is organized into the following four main titles:

1. **National Preparedness and Response, Leadership, Organization, and Planning**: This title makes the HHS secretary the lead person for all public health and medical responses to emergencies covered by the National Response Framework (the act actually refers to the National Response Plan, which was later updated and renamed the National Response Framework). It also established the position of assistant secretary for preparedness and response at HHS and required HHS to create a National Health Security Strategy.

2. **Public Health Security Preparedness**: This section of the act focuses on developing preparedness infrastructure, primarily at the state and local levels, to include pandemic plans, interoperable networks for data sharing, and telehealth capabilities. It also addresses laboratory security and the need to ensure readiness of the Commissioned Corps of the Public Health Service to respond to public health emergencies.

3. **All-Hazards Medical Surge Capacity**: This title has several key provisions, including the transfer of the NDMS back to HHS from Department of Homeland Security (DHS). HHS is responsible for evaluating capacity for a medical patient surge during a public health emergency, and is required to establish a Medical Reserve Corps of volunteers to assist during such emergencies. Title III also requires HHS to develop public health preparedness curricula and establish centers for preparedness at schools of public health.

4. **Pandemic and Biodefense Vaccine and Drug Development**: The final title of PAHPA builds on the Bioshield Act of 2004 by requiring the establishment of the Biomedical Advanced Research and Development Authority (BARDA) within HHS to coordinate countermeasure research and development. Although the Bioshield Act enticed manufacturers to develop countermeasures, it did not do enough to assist companies during the expensive years of product research and development. Through payment structure reform, Title IV permits BARDA to better enable countermeasure development and production.

Pandemic and All-Hazards Preparedness Reauthorization Act of 2013 (Public Law 113-5)

PAHPA was reauthorized in 2013 as the Pandemic and All-Hazards Preparedness Reauthorization Act (PAHPRA). PAHPRA is organized into the following four main titles:

1. Strengthening National Preparedness and Response for Public Health Emergencies
2. Optimizing State and Local All-Hazards Preparedness and Response
3. Enhancing Medical Countermeasures Review
4. Accelerating Medical Countermeasure Advanced Research and Development

Implementing Recommendations of the 9/11 Commission Act of 2007 (Public Law 110-53)

In August 2007, Congress passed the Implementing Recommendations of the 9/11 Commission Act, which, as the title suggests, focuses on implementing the recommendations from the 9/11 Commission Report. The act includes numerous specific provisions pertaining to preparedness, such as preparedness grants to state and local entities, improving the incident command system, improving the sharing of intelligence information across the federal government, enhancing efforts to prevent terrorists from gaining entry into the United States, increasing the safety of transportation, and improving generally the preparedness infrastructure. It also includes sections on diplomatic engagement and advancing democratic values abroad. Specific to public health, Title XI of the act addresses enhanced defenses against weapons of mass destruction (WMD), particularly the need to maintain a National Biosurveillance Integration Center that reports to Congress on the "state of . . . biosurveillance efforts."[5]

The National Defense Authorization Act for Fiscal Year 2017 (Public Law 114-328)

The National Defense Authorization Act (NDAA) was signed into law in December 2016. It has a multitude of requirements, but includes language requiring a review of existing policies and strategies associated with biodefense, and calls for the creation of a new National Biodefense Strategy and implementation plan. The legislation specifically tasked the Department of Defense (DoD), DHS, HHS, and Agriculture to review and assess all biodefense policies, practices, and programs; to devise a strategy; and to revise the strategy biennially.

🔎 CASE STUDY: Passage of the Pandemic and All-Hazards Preparedness Act of 2006

By Jennifer Bryning Alton

Introduction

Congress passed PAHPA on a bipartisan basis in December 2006 and President George W. Bush signed it into law later that month. PAHPA established a new preparedness framework that significantly advanced America's emergency public health and medical response capabilities. It has subsequently been reauthorized by Congress and is scheduled for reauthorization again in 2018. Ten years after its initial passage, this case study examines the factors that created the conditions to enable passage of this important law.

Background

The 109th Congress began in January 2005, three and a half years after the 9/11 terrorist and anthrax letter attacks of 2001. The anthrax letters killed only 5 people and sickened 22, but cost over $1 billion in damages and cleanup. The fear they generated gripped the nation and demonstrated the grave threat from biological weapons.

Starting in 2000, Congress passed several laws to improve the country's ability to respond to acts of biological terrorism (see previous section of chapter). However, Congress was still dissatisfied with the state of the country's public health and medical preparedness. During the fall of 2005, they saw firsthand how ill-prepared the country was when Hurricane Katrina devastated the Gulf Coast and H5N1 avian influenza virus threatened a global pandemic.

At the start of the 109th Congress, Senate leadership, led by physician Senator Bill Frist (R-TN), established a new Subcommittee on Bioterrorism and Public Health Preparedness, under the Senate Committee on Health, Education, Labor and Pensions (HELP). Frist chose then-freshman Senator Richard Burr (R-NC) as the subcommittee chairman. Paired with Burr was Senator Edward Kennedy (D-MA) as the subcommittee ranking member.

The subcommittee was tasked with drafting legislation to further improve America's public health and medical preparedness and response capabilities. Under Burr's leadership, the subcommittee set out to methodically evaluate gaps in current government efforts and build on existing laws.

Timeline

The process of evaluating existing programs and laws, drafting, negotiating, and passing PAHPA through the Senate and House occurred over a two-year period: January 2005–December 2006. During those two years, the Senate subcommittee held 13 public hearings and roundtables, including a field hearing in New Orleans to discuss Hurricane Katrina, and a member level bioterrorism tabletop exercise at the National Defense University in Washington, D.C.

Members first introduced a bill to address deficiencies in medical countermeasures development. The Biodefense and Pandemic Vaccine and Drug Development Act (S. 1873) was introduced by Senator Burr and five Republican cosponsors and passed by the HELP committee in October 2005. After taking into account concerns about excessive secrecy and drug safety, and removing provisions dealing with liability and compensation that had been passed separately in a different bill, the senators revised and reintroduced the bill (S. 2564) in April 2006. Representatives Mike Rogers (R-MI) and Anna Eshoo (D-CA) introduced a companion bill in the House in June 2006. The House passed its bipartisan bill (H.R. 5533) in September 2006, but medical countermeasure legislation still awaited a vote in the Senate.

Senators Burr and Kennedy and five other bipartisan cosponsors meanwhile introduced the PAHPA (S. 3678) in July 2006. This new bill addressed many additional elements of preparedness beyond medical countermeasure development. The Senate HELP committee passed the bill that same month. The bill sponsors then agreed to add the Biodefense and Pandemic Vaccine and Drug Development Act to PAHPA after it passed the committee. The combined PAHPA legislation passed the Senate by unanimous consent on December 5, passed the House without objection on December 9, and was signed into law by President George W. Bush on December 19, 2006.

(continues)

The Public Health Implications

During 2005, the United States faced two public health emergencies—(1) Hurricanes Katrina and Rita and (2) a potential influenza pandemic from H5N1. These two events highlighted different sets of issues that needed to be addressed to enhance preparedness for future emergencies.

Local, state, and federal public health and medical responses to Hurricanes Katrina and Rita were inadequate and uncoordinated; respective roles and responsibilities were ill defined; and Americans died. The White House performed an after action report and stated that HHS should "lead a unified and strengthened public health and medical command for Federal disaster response. . . . Public health professionals and emergency medical responses should be managed and overseen by HHS, which has the greatest health experience and expertise."[6(Appendix A)] The designation of HHS as the lead for public health and medical emergency responses was a fundamental shift from the previous reliance on the DHS.

Later in 2005, the emergence of H5N1 avian influenza and the potential for a human pandemic highlighted the risk of infectious disease threats and the shortcomings in government programs and efforts to develop vaccines and drugs against such high-consequence events. Many experimental but promising medical countermeasures were failing in later stages of development due in part to a lack of research funding and support from the U.S. government. Further, the process of human drug and vaccine development typically takes a decade, which is too long to combat an emerging threat that may occur without warning and spread rapidly.

To address these challenges, PAHPA made important changes to law and government structure in order to

- *Put someone in charge.* It designated the secretary of HHS as the lead official for public health and medical responses to public health emergencies, created the assistant secretary for preparedness and response (ASPR) to coordinate these activities, and moved the NDMS from DHS back to HHS.
- *Streamline preparedness spending.* It reauthorized over $1 billion per year of HHS funding for state and local public health and medical preparedness from the PHEP grants and Hospital Preparedness Programs (HPP).
- *Enhance medical surge response.* It established a process for registering and organizing volunteers, improving training and support for volunteers, and promoting the use of mobile medical assets and alternative federal facilities to increase surge capacity during an emergency.
- *Promote uniformity of performance.* It required establishment of overarching preparedness goals and essential public health security functions to ensure uniform standards of preparedness from state to state.
- *Expedite the development of medical countermeasures.* It established the HHS BARDA to partner with biopharmaceutical companies to develop the diagnostics, vaccines, and drugs needed to protect Americans from deliberate and natural threats.

The Solution—The Policy Window for PAHPA

In the 109th Congress, 10,703 bills were introduced and only 482 of those, or less than 5%, became law.[7] What contributes to whether a piece of legislation will be one of the successful 4%–5%?

In his text, *Agendas, Alternatives, and Public Policies*, John Kingdon presents a useful framework for considering this question.[8] Kingdon's conclusion is that policy windows open, thereby elevating an issue on the decision agenda and enabling important policy changes, when three different process streams converge—problems, policies, and politics. These policy windows are leveraged by ambitious policy entrepreneurs to push policy changes across the finish line. This is what happened with PAHPA.

A window opened for PAHPA due to changes in the political stream. It became a key political priority for Republican Senate leadership, due to a belief in the threat of bioterrorism and Senator Frist's experience as a medical doctor. Senate leadership demonstrated this priority by establishing a dedicated subcommittee and introducing in January 2005 one of 10 initial messaging bills for the 109th Congress—S.3, the Protecting America in the War on Terror Act.

The window opened further due to a predictable change in the policy stream, triggered by the need to reauthorize several public health and medical preparedness programs that would expire in September 2006. While the PHEP and HPP programs could continue to be funded without reauthorization, this potential expiration was a forcing function for policymakers and staff who are pressured to manage competing priorities with time constraints. The subcommittee staff conducted a very inclusive process with the bipartisan HELP committee staff, as well as solicited input and policy proposals from a variety of external stakeholders and advocacy organizations. This approach resulted in 14 bipartisan Senate cosponsors and 21 letters of support from outside organizations.

The political and policy streams might not have been sufficient to ensure PAHPA's success, but the window opened wider with changes in the problem stream. Poor governmental responses to Hurricanes Katrina and Rita as well as the country's lack of preparedness for a potential avian flu pandemic focused the attention of the public and government officials on the need for congressional action.

In addition to the joining of these three streams, the new subcommittee chairman, Senator Burr, was a powerful "policy entrepreneur," as defined by Kingdon, who seized the opportunity and advanced an ambitious, thorough, and assertive campaign to get PAHPA signed into law. He had just been elected to the Senate after 10 years in the House of Representatives and his subcommittee was extremely active, which is unusual in the Senate. Due to his subcommittee chairmanship, Burr and his staff had the standing needed to convene hearings and demand action. He and his staff were totally engaged, were good negotiators, and perhaps most importantly were doggedly persistent.

As an example, Burr personally briefed members and staff on the need for the legislation and dropped in on staff-level negotiations to weigh in and support his staff's position. After PAHPA passed the Senate, he personally went to the House floor and talked with members to address concerns and convince them to support final passage of the bill. This level of personal engagement and tenacity ensured the success of PAHPA.

There were certainly many other key players who contributed to this achievement, including Senators Kennedy, Frist, Mike Enzi (R-WY), Tom Harkin (D-IA), Judd Gregg (R-NH), and Barbara Mikulski (D-MD); Representatives Rogers and Eshoo; and their respective legislative staffs. In addition, the White House Homeland Security Council staff was supportive of the bill and helped overcome resistance at some of the executive branch agencies.

Conclusion

Incrementally building on the legislative accomplishments of previous Congresses, the PAHPA made important improvements to the U.S. government's biodefense structure and public health preparedness programs. Looking back 10 years after its initial passage in 2006, it is even clearer that the confluence of the political, policy, and problem streams, as well as the perseverance of Senator Burr and his subcommittee staff enabled this bill to pass the Senate by unanimous consent, pass the House without objection, and be signed into law by the president.

▶ Presidential Directives

In previous chapters, we have looked at presidential directives, primarily as they directly applied to creating the preparedness infrastructure [e.g., Homeland Security Presidential Directive (HSPD) 5 and 8]. Here, we examine five more presidential directives that helped form the policy guidance and regulations for public health preparedness.

Biodefense for the 21st Century: National Security Presidential Directive 33/Homeland Security Presidential Directive 10 (April 2004)

In 2004, the Bush administration released HSPD 10, which provided a strategic overview of the biological weapons threat and the administration's approach to framing biodefense initiatives. The directive described four essential pillars of the national biodefense program: threat awareness, prevention and protection, surveillance and detection, and response and recovery. This document remained the primary policy directive concerning biodefense until the National Strategy for Countering Biological Threats was released in late 2009.

Medical Countermeasures Against Weapons of Mass Destruction: Homeland Security Presidential Directive 18 (January 2017)

HSPD 18 was released early in 2007, and it pertained to the development of medical countermeasures to counter WMD. HSPD 18 gave lead to HHS but with DoD retaining control over development of medical countermeasures specific to the armed forces.

Public Health and Medical Preparedness: Homeland Security Presidential Directive 21 (October 2007)

Building upon HSPD 10 and in accordance with HSPD 18, HSPD 21 was released in the fall of 2007 and defines four critical components of public health and medical preparedness. The four components are a robust and integrated biosurveillance system, the ability to stockpile and distribute medical countermeasures, the capacity to engage in mass casualty care in emergency situations, and building resilient communities at the state and local levels. The directive also mandates the creation of task forces, studies, and plans to meet public health and medical preparedness needs.

Establishing Federal Capability for the Timely Provision of Medical Countermeasures Following a Biological Attack: Executive Order 13527 (December 2009)

In the last days of 2009, President Obama released Executive Order 13527, establishing a policy of timely provision of medical countermeasures in the event of a biological attack and tasking the federal government with assisting state and local entities in this endeavor. The order also spells out the role of the U.S. Postal Service in the delivery of medical countermeasures and calls on HHS to develop continuity of operations plans in the event of a large-scale biological attack.

National Strategy for Countering Biological Threats: Presidential Policy Directive 2 (November 2009)

The National Strategy for Countering Biological Threats was released in time for Undersecretary of State Ellen Tauscher to share it with the international community at the December 2009 Meeting of States Parties of the Biological Weapons Convention.[9] The strategy, the first major policy statement by the Obama administration on the topic of biological threats, spells out seven major objectives:

1. Promote global health security
2. Reinforce norms of safe and responsible conduct
3. Obtain timely and accurate insight on current and emerging risks
4. Take reasonable steps to reduce the potential for exploitation
5. Expand our capability to prevent, attribute, and apprehend
6. Communicate effectively with all stakeholders
7. Transform the international dialogue on biological threats[10,11]

While many of the Bush administration directives focused on policies for responding to a biological threat, the Obama strategy directive placed more emphasis on prevention, with particular stress on the importance of working with international partners, reinforcing norms of responsible scientific conduct, and engaging scientists so that they can continue beneficial work in the life sciences (**FIGURE 5-1**).

National Preparedness: Presidential Policy Directive 8 (March 2011)

In early 2011, the Obama administration released Presidential Policy Directive (PPD) 8, replacing HSPD 8. The PPD required the development of a National Preparedness Goal (as did HSPD 8) and the creation of a National Preparedness System to integrate guidance,

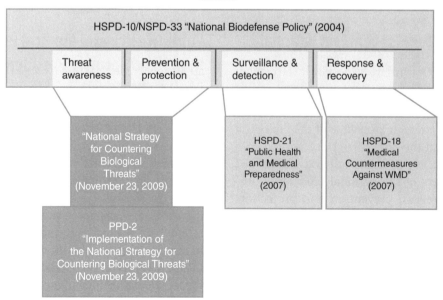

FIGURE 5-1 Select U.S. National policies to address biological threats

programs, and processes to build and sustain capabilities essential for preparedness. PPD 8 takes an "all-of-Nation" approach, identifying the importance of collaboration between governments at all levels and the private and not-for-profit sectors as well as the public in order to enhance resilience,[12] which the directive defines as "the ability to adapt to changing conditions and withstand and rapidly recover from disruption due to emergencies."[13]

Advancing the Global Health Security Agenda to Achieve a World Safe and Secure from Infectious Disease Threats, Executive Order (November 4, 2016)

The Obama administration issued an executive order in the last months of his administration aimed at solidifying the Global Health Security Agenda (GHSA). The executive order calls for an interagency review council and provides specific guidance on the roles and responsibilities of the different executive branch departments and agencies.

▶ Model Legislation

During a "public" health emergency, it is essential to have legal authorities in place that allow the government to mount an effective response, mitigate the consequences of the event, and save lives. Public health authority is primarily a power left to the state and local governments, but many states do not have appropriate legislation in place to effectively deal with a public health crises. In fact, some states have public health laws that are inconsistent, complicated, and often outdated.[14(Amend. X),15] With the shift in thinking regarding public health emergencies as potential national security concerns, legal experts embarked on an exercise to provide model legislation to enable states to revisit their legislative toolkit. In December 2001, Professor Lawrence Gostin, funded by the CDC, released the Model State Emergency Health Powers Act (MSEHPA).[16]

The MSEHPA was designed to allow state and local health authorities to effectively respond to public health emergencies, and is structured into five basic public health functions: (1) preparedness, (2) surveillance, (3) management of property, (4) protection of persons (including compelling vaccination, treatment, isolation, and quarantine), and (5) communication. The model law tries to balance the need to provide state and local authorities with the ability to manage a public health emergency with the need to protect civil liberties and safeguard personal rights. The model law prompted

much debate about the role of the federal government in responding to emergencies versus state responsibilities, the fear of abuse of power, personal and economic liberties during an emergency, and safeguarding of property. It also brought strong opposition from individuals and groups not comfortable with a government entity forcing vaccination, medical examination, quarantine, rapid burials, and takeover of private property, even if in response to an emergency. Some felt this was too much of an affront to civil liberties and not worth the sacrifice for the common good. Others were concerned that such powers might be abused by state authorities and applied in nonemergent situations.

As of 2011, 40 states had passed bills or resolutions that contain at least one provision from the model law.[17] States continue to update their laws, particularly as they concern quarantine and isolation. Ten states revised their quarantine laws following the 2014 Ebola outbreak.[18]

▶ International Law and Regulations

Early Agreements

There have been a series of international agreements about security and weapons of war aimed at addressing what we now term weapons of mass destruction. On April 24, 1863, the U.S. War Department issued General Orders 100, which declared "the use of poison in any manner, be it to poison wells, or foods, or arms, is wholly excluded from modern warfare."[19] More than 30 years later, the 1899 Hague Convention (II) declared "it is especially prohibited . . . [t]o employ poison or poisoned arms."[20]

The 1907 Hague Convention repeated this same text, and in 1925, the first agreement on chemical and biological weapons was signed that is still considered applicable under customary international law.[21] On June 17, 1925, 38 nations signed the Geneva Protocol for the Prohibition of the Use in War of Asphyxiating, Poisonous or Other Gases, and of Bacteriological Methods of Warfare, known as the Geneva Protocol (**BOX 5-2**).[22] (The United States signed the Geneva Protocol, but did not ratify it until 1975.) This agreement, developed in the aftermath of wide-scale chemical weapons use during World War I, does not ban the possession of chemical or biological weapons (CBW), but prohibits using them in war. In actuality, this is a "no first use" agreement, as many nations interpreted it to mean that they would not use CBW in war, but if used against a nation, they would—and could— retaliate in kind.

Protocol for the Prohibition of the Use in War of Asphyxiating, Poisonous or Other Gases, and of Bacteriological Methods of Warfare, Signed at Geneva, June 17, 1925

The Undersigned Plenipotentiaries, in the name of their respective Governments:

Whereas the use in war of asphyxiating, poisonous or other gases, and of all analogous liquids, materials or devices, has been justly condemned by the general opinion of the civilized world; and

Whereas the prohibition of such use has been declared in Treaties to which the majority of Powers of the World are Parties; and

To the end that this prohibition shall be universally accepted as a part of international law, binding alike the conscience and the practice of nations;

Declare:

That the High Contracting Parties, so far as they are not already Parties to Treaties prohibiting such use, accept this prohibition, agree to extend this prohibition to the use of bacteriological methods of warfare and agree to be bound as between themselves according to the terms of this declaration.

The High Contracting Parties will exert every effort to induce other States to accede to the present Protocol. Such accession will be notified to the Government of the French Republic, and by the latter to all signatory and acceding Powers, and will take effect on the date of the notification by the Government of the French Republic.

The present Protocol, of which the French and English texts are both authentic, shall be ratified as soon as possible. It shall bear today's date.

The ratifications of the present Protocol shall be addressed to the Government of the French Republic, which will at once notify the deposit of such ratification to each of the signatory and acceding Powers.

The instruments of ratification of and accession to the present Protocol will remain deposited in the archives of the Government of the French Republic.

The present Protocol will come into force for each signatory Power as from the date of deposit of its ratification, and, from that moment, each Power will be bound as regards other powers which have already deposited their ratifications.

Chemical Weapons Convention

The Chemical Weapons Convention (CWC) was concluded in 1993 and entered into force in 1997. As of December 2015, there were 192 states parties.[23] Building on the Geneva Protocol, the CWC explicitly prohibits the use of chemical weapons and bans the development, production, stockpile, and transfer of such agents. Under the agreement, states are required to declare any past chemical weapons program that existed after January 1, 1946, and obligates states that had chemical weapons to destroy their stockpiles within 10 years. The destruction of chemical weapons is a complicated and expensive endeavor, and this total destruction has not yet been completed.

The CWC established the Organization for the Prohibition of Chemical Weapons (OPCW), based in The Hague, which conducts inspections, ensures compliance with the treaty, and provides a forum for cooperation and consultation. (OPCW will be discussed in more detail in Chapter 9.)

Nuclear Non-Proliferation Treaty

The Treaty on the Non-proliferation of Nuclear Weapons (known as the Nuclear Non-proliferation Treaty or NPT) was signed in 1968 and entered into force in March 1970. There are 93 signatories, 5 of whom are known to have nuclear weapons (the United States, the United Kingdom, France, Russia, and China).[24] Only four nations, all of whom are known or suspected of having or wanting nuclear weapons, are not signatories: India, Pakistan, Israel, and North Korea, which withdrew from the treaty in 2003.

The purpose of the NPT is to limit the spread of nuclear weapons, encourage disarmament, and foster the right to peacefully use nuclear technology. While acknowledging that nations have nuclear weapons, the purpose of this treaty is to keep these weapons from spreading into the hands of other nations and make certain that nations with the knowledge to build such weapons refrain from doing so.

U.N. Security Council Resolution 1540

In 2004, the U.N. Security Council adopted Resolution (UNSCR) 1540, obligating U.N. member states to ensure they do not support non state actors in their efforts to develop, acquire, possess, or use nuclear, chemical, or biological weapons. To do this, the resolution obligates states to create or modify domestic legislation to criminalize the proliferation or use of WMD by non state actors. Not only must countries have appropriate legislation in place, but there also must be a means to enforce the legislation to prevent proliferation and use of chemical, biological, or nuclear weapons.

UNSCR 1540 is designed to complement other international regimes. The NPT and the International Atomic Energy Agency (IAEA) have programs supportive of 1540, including providing legislative and technical assistance. The resolution is also in line with CWC obligations and OPCW action plans. A 1540 Committee, established by the resolution, monitors global implementation, which contributes to compliance assessments of the Biological Weapons Convention (BWC).

Australia Group

While not a formal international agreement, there is an informal group of countries (and the European Commission) known as the Australia Group. Established in 1985, this group creates a list of items it believes has the potential to help "would-be proliferators" develop or acquire CBW.[25] Those items are then subject to export controls. While this group's efforts are not legally binding, they are supportive of obligations under the BWC and CWC.

Biological Weapons Convention

In 1972, nations around the world agreed to the BWC. As of September 2017, 169 nations have become party to the agreement. Under the BWC, nations agree never to develop, produce, stockpile, acquire, or retain any biological agent for other than peaceful purposes. The agreement also obliges parties to facilitate the exchange of equipment, materials, and information related to biological agents for peaceful purposes.

The BWC consists of a preamble and 15 articles:

- *Preamble:* This article cites the Geneva Protocol and reaffirms adherence to those principles, in essence pointing to the previous agreement not to use biological weapons and stating that such use would "be repugnant to the conscience of mankind."
- *Article I:* Never in any circumstances should a state develop, produce, stockpile, or otherwise acquire or retain biological agents or toxins, or weapons, equipment, or means to deliver such agents for hostile purposes.
- *Article II:* If a state has such agents or toxins, it must be destroyed immediately or diverted for peaceful purposes.

- *Article III:* No state will transfer, assist, encourage, or induce any other state or entity to manufacture or acquire any agent, toxin, weapons, or delivery mechanisms.
- *Article IV:* Each state must take necessary measures to prohibit and prevent the development, acquisition, or retention of biological agents or toxins or delivery mechanisms in all areas under its jurisdiction.
- *Article V:* All states parties must work with each other to solve any problems associated with the agreement, and can use appropriate international procedures.
- *Article VI:* If a state finds another state to be in breach of its obligations under the BWC, the state can lodge a complaint with the U.N. Security Council. States should cooperate with the Security Council if it wishes to carry out an investigation.
- *Article VII:* States will provide assistance and support to a nation that requests aid as a result of being exposed to danger per a violation of the BWC.
- *Article VIII:* Nothing in the BWC should be interpreted as limiting or detracting from the Geneva Protocol.
- *Article IX:* Each state recognizes the importance of prohibiting chemical weapons use and agrees to negotiate to reach a separate agreement on chemical weapons. (Note: The CWC came about almost 20 years after the BWC.)
- *Article X:* This article reaffirms the right of states parties to participate in the peaceful exchange of equipment, material, and technology related to biological and toxin agents. Here it declares that parties with resources should help those with less.
- *Articles XI–XV:* These are procedural regarding amendments, entry into force, duration, ratification, and translation.[26]

Unlike the CWC, the BWC does not have a verification mechanism, meaning that there is no means under the treaty for countries to inspect and verify that another nation is either compliant with or in violation of its treaty obligations. During the 1990s, such a mechanism was proposed, debated, and negotiated. In 2001, however, after almost a decade of discussion, the United States pulled out, stating that advances in technology and other factors made the BWC virtually unverifiable and, therefore, the proposed mechanisms would not be effective. With the departure of the United States from the negotiations, the verification protocol was dropped. The United States, however, remained committed to the BWC and proposed what was called a "work program," in which states parties meet each year to discuss topics relevant to the BWC, using the treaty as a forum for sharing ideas, forming collaborations, and advancing knowledge on a range of topics. This program was adopted and was used through the 2016 Review Conference to discuss biosecurity, codes of conduct, disease surveillance, technology transfer, investigating allegations of use, and a variety of topics directly related to the BWC.

It is worth noting that Article VII of the BWC is the "preparedness and response" article. Because states parties are obligated under this article to provide assistance to other states in the event of a violation of the treaty, it means the following:

1. States should have the ability to detect when there has been a violation (a biological weapons use event) and be able to differentiate a biological weapons use event from a naturally occurring event, if possible.
2. States should have procedures in place for requesting and receiving assistance.
3. States should have capacity to assist other states in containing and mitigating a biological weapons use event.

International Health Regulations 2005

In 2005, after almost a decade of negotiations, the World Health Assembly (WHA) of the World Health Organization (WHO) adopted the International Health Regulations (IHR) (2005). This agreement, binding on all member states of the WHA, revises previous international agreements, going back to 1891, which focused on international cooperation for containing a short, finite list of historically relevant diseases (**TABLE 5-1**). The updated version of the regulations recognizes the threat of emerging infectious diseases, the globalization of society, and the need for improved surveillance, response, communication, and coordination to effectively detect and respond to public health threats (**TABLE 5-2**).

IHR (2005) includes some major changes to the international regime for controlling communicable diseases. First, this version of the IHR addresses anything that may constitute a Public Health Emergency of International Concern (PHEIC). A PHEIC is defined using a decision-making algorithm to determine if an event is unusual or unexpected, if the public health impact is serious, if there is a significant risk of international spread, and if the event might require travel and trade restrictions.[27] It requires countries to identify and report any potential PHEIC in a timely fashion to the WHO, and provides for an effective response through

evidence-based recommendations, assistance, transparency, and communication. Countries are obligated to develop basic core competencies for disease surveillance and response, and to have a focal point in place for communication to and from the WHO (**FIGURE 5-2**).

A primary purpose of IHR (2005) is to improve global health security through international collaboration and communication in order to detect and contain public health emergencies at the source Full implementation requires multisectoral engagement and resources.

Countries had until 2012 to become compliant with IHR (2005), but as the deadline approached, it became clear that most countries would require additional time. In fact, only 22% of countries claimed to have fully implemented the regulations in 2012. That number jumped to 33% in 2014. The WHO has now set 2019 as the goal for implementation for the neediest countries.

IHR (2005) was tested for the first time during the 2009–2010 H1N1 influenza pandemic and, overall, the international framework created by the regulations greatly assisted in enabling the WHO to be notified of the virus in a timely fashion, coordinate response to nations who needed assistance, and to communicate evidence-based recommendations globally. H1N1 was the first ever declared PHEIC. This was followed by polio in 2014, Ebola in 2014, and Zika in 2016. With each PHEIC comes new lessons for how the IHR should operate, how nations should operate, and how global governance of disease can and should be improved.

Pandemic Influenza Preparedness Framework

The Pandemic Influenza Preparedness (PIP) Framework was adopted in 2011 to promote a new system of equitable access to influenza samples and subsequent benefits, including vaccines. PIP evolved from a dispute that started in 2007, when the Indonesian government withheld H5N1 influenza samples from the WHO's Global Influenza Surveillance and Response System (GISRS) (although in 2007, it was called the Global Influenza Surveillance Network (GISN)). Indonesia invoked "viral sovereignty," claiming the influenza samples from their citizens belonged to the country. They claimed that the system for sample sharing was unjust and populations impacted by the disease were not able to benefit from the medical countermeasures developed from the virus samples. In response, the global community,

TABLE 5-1 Select Treaties for Global Governance of Multiple Diseases 1892–2005		
Year	Treaty	Focus
1892	International Sanitary Convention	Cholera
1893	International Sanitary Convention	Cholera
1894	International Sanitary Convention	Cholera
1897	International Sanitary Convention	Plague
1903	International Sanitary Convention (replaces previous four versions)	Cholera and plague
1905	Inter-American Sanitary Convention	Governance
1912	International Sanitary Convention (replaces 1903 version)	Cholera, plague, and yellow fever
1924	Pan American Sanitary Code	Governance and plague, cholera, yellow fever, smallpox, typhus, epidemic cerebrospinal meningitis, acute epidemic poliomyelitis, epidemic lethargic encephalitis, influenza or epidemic la grippe, and typhoid and paratyphoid fevers
1926	International Sanitary Convention (modifying 1912 version)	Plague, cholera, yellow fever, smallpox, and typhus
1927	Protocol to the Pan American Sanitary Convention	Ratification
1938	International Sanitary Convention (amending 1926 version)	Plague, cholera, yellow fever, typhus, and smallpox; governance for Egypt, Suez Canal, and the Hajj
1944	International Sanitary Convention (modifying 1926 version)	Plague, cholera, yellow fever, typhus, and smallpox, as well as "outbreaks of such other communicable disease as . . . constitute a menace to other countries"; change of governance to U.N Relief and Rehabilitation Administration (UNRRA)
1946	Protocols to Prolong the 1944 International Sanitary Convention	Governance still with UNRRA
1951	International Sanitary Regulation	Governance with WHO; plague, cholera, yellow fever, smallpox, typhus, and relapsing fever
1969	International Health Regulations (1969) (International Sanitary Regulations Renamed)	Cholera, plague, yellow fever, smallpox, relapsing fever, and typhus
1973	International Health Regulations (modifying 1969 version)	Cholera, plague, yellow fever, smallpox. Requirement for cholera vaccination dropped
1981	International Health Regulations (modifying 1969 version)	Smallpox removed post eradication. Back to cholera, plague, and yellow fever
2005	International Health Regulations (2005)	Any public health emergency of international concern

TABLE 5-2 Evolution of the International Health Regulations, 2007 to the Present

IHR Component	2007–Present
Scope	Any PHEIC
Communication	National IHR Focal Point (NFP)
Notification	Report to World Health Organization (WHO) within 24 hours (72 hours to respond to follow up requests)
Coordinated response	Assistance in response/recommended measures
Authority	WHO can initiate requests for information, including on basis of unofficial sources
National capacity	Provide disease inspection and controls at ports of entry, and meet minimum core capacity for detection, assessment, reporting, and response

Data from Fischer J, Katz R. The Revised International Health Regulations: A Framework for Global Pandemic Response. *Global Health Governance*. 2010; III(2). Available at: www.ghgj.org /Katz%20and%20Fischer_The%20Revised%20International%20Health%20Regulations.pdf. Accessed May 2017.

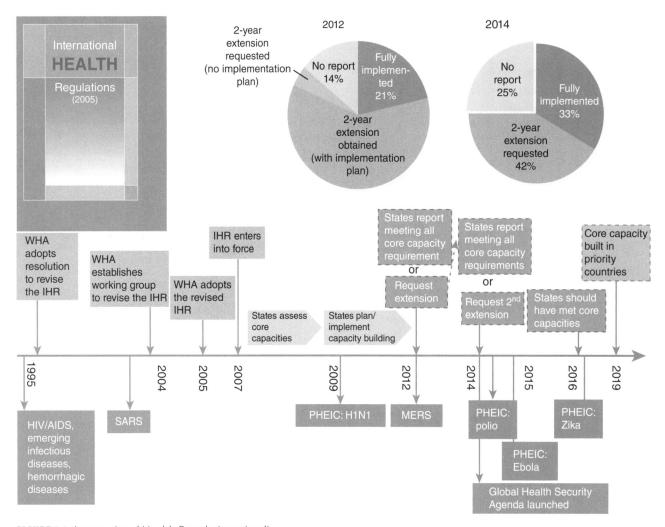

FIGURE 5-2 International Health Regulations timeline

under the auspices of the WHO, negotiated what became the PIP Framework, to enable sample sharing of influenza viruses, while insuring that pharmaceutical companies, diagnostic companies, and other researchers commit to equitable access to vaccines and other supplies during a pandemic.

Global Health Security Agenda

In early 2014, the United States along with over two dozen partner countries and three international organizations (WHO, Organization for Animal Health (OIE), and Food and Agriculture Organization (FAO)) launched the GHSA. GHSA is a multilateral partnership, now with approximately 55 nations, designed to accelerate progress in global health security. It aimed to address infectious disease threats by marshaling resources toward IHR implementation, securing concrete commitments to help nations build core capacities, and to bring

global health security issues to the attention of world leaders.

GHSA is organized around 11 action packages, covering prevent, detect, and respond (**TABLE 5-3**). The action packages roughly correspond to core capacities under the IHR, and these action packages have now been incorporated into an external assessment tool. The Joint External Evaluation Tool (JEE) has been adopted by the WHO to be used to assess IHR implementation and country progress toward being able to prevent, detect, and respond to public health threats. Countries voluntary sign up to have external evaluators assess national core capacities. This process is then supposed to be followed by "country action plans" designed to create road map toward capacity building, including financing.

The United States committed to supporting two sets of countries under the GHSA. The government made a financial commitment of approximately $1 billion over 5 years to support 17 countries, called GHSA

TABLE 5-3 Action Packages	
Action Packages—Prevent	
Prevent 1	Combat antimicrobial resistance
Prevent 2	Minimize spillover of zoonotic diseases into humans
Prevent 3	National biosafety and biosecurity system
Prevent 4	National vaccine delivery system
Action Packages—Detect	
Detect 1	National laboratory system
Detect 2 & 3	Indicator and event-based surveillance systems
Detect 4	Disease reporting consistent with WHO, OIE, and FAO requirements
Detect 5	Workforce development to meet International Health Regulations and Performance of Veterinary Services core competencies
Action Packages—Respond	
Respond 1	Emergency Operations Centers
Respond 2	Linking public health with law and multisectoral rapid response
Respond 3	Deployment of medical countermeasures and medical personnel

Data from CDC. Global Health Security Agenda: Action Packages. *Global Health*. Available at: https://www.cdc.gov/globalhealth/security/actionpackages/. Accessed May 2017.

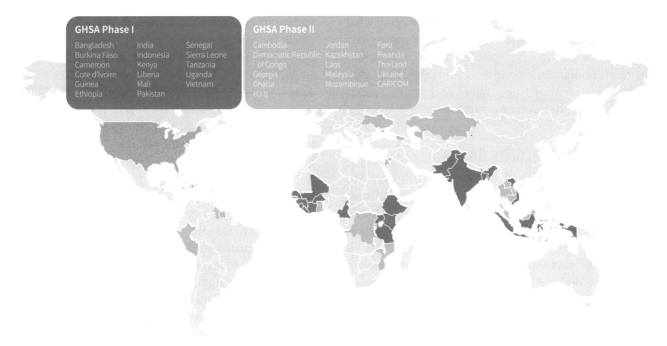

FIGURE 5-3 Global Health Security Agenda Phases I and II partner countires

Reproduced from Global Health Security Agenda. *Advancing the Global Health Security Agenda: Progress and Early Impact from U.S. Investment.* December 2016. Available at: https://www.ghsagenda.org/docs/default-source/default-document-library/ghsa-legacy-report .pdf?sfvrsn=12. Accessed May 2017.

Phase 1. The rest of the countries (labeled GHSA Phase II) were identified to receive technical assistance or possibly funding from non-GHSA-specific appropriations (**FIGURE 5-3**). Other nations also made financial commitments and the G7 committed to funding GHSA action packages in 76 countries.

▶ The Functionality of International Agreements

Some argue that international agreements are not a good way to force nations to act a particular way, to promote an agenda, or to facilitate cooperation. This argument is based on the concept that nations are sovereign states, and regardless of what document they may have signed, they will do whatever they see as in their national interests. Because of this concern, many agreements have associated penalties for violations. In some cases, those violations may be official U.N. sanctions, with economic and political consequences. In other cases, the enforcement mechanism may be less formal, such as travel and trade recommendations made by the WHO that might result in economic losses for a noncompliant country.

Even in the absence of an enforcement mechanism, it can be argued that international agreements are vital tools in preparedness and prevention. They create an important forum for international dialogue, for information exchange, and for addressing serious global challenges. In some cases, this dialogue may be at a very high political level, and in other cases, these foras become opportunities for pragmatic cooperation leading to measurable changes.

While perceptions of the importance of international agreements may vary, it is clear that they are important tools both internationally and domestically in shaping policy and global interactions.

Key Words

Australia Group
Biological Weapons Convention
Chemical Weapons Convention
Geneva Protocol
Global Health Security Agenda

International agreements
International Health Regulations
Legislation
Model legislation
National Strategy

Nuclear Non-Proliferation Treaty
Pandemic and All-Hazards
    Preparedness Act
Presidential directives
UNSCR 1540

Discussion Questions

1. How do legislation and regulations support public health preparedness?
2. What would happen if these laws were not in place?
3. What is missing in the legal landscape of public health preparedness?
4. Is there one particular law, regulation, or directive that you think is most important? Why?
5. The PAHPRA of 2013 included changes to each of the four main titles of the previous PAHPA law. Looking back at PAHPA 2006, how significant do you think these changes were and what might have been the rationale behind the revisions?
6. What are the distinct roles of local, state, federal, and international governments and organizations in managing a PHEIC?
7. In addition to those described, what other factors could have contributed to the policy window that opened for PAHPA? What could be done to create such an opportunity again for dealing with persistent public health security challenges?
8. Are all three elements of a policy window of equal impact (politics, policy, and problems) or does one tend to outweigh the others?
9. Would it be harder to pass the PAHPA today than it was in 2006? If so, why?
10. In light of the recent emerging infectious disease outbreaks, including Ebola and Zika, what policy changes should be considered during the next PAHPA reauthorization in 2018?
11. Describe the federal preparedness infrastructure that evolved after 9/11. Are there things about the departments, agencies, and offices that to you represent improvements over the pre-9/11 infrastructure? Are there aspects that seem redundant or misplaced?
12. How would you balance civil liberties and common good during a public health emergency?
13. What are the major differences between the Geneva Protocol, the BWC, and the CWC?
14. In your opinion, are international agreements useful? Why or why not?
15. Does the international community require a new treaty for public health preparedness? If so, what would it say?

References

1. Portions of this chapter come from Katz, R and Standley, C. Public health preparedness policy. In: Teitelbaum, JB ed. *Essentials of Health Policy & Law,* 3rd ed. Burlington, MA: Jones & Bartlett Learning: 2017: 253–270.
2. Kates K, Katz R. The Henry J Kaiser Family Foundation. *U.S. Participation in International Health Treaties, Commitments, Partnerships, and Other Agreements.* September 2010. Available at: https://kaiserfamilyfoundation.files.wordpress.com/2013/01/8099.pdf. Accessed May 2017.
3. Uniting and Strengthening America by Providing Appropriate Tools Required to Intercept and Obstruct Terrorism (USA PATRIOT) Act of 2001, P.L. 107-56 § 1013.
4. Public Health Security and Bioterrorism Preparedness and Response Act of 2002, P.L. 107-188 title 1 subtitle B.
5. Implementing Recommendations of the 9/11 Commission Act of 2007, P.L. 110-53 §1102.
6. The White House. *The Federal Response to Hurricane Katrina: Lessons Learned.* Available at: https://georgewbush-whitehouse.archives.gov/reports/katrina-lessons-learned/. Accessed May 2017.
7. The Brookings Institution, The American Enterprise Institute. *Vital Statistics on Congress.* January 9, 2017. Available at: www.brookings.edu/vitalstats. Accessed May 2017.
8. Kingdon J. *Agendas, Alternatives, and Public Policies.* New York: HarperCollins College Publishers; 1995.
9. Tauscher EO. Address presented at: Annual Meeting of the States Parties to the Biological Weapons Convention; December 9, 2009; Geneva, Switzerland. Available at: http://geneva.usmission.gov/2009/12/09/tauscher-bwc/. Accessed May 2017.
10. National Security Council. *National Strategy for Countering Biological Threats.* November 2009. Available at: http://geneva.usmission.gov/wp-content/uploads/2009/12/Natl-Strategy-for-Countering-BioThreats.pdf. Accessed May 2017.
11. Miller JE. National Strategy for Countering Biological Threats. In: Katz R, Zilinskas R, eds. *Encyclopedia of Bioterrorism Defense.* 2nd ed. Hoboken, NJ: Wiley and Sons, 2011.
12. Balboni M, Kaniewski D, Paulison RD. *Preparedness, Response, and Resilience Task Force: Interim Task Force Report on Resilience.* Washington, DC: The George Washington University Homeland Security Policy Institute. May 16, 2011. Available at: http://www.nasemso.org/Projects/DomesticPreparedness/documents/DHSresiliencereport_Resilience1.pdf. Accessed July 8, 2015.
13. Department of Homeland Security. *Presidential Policy Directive 8: National Preparedness.* March 30, 2011. Available at: https://www.dhs.gov/presidential-policy-directive-8-national-preparedness. Accessed May 2017.
14. Constitution of the United States of America.
15. Hodge JG, Gostin LO, Gebbie K, et al. Transforming Public Health Law: The Turning Point Model State Public Health Act. *Journal of Law, Medicine & Ethics.* Spring 2006;34(1):77–84.
16. Gostin LO. *The Model State Emergency Health Powers Act.* The Centers for Law & the Public's Health. December 21, 2001. Available at: http://www.publichealthlaw.net/MSEHPA/MSEHPA.pdf. Accessed September 10, 2010.

17. The Network for Public Health Law. *The Model State Emergency Health Powers Act.* June 2012. Available at: https://www.networkforphl.org/_asset/80p3y7/MSEHPA -States-Table-022812.pdf. Accessed May 2017.

18. Katz R, Vaught A, Formentos A, Capizola J. Raising the Yellow Flag: State Variation in Quarantine Laws. (Forthcoming, *Journal of Public Health Management and Practice*)

19. Instructions for the Government of Armies of the United States in the Field, Sec. III Article 70 (1863). Available at: http://avalon.law.yale.edu/19th_century/lieber.asp#art70.

20. Convention (II) With Respect to the Laws and Customs of War on Land and its annex: Regulations concerning the Laws and Customs of War on Land, Sec.2 Chap.3 Art. 23 (1899). Available at: http://avalon.law.yale.edu/19th_century /hague02.asp

21. Convention (IV) respecting the Laws and Customs of War on Land and its annex: Regulations concerning the Laws and Customs of War on Land, (1907). Available at: https://ihl -databases.icrc.org/ihl/INTRO/195

22. League of Nations. *Geneva Protocol: Protocol for the Prohibition of the Use of War of Asphyxiating, Poisonous or Other Gases, and of Bacteriological Methods of Warfare.* June 17, 1925. Available at: https://www .state.gov/t/isn/4784.htm#treaty. Accessed May 2017.

23. OPCW, Technical Secretariat. *Status of Participation in the Chemical Weapons Convention* as at 17 October 2015. Available at: https://www.opcw.org/fileadmin/OPCW/S _series/2015/en/s-1315-2015_e_.pdf. Accessed May 2017.

24. UNODA. *Treaty on the Nonproliferation of Nuclear Weapons.* March 5, 1970. Available at: http://disarmament.un.org /treaties/t/npt. Accessed May 2017.

25. The Australia Group. *Introduction.* 2007. Available at: http://www.australiagroup.net/en/introduction.html. Accessed May 2017.

26. United Nations. *Convention on the Prohibition of the Development, Production and Stockpiling of Bacteriological (Biological) and Toxin Weapons and on their Destruction.* March 1975. Available at: https://www.un.org/disarmament /wmd/bio/. Accessed May 2017.

27. World Health Organization. *WHO Technical Consultation on the Implementation and Evaluation of Annex 2 of the International Health Regulations (2005).* October 2008. Available at: http://www.who.int/ihr/summary_report _annex2.pdf?ua=1. Accessed May 2017.

© f00sion/E+/Getty

PART IV
Solving Problems

CHAPTER 6

Biosecurity

▶ Introduction

In previous chapters, we looked at the public health threats from both weapons of mass destruction (WMD) and naturally occurring disease. We have examined the infrastructure and legislative and regulatory environments that have evolved over the past decade that support public health preparedness. In this part of the text, we start to look at how some of the challenges and threats are being addressed in an attempt to "solve problems." This chapter examines biosecurity and biosafety, discusses the dual use dilemma in scientific research, and describes the policy positions and guidance that have evolved around research, publications, and the control of dangerous pathogens. We also look at some of the programs adopted by the U.S. government to reduce the threat posed by WMD.

Biosecurity is a process to reduce or eliminate the ability of a biological agent to adversely affect human, animal, or plant health, as well as the economy or the environment. It is the management of biological and environmental risks, whether the risks come from the agents themselves, infectious diseases, invasive species, or biological weapons. It is also the protection of agents or facilities "against the theft or diversion of high-consequence microbial agents, which could be used by someone who maliciously intends to conduct bioterrorism or pursue biological weapons proliferation."[1(p7)] Achieving biosecurity, or in the case of protection of agents, pathogen security, involves physically protecting agents (i.e., locking them up and securing facilities), ensuring the staff working with these agents take responsibility for the safety and security of the agents themselves, and implementing other administrative measures to enhance accountability, security, and oversight.

Biosafety, often mistakenly used interchangeably with biosecurity (and in some languages, they are the same word), is the process used to prevent people and the environment from being exposed to hazardous biological agents. It is about safely handling infectious agents, through the application of proper techniques, equipment, and personal behavior (TABLE 6-1). The simple phrase used to distinguish biosafety from biosecurity is, "Biosafety is about protecting people from bad bugs; biosecurity is about protecting bugs from bad people."[2(p27)]

TABLE 6-1 Biosafety Levels (BSL) for Infectious Agents

BSL	Agents	Equipment and Facilities for Appropriate Barriers
1	These do not usually lead to disease in healthy adults (e.g., nonpathogenic *Escherichia coli*).	■ Lab coats and gloves ■ Face and eye protection as needed ■ Laboratory bench and sink
2	These cause disease, but not through inhalation (e.g., HIV or *Yersinia pestis*).	■ Lab coats and gloves ■ Face and eye protection as needed ■ Physical containment devices for manipulations of agents that cause splashes or aerosols of agents ■ BSL-1 facilities + autoclave
3	These cause serious or potentially lethal disease through inhalation (e.g., tuberculosis or St. Louis encephalitis).	■ Protective lab clothing and gloves ■ Face, eye, and respiratory protection as needed ■ Physical containment devices for all open manipulations of agents ■ BSL-2 facilities + physical separation from access corridors, double-door access, negative airflow, entry through air lock or anteroom, and handwashing sink near lab exit
4	These are dangerous or exotic, are frequently fatal, and for which there are no vaccines or treatments. These agents may have an unknown risk of transmission or have a high risk of aerosol transmission (e.g., Ebola).	■ All primary barriers, equipment, and procedures conducted in BSL-3, or procedures conducted with equipment from BSL-1 and BSL-2 in combination with a full-body, air-supplied, positive pressure suit ■ BSL-3 facilities + separate building or isolated areas, dedicated supply and exhaust, vacuum and decontamination system, and other specified safety requirements

Notes: Depending on the type of agent one is working with, there are recommended biosafety measures that should be taken. These measures range from best practices by the laboratorian to the infrastructure necessary to work safely with agents. There are four biosafety levels that prescribe how to work with increasingly dangerous infectious agents.

Data from CDC. Section IV—Laboratory Biosafety Level Criteria. *Biosafety in Microbiological and Biomedical Laboratories*. 2009. p 59. Available at: https://www.cdc.gov/biosafety/publications/bmbl5/bmbl.pdf. Accessed May 2017.

Biorisk is the name given to the chance that any type of adverse event leading to potential harm will occur—be it an accidental infection within the laboratory or the loss, theft, unauthorized access, or intentional release of an agent.[3] Biorisk management is then the development of strategies incorporating both biosafety and biosecurity techniques to minimize the occurrences of biorisks and manage the consequences. This integrated approach to biological threats within the laboratory environment is the responsibility of individual laboratories.[3]

The technical aspects of biosafety are outside the purview of this text, but we focus here on some aspects of biosecurity, the problems for science posed by the dual use dilemma, the debate over codes of conduct for life science researchers, and efforts to regulate biosecurity.

▶ The Dual Use Dilemma

Within the life sciences, "dual use" refers to research, agents, technologies, equipment, or information that can be used both for legitimate scientific purposes and for malevolent use to threaten public health or security.[4] The U.S. National Science Advisory Board for Biosecurity (NSABB) defined dual use research of concern (DURC) specifically as follows:

Research that, based on current understanding, can be reasonably anticipated to provide knowledge, products, or technologies that could be directly misapplied by others to pose a threat to public health and safety, agricultural crops and other plants, animals, the environment, or materiel.[5(p2)]

Life science research, particularly biological research, is grounded in the idea that research is good; it advances science and, thus, mankind; it saves lives; and in order to grow and develop, there must be open communication among researchers. This openness, however, becomes complicated when security is at risk. Scientists and security experts have struggled for decades to determine the right balance to ensure advances in life sciences, while being aware of and mitigating the threat posed by the same research. This tension goes back to the 1940s in the post–World War II society. The 1947 President's Scientific Research Board report on science and public policy wrote, "However important secrecy about military weapons may be, the fundamental discoveries of researchers must circulate freely to have full beneficial effect. . . . Security regulations, therefore, should be applied only when strictly necessary."[6,7] This concept was echoed by President Harry S. Truman in 1948, when he said, "Continuous research by our best scientists is the key to American scientific leadership and true national security."[8] This position, although not always easy—particularly in physics, where technology was being used to make nuclear weapons and other weapons systems—remained the position of the government and researchers alike. This sentiment, however, began to change in the 1980s at the height of the Cold War. Advanced technology was acquired from U.S. universities and government national laboratories by adversarial nations.[9] In 1980, the National Academies suspended its bilateral exchanges with the USSR.[10(p31)]

In 1982, Executive Order 12356 broadened authorities to classify information, but reiterated that "basic scientific research information not clearly related to national security may not be classified."[11] The same year, the National Academy of Sciences was asked to examine whether scientific information need to be controlled. The subsequent report, Scientific Communication and National Security (also known as the Corson Report), had several major findings: that security by secrecy would weaken the United States; that there is no practical way to restrict international scientific communication; and that, while there has been a significant transfer of scientific information from the United States to adversarial countries, transfers of information from universities and through the publication of fundamental research was very small.[12]

In 1985, the Reagan administration released National Security Decision Directive (NSDD) 189, which stated:

It is the policy of this Administration that, to the maximum extent possible, the products of fundamental research remain unrestricted... that, where the national security requires control, the mechanism for control of information generated during federally-funded fundamental research in science, technology and engineering at colleges, universities, and laboratories is classification.[13]

The responsibility for classification of research was given to the federal governmental agencies that provide the research grants, and no restrictions were allowed on the conduct or reporting of the research that did not receive a national security classification.[13]

This policy from 1985 was reiterated right after 9/11. In a letter from Dr. Condoleezza Rice, then–National Security advisor, and reaffirmed by Dr. John Marburger, science advisor in congressional testimony, the administration confirmed that "the policy on the transfer of scientific, technical, and engineering information set forth in NSDD-189 shall remain in effect, and we will ensure that this policy is followed."[14,15]

▶ Mousepox and Other Research of Concern

In 2001, a team of Australian researchers inserted the gene for interleukin-4 (IL-4) into the mousepox virus. The purpose of the study was to try to alter the virus so that it would make mice infertile, and thus become a pest control method. They found that the recombinant virus killed mice genetically resistant to mousepox as well as mice that had been immunized. When the researchers published their findings, scientists around the world voiced concerns that the researchers had published a road map for increasing the lethality of mousepox by showing how to kill mice even after they had been immunized, and by extension, demonstrating how to increase the lethality of smallpox.[16] Critics quickly claimed that the article should never have been published and this "dual use" research could easily be picked up by terrorists and used to make a biological weapon that would circumvent our medical countermeasures.[17]

The publication of this mousepox experiment raised a series of questions for the scientific community. Should the experiment have been done in the first place if researchers recognized the possible implications of the research? Should the research have been publicized given the findings? Should any journal have published it? These questions went beyond this particular experiment to the larger problem being posed for science. Other articles were being published that sparked similar concerns.[18,19] The community had to decide if scientists should be constrained as to the research questions they could ask. Scientific journals had to determine their responsibility for publishing manuscripts with potentially sensitive information. And the security community in the United States began to question the number of foreign students and scholars being trained and working in domestic universities and research environments.

In 2003, the journal editors responded: 32 largely American-based scientific journals agreed to guidelines for reviewing, modifying, and even rejecting research articles where the potential harm of publication might outweigh the potential for societal benefits (**BOX 6-1**).[20]

The same year, the National Academies published Biotechnology Research in an Age of Terrorism, also known as the Fink Report. The purpose of the Fink

---

BOX 6-1 Statement on Scientific Publication and Security by Journal Editors

Preamble

The process of scientific publication, through which new findings are reviewed for quality and then presented to the rest of the scientific community and the public, is a vital element in our national life. New discoveries reported in research papers have helped improve the human condition in myriad ways: protecting public health, multiplying agricultural yields, fostering technological development and economic growth, and enhancing global stability and security.

But new science, as we know, may sometimes have costs as well as benefits. The prospect that weapons of mass destruction might find their way into the hands of terrorists did not suddenly appear on September 11, 2001. A policy focus on nuclear proliferation, no stranger to the physics community, has been with us for many years. But the events of September 11 brought a new understanding of the urgency of dealing with terrorism. And the subsequent harmful use of infectious agents brought a new set of issues to the life sciences. As a result, questions have been asked by the scientists themselves and by some political leaders about the possibility that new information published in research journals might give aid to those with malevolent ends.

Journals that dealt especially with microbiology, infectious agents, public health, and plant and agricultural systems faced these issues earlier than some others, and have attempted to deal with them. The American Society of Microbiology, in particular, urged the National Academy of Sciences to take an active role in organizing a meeting of publishers, scientists, security experts, and government officials to explore the issues and discuss what steps might be taken to resolve them. In a one-day workshop at the Academy in Washington on January 9, 2003, an open forum was held for that purpose. A day later, a group of journal editors, augmented by scientist-authors, government officials, and others, held a separate meeting designed to explore possible approaches.

What follows reflects some outcomes of that preliminary discussion. Fundamental is a view, shared by nearly all, that there is information that, although we cannot now capture it with lists or definitions, presents enough risk of use by terrorists that it should not be published. How and by what processes it might be identified will continue to challenge us, because—as all present acknowledged—it is also true that open publication brings benefits not only to public health but also to efforts to combat terrorism.

The Statements Follow:

FIRST: The scientific information published in peer-reviewed research journals carries special status, and confers unique responsibilities on editors and authors. We must protect the integrity of the scientific process by publishing manuscripts of high quality, in sufficient detail to permit reproducibility. Without independent verification—a requirement for scientific progress—we can neither advance biomedical research nor provide the knowledge base for building a strong biodefense system.

SECOND: We recognize that the prospect of bioterrorism has raised legitimate concerns about the potential abuse of published information, but also recognize that research in the very same fields will be critical to society in meeting the challenges of defense. We are committed to dealing responsibly and effectively with safety and security issues that may be raised by papers submitted for publication, and to increasing our capacity to identify such issues as they arise.

THIRD: Scientists and their journals should consider the appropriate level and design of processes to accomplish effective review of papers that raise such security issues. Journals in disciplines that have attracted numbers of such papers have already devised procedures that might be employed as models in considering process design. Some of us represent some of those journals; others among us are committed to the timely implementation of such processes, about which we will notify our readers and authors.

FOURTH: We recognize that on occasion an editor may conclude that the potential harm of publication outweighs the potential societal benefits. Under such circumstances, the paper should be modified or not be published. Scientific information is also communicated by other means: seminars, meetings, electronic posting, etc. Journals and scientific societies can play an important role in encouraging investigators to communicate results of research in ways that maximize public benefits and minimize risks of misuse.

Report was to develop a system to help reduce the threat of misuse of the life sciences, while protecting scientific research and communication to the maximum extent possible. The report proposed a system, based mostly on voluntary self-governance by the scientific community, which would have experiments reviewed at several stages to evaluate for dual use concerns. The proposed system of review included a review at the university level through an Institutional Biosafety Committee (IBC), followed by review at National Institutes of Health (NIH)-assuming NIH supported the research- through the NIH Recombinant Advisory Committee. The research would then be evaluated by the journal editors, followed by a proposed National Science Advisory Board for Biodefense to provide advice, guidance, and leadership on whether research should be published. The report identified seven types of "experiments of concern" that should be evaluated. The question posed was whether proceeding with the experiment would:

- Render a vaccine to a pathogen ineffective
- Confer antibiotic resistance to a pathogen so as to decrease the effectiveness of a countermeasure
- Increase the virulence of a pathogen
- Increase the transmissibility of a pathogen
- Increase the host range/tropism of a pathogen
- Enable evasion of diagnostic/detection capabilities
- Demonstrate weaponization of a pathogen[21]

If an experiment met any of these criteria, it would require review. The government took these recommendations seriously and created the National Science Advisory Board for Biosecurity (NSABB). NSABB is an advisory board to the secretary of Health and Human Services made up of scientists and ex-officio members from across the federal government. In addition to recommendations on criteria for identifying DURC, NSABB provides national guidelines for oversight of dual use research and advises on educational programs, codes of conduct for scientists, guidelines for dissemination of research methodologies and results, and strategies for international dialogues on dual use research.

The first article submitted to NSABB was the complete genetic sequencing of the 1918 influenza virus. Some argued that the data was important for better understanding of flu and thus enabling current researchers to more adequately prepare for a future pandemic.[22] Others argued that "the genome is essentially the design of a weapon of mass destruction" and should not have been published.[23]

Another controversial article, which provided a detailed description of how to contaminate the milk supply with Botulinum toxin, was published by the *Proceedings of the National Academies of Science* (*PNAS*).[24] The authors argued that the paper was a wake-up call to enhance preparedness activities. Critics, however, saw it as a road map for bioterrorism. The paper was initially published online by *PNAS*, but then pulled for review by NSABB. When it was finally published in the journal, some details had been removed from the article to make it less of a "how-to" for terrorists. Additional papers on H5N1 influenza were reviewed by NSABB in 2011—the details of these papers are described in the case study in this chapter.

Today, we still do not really know how best to handle the dangerous aspects of science. At the same time, we do not want to constrain scientific advancement. Much of the current discussion is around setting up voluntary "codes of conduct" for scientists to follow, giving them self-policing power to ensure the science they produce cannot be used for malevolent purposes. There is discussion about making this a part of the Responsible Conduct of Research—ethical guidelines for life science researchers.[25] The debate, though, continues to be waged regarding whether the control of dual use research is a personal level decision, a discipline wide commitment, or a situation requiring government regulation or legal frameworks.

🔍 CASE STUDY: The H5N1 Transmission Papers—Reinvigorating the Dual Use Dilemma

By Erin Sorrell

Public Health Threat of H5N1

Since its first detection in 1997, highly pathogenic avian influenza (HPAI) H5N1 virus has impacted the global poultry industry, leading to the direct transmission of virus from avian species to humans. As of December 2016, there have been 856 documented human cases of infection, of which 452 were fatal.[26] While sustained human-to-human transmission of HPAI H5N1 has not yet been reported, the risk of an H5 pandemic has spurred the development of preparedness plans and response strategies.[27] Experts have argued that an aerosol-transmissible H5N1 virus would probably be less virulent than the currently circulating HPAI H5N1 viruses; however, there is no scientific evidence to support this assumption. As such, the impact of an H5N1 pandemic has become a matter of debate among researchers

(continues)

and across public health and preparedness communities. Since the early 2000s, U.S. government (USG) agencies have been funding research to elucidate mechanisms for the transmission of avian influenza to humans.

What Is the Dual Use Research of Concern?

DURC is legitimate life sciences research that is intended for benefit (developed for beneficial purposes), but which might yield information and technology that can easily be misapplied for malevolent purposes. Advances in life science and biotechnology (genetic engineering, genomics and proteomics, vaccine development, and antiviral therapies) have led to significant advances in the prevention, diagnosis, and treatment of diseases. These advances present new challenges in the field of bioethics and of equitable access to life sciences research and have been the subject of dual use debates.[28]

The H5 Experiments

In 2005, the National Institute of Allergy and Infectious Diseases (NIAID) within the NIH issued a Broad Agency Announcement (BAA; NIH-NIAID-DMID-07-20) to support the research agenda of the U.S. Department of Health and Human Services (HHS) Pandemic Influenza Plan. Many research groups submitted proposals to support this work; two groups in particular were Ron Fouchier's team at Erasmus Medical Center (EMC) in the Netherlands and another was Yoshi Kawaoka's group at University of Wisconsin, Madison (UW). Both teams, highly qualified and respected as leading influenza research teams, were successfully funded as part of the Centers of Excellence for Influenza Research and Surveillance, Center for Research on Influenza Pathogenesis.[29]

In the summer of 2011, both the EMC and UW research teams submitted original research articles to *Science* and *Nature*, respectively, presenting data on aerosol-transmitted H5N1 viruses, highlighting key amino acids that could play a role in the evolution of current avian strains to human potentially pandemic viruses. The teams used different techniques to arrive at the same conclusion: There is a key combination of mutations that create a viable, aerosol-transmissible H5N1 virus, highlighting implications for future vaccines and surveillance strategies. After initial editorial and peer review, the editors of both *Science* and *Nature* submitted a request for the NSABB to review each of the manuscripts, noting concern about the potential dual use implications of the results. In December 2011, the NSABB recommended that the general conclusions of both papers be published; however, the manuscripts should not report the methodological detail necessary to replicate the reported experiments and include potential public health benefits of the research as well as the safety and security measures taken to protect laboratory workers and the public.[30,31] In response to NSABB recommendations, the authors, along with 37 other prominent influenza researchers, published letters in both *Nature* and *Science* calling for an international forum to bring the scientific community together to discuss key issues and concerns.[32,33] In doing so, the researchers called for a voluntary 60-day moratorium on any research involving highly pathogenic avian influenza H5N1 viruses leading to the generation of viruses that are more transmissible in mammals in order to find the time for all relevant stakeholders to organize and meet.

In February 2012, the World Health Organization (WHO) convened a stakeholders meeting in Geneva, attended by the lead researchers from EMC and UW, representatives of *Science* and *Nature*, and bioethicists and directors from several WHO collaborating-center laboratories specializing in influenza. The symposium reached consensus on two issues: the temporary moratorium on research with newly modified H5N1 viruses must continue, while allowing research on naturally occurring H5N1 influenza virus to proceed; and delaying publication of the entire manuscripts in place of the partial articles. After some review and additional studies, the NSABB approved the manuscripts; Kawaoka's paper was published in *Nature* in May 2012 and Fouchier's in *Science* in June 2012, close to a year after the original submission.[34,35] In February 2013, a year after the WHO meeting, influenza researchers called for a lift of the moratorium.[36] They noted that scientists working in nations that finalized funding and laboratory safety rules should now be free to resume experiments; this did not include the United States or U.S.-funded research in other countries.

The Dual Use Dilemma

This was not the first time advances in science and basic research sparked controversy on potential dangers of its use and it will certainly not be the last. In 1974, in response to concerns about recombinant DNA technology, Paul Berg, chairman of the U.S. National Academy of Science's Committee on Recombinant DNA Molecules Assembly of Life Sciences, called for a voluntary moratorium on certain recombinant DNA experiments which the committee deemed to be potentially dangerous—calling for an international forum to discuss the potential biohazards.[37] It was agreed at the meeting (which included media, lawyers, and scientists) that the moratorium should be lifted. The recommendations from the meeting, issued in 1976, laid the foundation for official U.S. guidelines on research on recombinant DNA technology to this day.[38,39]

In 2002, researchers created a whole poliovirus genome using synthetic chemical oligonucleotides and a map of the polio genome that had been published on the Internet. The rescued virus was effective in causing paralysis in mice and the paper, including all methods and results, was published in *Science* in 2002.[40] Three years later, researchers recreated the 1918 pandemic influenza strain using reverse genetics. While the NSABB was convened, the paper, eventually published in *Science*, included the complete genome sequence.[41] Even after the H5 debate in January 2012, a report by Li-Mei Chen et al. (published in full in *Virology*)[42] mimicked some of the techniques and results from Fouchier and Kawaoka, describing mutations in an H5N1 virus which confer airborne transmissibility between ferrets.

Public Health Impact

There is much debate among the scientific research community as well as across public health professionals and policy makers as to whether the knowledge gained from the H5 research will help prepare for a potential pandemic and whether the information generated from the research outweighs any risks. The cons are quite clear and have been continually raised in public policy and security forums: terrorist misuse of the information, risk of accidental exposure or release from the laboratory, and creation of a novel pathogen. Support for the research includes the basic principles of scientific research and the importance of not censoring. Openness and knowledge sharing is the cornerstone of scientific development. The techniques used in both papers are methods freely available from the scientific literature, not new to these papers or their publication. Many argue restriction and prescreening would discourage frontier research in molecular biology and the life sciences. In addition, the information gained may help predict pandemics, identifying key mutations can assist in more aggressive control programs and assist in a better understanding of influenza host–pathogen interactions, transmission, and pathogenicity. It is evident there are many arguments and valid concerns on each side of the debate, one that will continue to evolve with influenza and other infectious pathogens.

DURC Policies

In response to the H5 debate, U.S. policymakers released the USG Policy for Oversight of Life Sciences Dual Use Research Concern on March 29, 2012 with the intent to preserve the benefits of life sciences research, while minimizing the risk of misuse of the knowledge, information, products or technologies provided by such research.[43] In addition, the USG released the USG Policy for Institutional Oversight of Life Science Dual Use Research of Concern on September 24, 2014.[44] This policy, effective September 24, 2015, addresses institutional oversight of DURC, including policies, practices, and procedures to ensure DURC is identified and risk mitigation measures are implemented, where applicable. The policy delineates the roles and responsibilities of USG funding agencies, research institutions, and life scientists, and provides requirements and performance standards for review of life sciences research, identification of potential DURC, and development and implementation of risk mitigation measures for DURC, where applicable. In addition, during the 2012, moratorium policymakers considered whether certain gain-of-function (GOF; **BOX 6-2**) studies should be conducted using federal funds, and if so, how those studies could be safely conducted. In response, Centers for Disease Control and Prevention (CDC) and NIH issued new biosafety guidelines for working with highly pathogenic avian influenza strains, and the HHS developed a framework (released February 2013) for guiding its funding decisions about projects that may generate highly pathogenic H5N1 viruses that are transmissible between mammals by respiratory droplets.[45]

BOX 6-2   Gain of Function

Gain of function refers to any modification of a biological agent that confers new or enhanced activity. Typically, researchers mutate or alter genes and examine the impact of these modifications on a particular property or trait of the organism. Some gain-of-function studies may entail biosafety and biosecurity risks that require unique risk assessment and mitigation measures.

On October 16, 2014, the White House announced a USG deliberative process to assess the risks and benefits of certain GOF experiments, leading to the moratorium for USG departments and agencies to hold the release of federal funding for GOF studies that enhances the pathogenicity or transmissibility among mammals by respiratory droplets of influenza, Middle East Respiratory Syndrome (MERS), or Severe Acute Respiratory Syndrome (SARS). At the writing of this case study (December 2016), the National Research Council and the Institute of Medicine of the National Academies were in the process of convening forums to engage the life sciences community as well as to solicit feedback from scientists and the public on optimal approaches to ensure effective federal oversight of GOF research. These forums involve discussion of principles important for the design of risk and benefit assessments of GOF research and of NSABB draft recommendations.[46]

▶ Select Agents

Since 1996, the government has tried to legislate on how to handle potentially dangerous pathogens so they do not fall into the hands of people wishing to do harm. The first such legislation was the Antiterrorism and Effective Death Penalty Act of 1996.[47] The act identified certain biological agents as posing a threat to society and provided that the transfer and possession of such agents should be regulated to protect public health and safety, so only those with legitimate purposes would have access to the agents.[47(p511)] HHS was to establish a list of "select agents" for regulation, including those agents that cause significant morbidity and mortality, are contagious, or may not have medical countermeasures available. The authority to regulate the select agents was delegated to the CDC, and CDC then required any laboratory-transferring select agents to register and report any transfer.[48] In 1997, the select agent list had 42 biological agents and toxins.

The Uniting and Strengthening America by Providing Appropriate Tools Required to Intercept and Obstruct Terrorism Act of 2001 furthered the 1996 law, so that it became an offense to possess select biological agents or toxins without reasonable justification.[49] The act also restricted possession or transfer of select agents to only approved individuals.

The Bioterrorism Act of 2002 added additional requirements for the possession or transfer of select agents, including requiring a background check by the Federal Bureau of Investigation (FBI). This act also made regulation of the select agents a shared responsibility between CDC, U.S. Department of Agriculture (USDA), and the FBI. CDC is in charge of regulating human pathogens, while USDA has the lead for animal and plant pathogens. FBI leads any criminal investigative actions.

In July 2010, the Obama administration released an executive order (EO) for optimizing the security of biological select agents and toxins in the United States.[50] The EO called for several things:

1. *Tiering and the potential reduction of the select agent list:* HHS and USDA will tier the list of select agents to separate out those agents that require the most stringent physical security and personnel reliability measures, so that other (less dangerous agents) can have fewer restrictions. They will change the regulations accordingly.
2. *Creating a security advisory panel made up of federal experts:* This panel will help with the tiering or reduction of the select agent list, as well as best practices for physical security and personnel reliability.

Part of the 2010 E.O. was to establish the Federal Experts Security Advisory Panel (FESAP), a collection of federal government experts organized to provide recommendations to the secretaries of HHS and DHS on select agents. FESAP released a series of recommendations in late 2010. In 2014, the group was renewed to look at biosafety and biosecurity in the United States. The call for the renewed FESAP efforts came after a series of biosecurity failures (see BOX 6-3), and the group was charged with not only identifying

---

BOX 6-3 U.S. Biosafety Incidents in 2014

Over the summer of 2014, three significant biosafety incidents occurred involving U.S. government facilities. The first incident took place in early June at CDC's Roybal Campus in Atlanta, Georgia. On June 5, a laboratory worker used an improper method to deactivate anthrax spores that were being transferred to several lower biocontainment laboratories on the same campus. The mistake was discovered over a week later, when culture plates left in the original laboratory showed signs of bacterial growth. As a result of this error, 35 staff and 67 visitors were considered at risk of exposure to anthrax.

The second incident also involved CDC. On July 9, it was discovered that a sample of low-pathogenic avian influenza shipped to the USDA from CDC was contaminated with highly pathogenic H5N1. Because the sample was assumed to be of low risk, safety and security precautions required for shipping of select agents were not carried out. All handling of the sample at both institutions took place under BSL-3 conditions, minimizing the risk of accidental exposure. The contamination was determined to have taken place at the CDC influenza laboratory, and the discovery was made by USDA on May 23. However, the incident was not reported for another 6 weeks.

The third incident occurred in mid-July, when several vials labeled as smallpox were discovered on the NIH campus in Bethesda, Maryland. The vials dated from the 1950s, when smallpox was still widespread, and are believed to have been part of a previous Food and Drug Administration facility on the site. While some of the viral contents were shown to still be viable, the vials were well sealed and the risk of exposure was deemed to be very low.

While no casualties resulted from any of these incidents, they serve to highlight the potential risks of accidental exposure to dangerous biological agents as a result of poor biorisk management practices.

Data from Katz R, Standley, C. Public Health Preparedness Policy. In: Teitelbaum J, Wilensky S. *Essentials of Health Policy and Law*. 2nd ed. Burlington, MA: Jones & Bartlett Learning; 2016: 253–270.

needs and gaps to improve biosafety and biosecurity for select agents, but also to determine the number of laboratories that should house select agents in the United States.[51]

The Federal Select Agents Program, which is run jointly by CDC and USDA, registers and inspects labs where select agents are handled, and ensures that appropriate biosafety and biosecurity procedures are in use (**FIGURE 6-1**). In 2016, it released the first annual report, documenting the oversight provided to laboratories as well as describing the plethora of work conducted throughout the country.[52]

The overall body of laws and regulations on select agents makes it difficult to acquire and work with certain agents. It also makes clear that there are responsibilities that come with working with such agents. The effort to tier the agents is not only an attempt to retain the strictest of regulations for the most dangerous agents, but to ease up on other agents so that it is easier for researchers to conduct their work. The nature of research, however, has forever changed and scientists must now take responsibility for the agents they work with.

▶ Synthetic Biology

Another area of concern for biosecurity is synthetic biology. This refers to the design and creation of biological components and systems that do not naturally exist.[53] What this means is that biologists and engineers, along with computer modelers and other experts, combine expertise to synthesize biological agents. These efforts can be rapid, relatively inexpensive, and efficient for the creation of drugs and other medical countermeasures. The process also, however, can be used to synthesize naturally occurring pathogens *de novo*, including pathogens that are difficult to obtain or have been eradicated. It is also possible to use this process to create novel biological agents with unique properties.

The U.S. government sees synthetic biology as an important scientific development, with potential applications for the advancement of health and technology. There is also a recognition, however, that there is a potential for misuse. The NSABB has released reports addressing the biosecurity concerns raised by synthetic biology, the National Academy of Science

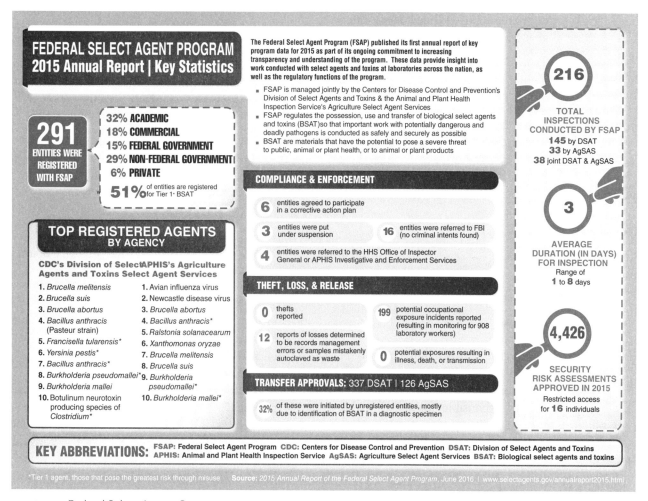

FIGURE 6-1 Federal Select Agents Program

Reproduced from CDC, USDA. *Federal Select Agent Program.* June 2016. Available at: https://www.selectagents.gov/resources/FSAP_Infographic_2015.pdf. Accessed May 2017.

has reviewed the topic, and the scientific and policy community continue to work on how best to address the dual use implications for synthetic bio.[54,55]

▶ Global Health Security Agenda Biosafety and Biosecurity Action Package and the Global Partnership Program

As discussed in previous chapters, the Global Health Security Agenda (GHSA) contains a series of action packages to guide global engagement in developing capacity to prevent, detect, and respond to biological threats. Prevent 3 (P3) is the action package devoted to building national biosafety and biosecurity systems. The intent of the action package is to ensure that governments develop systems to identify, secure, and monitor dangerous pathogens within their country; develop and conduct biological risk management training; and enact appropriate biosafety and biosecurity legislation.[56]

GHSA was initially intended to be a 5-year initiative, which is set to expire in 2019. While it is not clear at the writing of this text if GHSA will continue past the initial 5 years, the targets for biosecurity and biosafety have been adopted by multiple partners and may be integrated into national and international planning regardless of the future of GHSA. As of 2017, there were approximately 50 partnerships underway supporting the GHSA action package on biosecurity and biosafety. These include bilateral partnerships, partnerships supported by regional WHO offices, regional collaborations, and alignments with other international agreements.

One of the international agreements that are aligned with GHSA P3 is the Global Partnership Against the Spread of Weapons and Materials of Mass Destruction. This Global Partnership Program (GPP) was established in 2002 by the United States, Canada, France, the United Kingdom, Germany, Japan, Italy, and Russia (the Group of 8 (G8)) to collaborate on and implement projects around the world to counter WMD proliferation. Russia has since left the consortium, but there are now approximately 30 member countries of the GPP.[56] In 2010, the GPP created a Biosecurity Working Group (BSWG), prioritizing strengthening biological security as a key component of the partnership. The BSWG created five deliverable objectives for the GPP:

1. Secure and account for material that represents biological proliferation risks
2. Develop and maintain appropriate and effective measures to prevent, prepare for, and respond to the deliberate misuse of biological agents
3. Strengthen national and global networks to rapidly identify, confirm and respond to biological attacks
4. Reinforce and strengthen biological nonproliferation principles, practices and instruments
5. Reduce proliferation risks through the advancement and promotion of safe and responsible conduct in the biological sciences[57]

These five deliverables have served to guide investments on biosecurity round the world, while also aligning with other international agreements, including the Biological Weapons Convention.

Key Words

Biorisk management
Biosafety
Biosecurity

Dual use dilemma
Dual use research of concern

National Science Advisory Board
for Biosecurity
Select agents

Discussion Questions

1. What is the difference between biosecurity, biosafety, and biorisk management?
2. Explain the dual use dilemma.
3. Who should be responsible for policing the publication of scientific papers for potential dual use? Should there be any policing?
4. How should scientists and policymakers best manage advances in life sciences against the possible misuse of science?
5. If the EMC and UW experiments were performed with low-pathogenic avian influenza

viruses, do you believe the papers would have been reviewed by the NSABB? Would this paper elicit DURC discussions? Why or why not?
6. Should scientists be constrained to risk-averse research? How do you determine risk-averse research?
7. How does the research community conduct outreach to the government, private sector, and community to explain research and its benefits?
8. What mechanisms should be used to share sensitive DURC information that could assist in public health preparedness? Who decides how to share the information? Using which criteria and

mechanism? (*Note:* Consider research may be performed in high-resourced countries with policies for DURC, biosafety, and biosecurity on a pathogen that is endemic in a low-resourced country without the necessary resources to conduct research and diagnostic testing. For example, how do you share relevant information about transmission risks with countries where H5 is endemic?)

9. Consider the 2014–2015 Ebola virus disease outbreak. You are part of a research team capable of determining the key mechanisms for virulence of the outbreak strain in an effort to determine viral targets for vaccines or therapies. Would this be potential DURC?

References

1. Salerno RM, Koelm JG. *Biological Laboratory and Transportation Security and the Biological Weapons Convention.* Sandia National Laboratories. February 2002. Available at: http://www.sandia.gov/cooperative-monitoring-center/_assets/documents/sand2002-1067p.pdf. Accessed September 2017.

2. National Research Council of the National Academies, Committee on Laboratory Security and Personnel Reliability Assurance Systems for Laboratories Conducting Research on Biological Select Agents and Toxins. *Introduction: The Promise and Performance of BSAT Research. Responsible Research with Biological Select Agents and Toxins.* Washington, DC: The National Academies Press; 2009; Available at: http://books.nap.edu/openbook.php?record_id=12774&page=27.

3. World Health Organization. *Biorisk Management: Laboratory Biosecurity Guidance.* September 2006. Available at: http://www.who.int/csr/resources/publications/biosafety/WHO_CDS_EPR_2006_6.pdf. Accessed May 2017.

4. National Research Council of the National Academies, Committee on Education on Dual Use Issues in the Life Sciences. Introduction: The Life Sciences and Dual Use Issues. In: *Challenges and Opportunities for Education about Dual Use Issues in the Life Sciences.* Washington, DC: The National Academies Press; 2010.

5. National Institutes of Health, Office of Science Policy. Dual Use Research and Dual Use Research of Concern. *Biosecurity.* Available at: http://osp.od.nih.gov/office-biotechnology-activities/biosecurity/nsabb/faq. Accessed May 2017.

6. Steelman JR. President's Scientific Research Board. *Science and Public Policy.* Washington DC: U.S. Government Printing Office; 1947.

7. Kerr L. National Institutes of Health. Integrating Science and Security: Making Intelligent Decisions [Webcast]. September 28, 2006. Available at: http://videocast.nih.gov/Summary.asp?File=13387. Accessed September 20, 2010.

8. Truman HS. Address to the The Centennial Anniversary AAAS Meeting; September 1948; Washington, DC. Available at: http://www.nsf.gov/about/history/nsf50/truman1948_address.jsp. Accessed September 19, 2010.

9. National Research Council of the National Academies, Committee on a New Government-University Partnership for Science and Security, Committee on Science, Technology, Law, Policy, and Global Affairs. *Science and Security in a Post 9/11 World: A Report Based on Regional Discussions Between the Science and Security Communities.* Washington, DC: The National Academies Press; 2007.

10. Schweitzer G. Who Wins in U.S.-Soviet Science Ventures? *Bulletin of the Atomic Scientists.* October 1988;5(8):28–32.

11. The President. *Executive Order 12356—National Security Information.* April 2, 1982. Available at: http://www.dod.mil/pubs/foi/Reading_Room/Administration_and_Management/152.pdf. Accessed May 2017.

12. National Academy of Sciences, National Academy of Engineering, Institute of Medicine, Committee on Science, Engineering, and Public Policy, Panel on Scientific Communication and National Security. *Scientific Communication and National Security.* Washington, DC: National Academy Press; 1982.

13. Federation of American Scientists. *National Policy on the Transfer of Scientific, Technical and Engineering Information.* September 21, 1985. Available at: http://www.fas.org/irp/offdocs/nsdd/nsdd-189.htm. Accessed September 19, 2010.

14. Marburger JH. Executive Office of the White House, Director of the Office of Science and Technology Policy. *Conducting Research during the War on Terrorism: Balancing Openness and Security: Hearing before the Committee on Science, House of Representatives, One Hundred Seventh Congress, Second Session.* October 10, 2002. Washington, DC: US Government Printing Office; 2003. Available at: https://www.loc.gov/item/2003628508/. Accessed May 2017.

15. Rice C. *Letter from National Security Advisor to CSIS.* Council on Governmental Relations. November 1, 2001. Available at: http://www.cogr.edu/sites/default/files/Letter_from_National_Security_Advisor_to_CSIS_.pdf. Accessed May 2017.

16. Jackson RJ, Ramsay AJ, Christensen CD, et al. Expression of Mouse Interleukin-4 by a Recombinant Ectromelia Virus Suppresses Cytolytic Lymphocyte Responses and Overcomes Genetic Resistance to Mousepox. *Journal of Virology.* February 2001;75(3):1205–1210.

17. Selgelid MJ, Weir L. The Mousepox Experience: An interview with Ronald Jackson and Ian Ramshaw on Dual-Use Research. *EMBO Reports.* January 2010;11(1):18–24.

18. Cello J, Paul AV, Wimmer E. Chemical Synthesis of Poliovirus cDNA: Generation of Infectious Virus in the Absence of Natural Template. *Science.* August 2002;297(5583):1016–1018.

19. Parkhill J, Wren BW, Thomson NR, et al. Genome sequence of *Yersinia pestis*: The Causative Agent of Plague. *Nature.* October 2001;413(6855):523–527.

20. Shea DA. The Library of Congress. *CRS Report for Congress: Balancing Scientific Publication and National Security Concerns: Issues for Congress.* July 9, 2003. Available at: http://www.fas.org/irp/crs/RL31695.pdf. Accessed September 19, 2010.

21. The National Academics of Science and Engineering. *Biotechnology Research in the Age of Terrorism.* 2004. Available at: https://www.nap.edu/catalog/10827/biotechnology-research-in-an-age-of-terrorism.

22. Sharp PA. 1918 Flu and Responsible Science. *Science.* October 2005;310(5745):17.

23. Kurzweil R, Joy B. Recipe for Destruction. *The New York Times.* October 17, 2005. Available at: http://www.nytimes.com/2005/10/17/opinion/17kurzweiljoy.html. Accessed September 19, 2010.

24. Wein LM, Liu Y. Analyzing a Bioterror Attack on the Food Supply: The Case of Botulinum Toxin in Milk. *PNAS.* July 2005;102(28):9984–9989.

25. Steneck NH. HSS, Office of Research Integrity. *Introduction to the Responsible Conduct of Research.* August 2007. Available at: https://ori.hhs.gov/ori-introduction-responsible-conduct-research. Accessed May 2017.

26. WHO. *Cumulative Number of Confirmed Human Cases for Avian Influenza A(H5N1) Reported to WHO.* 2017. Available at: http://www.who.int/influenza/human_animal_interface /H5N1_cumulative_table_archives/en/. Accessed May 2017.

27. HHS. *Pandemic Influenza Plan.* November 2005. Available at: https://www.cdc.gov/flu/pdf/professionals/hhspandemicin fluenzaplan.pdf. Accessed May 2017.

28. National Research Council of the National Academies, Committee on Research Standards and Practices to Prevent the Destructive Application of Biotechnology. *Biotechnology Research in an Age of Terrorism.* Washington, DC: National Academies Press; 2004. Available at: https://www.nap.edu /catalog/10827/biotechnology-research-in-an-age-of -terrorism.

29. CEIRS Networks. Center for Research on Influenza Pathogenesis (CRIP). Available at: http://www.niaidceirs.org /centers/crip/. Accessed May 2017.

30. NIH. Press Statement on the NSABB Review of H5N1 Research [News Release]. Bethesda, MD: NIH Office of the Director; December 20, 2011. http://www.nih.gov/news /health/dec2011/od-20.htm. Accessed May 2017.

31. Keim PS. The NSABB Recommendations: Rationale, Impact, and Implications. *mBio.* 2012;3(1): e00021-12.

32. Fouchier RA, García-Sastre A, Kawaoka Y. Pause on Avian Flu Transmission Studies. *Nature.* January 20, 2012; 481(7382):443.

33. Fouchier RA, García-Sastre A, Kawaoka Y, et al. Pause on Avian Flu Transmission Research. *Science.* January 27, 2012; 335(6067):400–401.

34. Imai M, Watanabe T, Hatta M, et al. Experimental Adaptation of an Influenza H5 HA Confers Respiratory Droplet Transmission to a Reassortant H5 HA/H1N1 Virus in Ferrets. *Nature.* May 2, 2012;486(7403):420–428. doi:10.1038/nature10831.

35. Herfst S, Schrauwen EJ, Linster M, et al. Airborne Transmission of Influenza A/H5N1 Virus between Ferrets. *Science.* June 22, 2012; 336(6088):1534–1541. doi:10.1126 /science.1213362.

36. Fouchier RA, García-Sastre A, Kawaoka Y, et al. Transmission Studies Resume for Avian Flu. *Science.* February 1, 2013;339(6119):520–521. doi:10.1126/science.1235140.

37. National Academy of Sciences, Assembly of Life Sciences. *Summary Statement of the Asilomar Conference on Recombinant DNA Molecules.* 1975. Available at: http://www.dnai.org/b /asilomar/asilomar_paper.pdf. Accessed May 2017.

38. Berg P, Baltimore D, Boyer HW, et al. Letter: Potential Biohazards of Recombinant DNA Molecules. *Science.* July 26, 1974; 185(4148):303.

39. Whelan WJ. Asilomar: 20 Years on. *FASEB Journal.* March 1995;9(5):295.

40. Cello J, Paul AV, Wimmer E. Chemical Synthesis of Poliovirus cDNA: Generation of Infectious Virus in the Absence of Natural Template. *Science.* August 9, 2002;297(5583):1016–1018.

41. Tumpey TM, Basler CF, Aguilar PV, et al. Characterization of the Reconstructed 1918 Spanish Influenza Pandemic Virus. *Science.* October 7, 2005;310(5745):77–80.

42. Chen LM, Blixt O, Stevens J, et al. In Vitro Evolution of H5N1 Avian Influenza Virus Toward Human-Type Receptor Specificity. *Virology.* January 5, 2012;422(1):105–113.

43. USG. *United States Government Policy for Oversight of Life Sciences Dual Use Research of Concern.* Available at: https://www.phe.gov/s3/dualuse/Documents/us-policy -durc-032812.pdf. Accessed May 2017.

44. USG. *United States Government Policy for Institutional Oversight of Life Sciences Dual Use Research of Concern.* September 24, 2014. Available at: https://www.phe.gov/s3 /dualuse/Documents/durc-policy.pdf. Accessed May 2017.

45. HHS. *A Framework for Guiding U.S. Department of Health and Human Services Funding Decisions about Research Proposals with the Potential for Generating Highly Pathogenic Avian Influenza H5N1 Viruses that are Transmissible among Mammals by Respiratory Droplets.* February 2013. Available at: https://www.phe.gov/s3/dualuse/Documents/funding -hpai-h5n1.pdf. Accessed May 2017.

46. The National Academies. *Potential Risks and Benefits of Gain of Function Research: Summary of a Workshop.* 2015. Available at: http://dels.nas.edu/Workshop-Summary/Potential-Risks -Benefits-Gain/21666. Accessed May 2017.

47. Antiterrorism and Effective Death Penalty Act of 1996, Public Law No. 104-132.

48. National Academy of Sciences, National Academy of Engineering, Institute of Medicine, Committee on Science, Engineering, and Public Policy. *On Being a Scientist: Responsible Conduct in Research.* Washington, DC: National Academy Press; 1995.

49. Uniting and Strengthening America by Providing Appropriate Tools Required to Intercept and Obstruct Terrorism (USA PATRIOT) Act of 2001, Public Law No. 107-56.

50. The White House, Office of the Press Secretary. *Executive Order—Optimizing the Security of Biological Select Agents and Toxins in the United States.* July 2, 2010. Available at: https:// obamawhitehouse.archives.gov/the-press-office/executive -order-optimizing-security-biological-select-agents-and -toxins-united-stat. Accessed May 2017.

51. HHS. Federal Experts Security Advisory Panel (FESAP). *Public Health Emergency.* January 2017. Available at: https:// www.phe.gov/Preparedness/legal/boards/fesap/Pages /default.aspx. Accessed May 2017.

52. CDC, USDA. *Federal Select Agent Program.* 2017. Available at: https://www.selectagents.gov/regulations.html. Accessed May 2017.

53. *Synthetic Biology Community.* Synthetic Biology. Available at: http://syntheticbiology.org/. Accessed September 19, 2010.

54. National Science Advisory Board for Biosecurity (NSABB). *Addressing Biosecurity Concerns Related to Synthetic Biology.* April 2010. Available at: http://osp.od.nih.gov/sites/default /files/resources/NSABB%20SynBio%20DRAFT%20Report -FINAL%20%282%29_6-7-10.pdf. Accessed May 2017.

55. The National Academies, Committee on Science, Technology, and Law. *Opportunities and Challenges in the Emerging Field of Synthetic Biology: A Symposium.* July 9–10, 2009. Available at: http://sites.nationalacademies.org/pga/stl/PGA_050738. Accessed May 2017.

56. GHSA. *Global Health Security Agenda Prevent 3 Biosafety and Biosecurity Update.* Presented at: Action Package Coordination Meeting; August 23, 2016; Jakarta, Indonesia. Available at: https://www.ghsagenda.org/docs/default-source/default -document-library/archive-action-package-meeting /2---biosafety-and-biosecurity-ghsa-ap3---508.pdf. Accessed May 2017.

57. GHSA. *GHSA in a Broader Context: Linkages to the Global Partnership, BWC, and UNSCR 1540.* Available at: http://www.unog.ch/80256EDD006B8954/(httpAssets) /27D6C4813C627D18C125806C002FB666/$file/Presentation +for+APP3+Side+Event+US.pdf. Accessed May 2017.

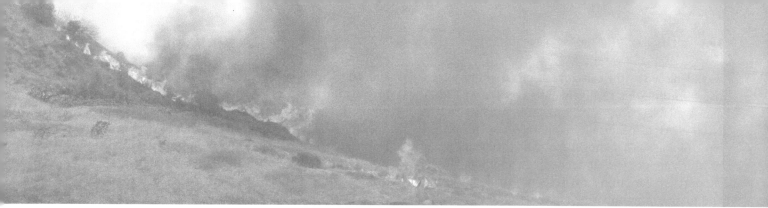

CHAPTER 7

The Research Agenda

▶ Introduction

Thus far, we have been examining the overall effort to defend against, prepare for, and respond to public health emergencies. In this chapter, we turn our attention to the research community. From basic scientific research to the development of medical countermeasures (MCMs), the scientific and pharmaceutical communities are integral components of public health preparedness. We look at each of the federal agencies engaged in supporting the preparedness research agenda. This chapter examines the infrastructure associated with supporting basic scientific research related to public health preparedness, including the types of laboratories necessary and the responsibilities of researchers. We also explore the programs in place to develop MCMs and related activities to document the policies and challenges associated with research, development, and distribution of drugs and vaccines that may be necessary in response to an emergency or public health disaster.

▶ Basic Scientific Research

Most of the basic scientific research in the United States in support of public health preparedness and addressing the chemical, biological, radiological, and nuclear (CBRN) threat is led through funding of grants and contracts by the National Institutes of Health (NIH), including the National Institute of Allergy and Infectious Diseases (NIAID), but also extending to other institutes including the Fogarty International Center. Through its intramural research program and extramural grants, NIH supports the advancement of scientific knowledge that can lead to better understanding of disease threats, as well as future treatments (therapeutics and vaccines) and diagnostics.

Research that might not obviously be linked to potential public health threats can often prove valuable. For example, NIH funded research into coronaviruses for years. When Severe Acute Respiratory Syndrome (SARS) emerged in 2003 and a coronavirus was identified as the causative agent, scientific expertise regarding this relatively obscure virus was ready and available because of long-term funding by the NIH. NIAID, specifically, supports research into the basic biology and pathogenesis of threat agents, many of which are not well understood. In addition, NIAID supports research on host response to threat agents and toxins, immunity, and cross-disciplinary research that can lead to vaccines, therapies, and diagnostics.[1] The focus of this research aims to use a more flexible, broad spectrum approach that enables development of MCMs that might be effective against a variety of agents, technology that could be applied to whole classes of products, and platforms that might reduce the time and expenses associated with creating products.[2]

In addition to federal support for basic research on biological organisms and toxins, NIAID also supports research that leads to MCMs for exposure to ionizing radiation and works with others parts of NIH to support efforts that lead to the development of MCMs for exposure to chemical threats (**BOX 7-1**).[3]

▶ Infrastructure for Research

To support the growing research agenda to address CBRN and naturally occurring threats, as well as to develop domestic diagnostic capacity, over the past 10 years, the U.S. government has invested in building laboratory infrastructure, including high-containment research laboratories, such as biosafety levels (BSL) 3s

and 4s. (See Table 6-1 for description of BSL laboratory distinctions.)

Both Department of Health and Human Services (HHS) (mostly through NIH) and Department of Homeland Security (DHS) have supported the expansion of the research infrastructure through support for BSL-3 and BSL-4 as well as Centers of Excellence (COE) around the country. There are currently 13 BSL-4 facilities in the United States (**FIGURES 7-1, 7-2**). In addition to these 13, the NIH has a BSL-4 laboratory in Bethesda, Maryland, but it is only being used as a BSL-3 facility.[4] The 13 BSL-4 facilities include the following:

- 2 Centers for Disease Control and Prevention (CDC) in Atlanta, Georgia (HHS/CDC facility)
- Robert E. Shope, MD Laboratory in Galveston, Texas (university facility)
- Galveston National Laboratory, Galveston, Texas (HHS/NIAID facility at University of Texas Medical Branch)
- U.S. Army Medical Research Institute for Infectious Diseases (USAMRIID), Frederick, Maryland (Department of Defense (DoD) facility)
- Southwest Foundation for Biomedical Research, San Antonio, Texas (private facility)
- Rocky Mountain Laboratories Integrated Research Facility (IRF), Hamilton, Montana (HHS/NIAID facility)
- Georgia State University, Atlanta, Georgia (university facility, not a full BSL-4 facility, glove box capability)

BOX 7-1 NIH and NIAID Research Strategies and Expert Reports for Biodefense, Chemical Defense, and Radiological Defense

Biodefense

- 2016 Public Health Emergency Medical Countermeasures Enterprise (PHEMCE) Strategy and Implementation Plan
- 2014 PHEMCE Strategy and Implementation Plan
- NIAID Strategic Plan for Biodefense Research, September 2007
- NIAID Biodefense Research Agenda for CDC Category A Agents, February 2002 (progress reports in 2003 and 2006)
- NIAID Biodefense Research Agenda for Category B and C Priority Pathogens, June 2004

Chemical and Toxin Defense

- NIH Strategic Plan and Research Agenda for Medical Countermeasures Against Chemical Threats, August 2007
- NIAID Expert Panel Review on Medical Chemical Defense, March 2003
- NIAID Expert Panel on Botulinum Toxins, November 2002
- NIAID Expert Panel on Botulinum Diagnostics, May 2003
- NIAID Expert Panel on Botulinum Neurotoxins Therapeutics, February 2004

Radiological and Nuclear Defense

- Strategic Plan and Research Agenda for Medical Countermeasures Against Radiological and Nuclear Threats Progress Reports (2005–2011) and Future Directions (2012–2016), June 2012
- NIH Strategic Plan and Research Agenda for Medical Countermeasures Against Radiological and Nuclear Threats, June 2005

Data from NIH, NIAID. *Biodefense & Strategic Plan*. August 7, 2015. Available at: https://www.niaid.nih.gov/research/biodefense-strategic-plan. Accessed May 2017.

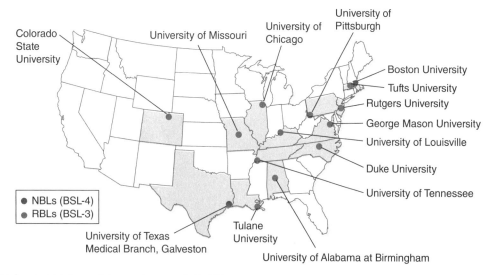

FIGURE 7-1 NIH-funded high-containment research facilities

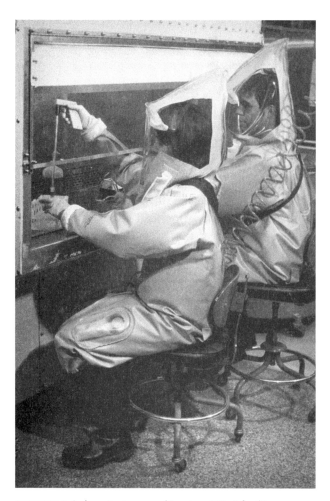

FIGURE 7-2 Laboratorians working in a BSL-4 facility

■ National Biodefense Analysis and Countermeasures Center (NBACC), Frederick, Maryland (DHS facility)

■ IRF, Ft. Detrick, Frederick, Maryland (HHS/NIAID facility)

■ Virginia Division of Consolidated Laboratory Services, Richmond, Virginia (Virginia Department of Health Facility, BSL-4 surge capacity)

■ National Bio and Agro-Defense Facility, Manhattan, Kansas (DHS facility)

■ National Biocontainment Laboratory, Boston, Massachusetts (HHS/NIAID facility at Boston University, not yet operational/planned facility)[5]

As part of an effort to build the national infrastructure for research, NIAID established the Centers of Excellence for Translational Research (CETR) in 2014 (**FIGURE 7-3**). NIAID also supports 2 biosafety level National Biocontainment Laboratories (BSL-4) and 12 Regional Biocontainment Laboratories (BSL 3), which are used for research, but are available to assist in public health emergencies. In addition to these extramurally funded research centers, NIAID has its own biocontainment labs—two BSL-4 and one BSL-3 labs.[6]

In addition to the research infrastructure funded by the NIH, multiple other federal agencies support research that contributes to public health preparedness. This includes work supported by the U.S. Department of Agriculture (USDA), the efforts of the DoD, both in the United States as well as in a network of overseas laboratories around the world, supported by both the navy and army. Additionally, the National Laboratories, part of the Department of Energy, conduct advanced research into a range of challenging arenas often requiring advanced technological solutions, including biological threats (**FIGURE 7-4**).[7]

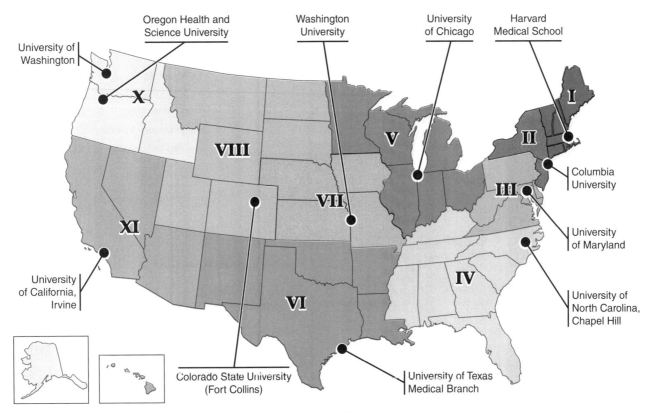

FIGURE 7-3 Map of the 11 NIH-supported regional Centers of Excellence

Data from the NIAID. *Regional Centers of Excellence for Biodefense and Emerging Infectious Diseases.*

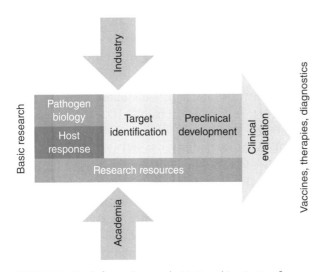

FIGURE 7-4 Biodefense Research: National Institute of Allergy and Infectious Diseases approach to how basic scientific research leads to vaccines, therapies, and diagnostics

Reproduced from NIH, NIAID. *Biodefense: Introduction to Biodefense Research.* Available at: https://www.niaid.nih.gov/research /biodefense-introduction. Accessed May 2017.

Much of the federal biodefense work is centralized at Fort Detrick in Frederick, Maryland. DHS centralizes its research at the National Biodefense Analysis and Countermeasures Center (NBACC) located on the Fort Detrick campus. The official mission of NBACC is to "provide the nation with the scientific basis for characterization of biological threats and bioforensic analysis to support attribution of their use against the American public."[8] This center focuses on activities that support threat characterization and bioforensic analysis to support attribution assessments of biocrimes and bioterrorism.[8] Also at Fort Detrick is the USAMRIID, a BSL-4 facility that has long engaged in biodefense work and basic scientific research, including research on dangerous pathogens, such as Ebola. USDA and the NIH/ National Cancer Institute (NCI) have also long had a presence on the campus. NIAID also constructed an IRF to direct, coordinate, and facilitate research in emerging infectious diseases and biodefense; to support countermeasure development; and to improve medical outcomes (**FIGURE 7-5**).[9]

DHS also supports a network of primarily university-based COE, funded by the Science and Technology Directorate, Office of Research and Development. Each COE has specific goals and objectives, including technology improvements, basic research, and multidisciplinary analysis (**BOX 7-2**).

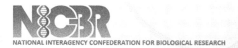

ABOUT THE NICBR

The National Interagency Confederation for Biological Research is a consortium of eight agencies with a common vision of Federal research partners working in synergy to achieve a healthier and more secure nation. It serves as a framework for facilitating and encouraging interaction among the NICBR member organizations where there are areas of mutual interest. Members collaborate and share technical expertise and scientific services. This multiagency confederation operates by consensus to ensure a balanced direction and focus. The eight members include elements of the Department of Defense, Health and Human Services, Agriculture, and Homeland Security.

Contact Us

For NICBR specific inquiries, please email us at: USArmy.Detrick.MEDCOM-USAMRMC.Other.NICBR-Support@mail.mil .

For agency specific inquiries, please contact the agencies listed below:

National Cancer Institute at Frederick ⬚

National Institute of Allergy and Infectious Diseases ⬚

US Army Medical Research and Materiel Command ⬚

US Department of Agriculture, Agricultural Research Service ⬚

National Biodefense Analysis and Countermeasures Centers ⬚

Centers for Disease Control and Prevention ⬚

Naval Medical Research Center ⬚

US Food and Drug Administration ⬚

FIGURE 7-5 National Interagency Confederation for Biological Research

Reproduced from Fitch, PJ; Laboratory Director NBACC. *Science-Based Biodefense Analysis in an Uncertain World*. Presented at: Science and Security Seminar Series Center for Strategic & International Studies; May 12, 2008; Washington, DC. Available at: https://csis-prod .s3.amazonaws.com/s3fs-public/legacy_files/files/attachments/080529_csis_fitch_presentation.pdf. Accessed May 2017.

▸ High-Containment Laboratories—The Debate

We just discussed the expansion of laboratory infrastructure in the past decade. While the government has invested in this infrastructure citing a need for more laboratory resources, enhanced research, and diagnostic facilities, others have pointed to a "proliferation of laboratories" and brought up security and environmental concerns associated with having so many high-containment laboratories. Questions arose as to the following:

- How much laboratory capacity is sufficient?
- Is or was there enough coordination among federal-funding agencies in determining where these labs should be built?
- Does increasing the number of labs increase the potential for intentional or accidental spread of dangerous pathogens?[10]

In September 2009, the House of Representatives Subcommittee on Oversight and Investigations, Committee on Energy and Commerce, held a hearing on federal oversight of high-containment biolaboratories. This was a follow-up hearing to one held 2 years prior in October 2007, and the main question of both of those hearings was: how many high-containment labs are there in the United States and how many are required to meet the research needs of the scientific community.

▸ Galveston and Boston

In 2002, NIAID hosted several Blue Ribbon panels of experts, who recommended expanding the research infrastructure to include the construction and renovation of BSL-3 and BSL-4 laboratories. NIAID decided to fund the construction of two National Biocontainment Laboratories, capable of doing BSL-4 research. In FY 2003, Boston University and the University of Texas Medical Branch (UTMB) at Galveston were selected in a national competitive process to be the sites of the two BSL-4 laboratories.[11]

What followed is an interesting case study in public relations, community engagement, and political support. Galveston, a location prone to hurricanes, made a strong argument about how hurricanes were predictable, a facility could be built to withstand them, and Galveston was—in fact—an ideal site for a facility. UTMB worked closely with the community, developed support for the project from the bottom up, and by 2010, had a fully functional facility that has already proven its ability to withstand hurricanes.

In Boston, university officials obtained support from high-level political officials for the location of the BSL-4 facility, but made only minimal effort to engage the community. Limited attention was paid to environmental assessments or to working with the local neighborhoods to educate them about the risks associated with having a BSL-4 facility in the middle of an urban community. The community reacted very

---

BOX 7-2   The Case of Thomas Butler

As the awareness and perception of the threat of biological agents changed post-9/11, the rules and regulations applicable to research changed. A new set of rules was instituted that were imposed on researchers who had previously operated in regulation-free environment. Many of the most renowned researchers working on dangerous pathogens were described as "disease cowboys." They went places most people did not travel to, took risks, and worked with dangerous diseases that the majority of their peers shied away from. They made incredible contributions to science and public health, but this small community of researchers were not used to having anyone look over their shoulder or be accountable to administrators outside of their fields. The new rules governing research on dangerous pathogens (including the rules discussed in Chapter 6 on select agents) were not easily adapted by the disease cowboys. The case of Thomas Butler highlights the consequences of this challenge.

In 2003, Thomas Butler, age 60 at the time, was a nationally recognized scientist at Texas Tech University Health Sciences Center in Lubbock, and had worked there for 15 years. He developed an interest in *Yersinia pestis* (plague) after spending time in Vietnam and witnessing tragic deaths as a result of the disease. He became one of the most prominent plague researchers in the world, traveling to distant sites to collect samples and further knowledge of the disease. During a 2001 trip to Tanzania, Butler collected samples of plague from patients who had contracted the disease and proceeded to bring the samples back into the United States the way he had always done so— without paperwork. He later claimed he was unaware of a Centers for Disease Control and Prevention policy on pathogen transport. He returned to Texas with his samples and proceeded to conduct research on them. In January 2002, however, Butler filed a report to his university claiming 30 of 150 vials of plague were missing from his lab. The university, concerned about a possible terrorist-backed theft, called the Federal Bureau of Investigation (FBI). With no signs of forced entry or foul play, investigators began to question Butler and his involvement in the case. After 2 days of interrogation, Butler admitted to destroying the vials himself and was then taken to a Lubbock jail and charged with lying to federal agents about the disappearance of the vials as well as illegally bringing samples of plague into the United States. Dr. Butler, denying a plea bargain, was charged with 18 counts of theft, fraud, and embezzlement; 13 counts of mail fraud; 13 counts of wire fraud; and 3 counts of unauthorized export. He was convicted and sentenced to 2 years in prison and over $50,000 in fines. He was stripped of his medical license and, despite pleas from prominent scientists around the world, he served his time in jail. His career was destroyed.

Whether the FBI was making an example out of Dr. Butler, whether foul play was involved, or whether the practices of disease researchers had to be amended in the post-9/11 world, this case was a wake-up call to researchers around the country. This case shook the scientific community into understanding that their roles and responsibilities as scientists has changed, and the consequences of non-adherence to the rules was significant.

Data from Chang K. 30 Plague Vials Put Career on Line. *The New York Times*. October 19, 2003. Available at: http://www.nytimes.com/2003/10/19/us/30-plague-vials-put-career-on-line.html. Accessed May 2017; Enserink M, Malakoff D. The Final Score 47 to 22. *Science*. 2003; 302(5654): 2062. DOI: 10.1126/science.302.5653.2062; Chang K. Scientist In Plague Case Is Sentenced To Two Years. *The New York Times*. March 11, 2004. Available at: http://www.nytimes.com/2004/03/11/us/scientist-in-plague-case-is-sentenced-to-two-years.html?_r=0. Accessed May 2017.

---

negatively and construction on the facility was blocked by court order. The facility has been constructed, but as of September 2017, it was still not operational as a BSL-4.

Increasing high-containment laboratory capacity has been described as a double-edged sword.[10] Building capacity allows for more research, more infrastructure for diagnostic testing, and advancement of scientific knowledge in general. On the other hand, increasing the number of labs means increasing the number of personnel working in these labs, which increases the opportunities for accidental exposures to pathogens, mistakes, or accidents that might lead to environmental release of pathogens; or

the opportunity for a research scientist to intentionally access a pathogen and use it for malevolent purposes; or share knowledge with an outside entity or person who then uses that knowledge for malevolent purposes.

These high-containment laboratories are heavily regulated in the United States. There are physical security measures as well as personal responsibilities, all aimed at limiting both accidents and potential intentional-use events. A similar debate is now playing out over "biobanking," the balance of enabling countries to safety and securely store pathogens of national importance for research purposes, and the potential threat these facilities may cause.

🔍 *CASE STUDY: Epidemics and Biobanking*

By Claire Standley

Summary

During outbreaks of infectious disease, patient samples are often critical resources for the development of new treatments, vaccines, and other countermeasures. Data derived from these specimens may also be important for understanding the epidemiology of the outbreak, its origin, or even the evolution of the etiological agent; all factors that can drive decision-making during the outbreak. After the outbreak, samples may be stored long term in "biobanks," where they are managed for future research use. Such samples may be especially important for preparedness and response to future outbreaks. However, the establishment and use of biobanks, particularly in the context of epidemics, is not without controversy, including ethical concerns over access, equity of benefit, and sovereignty, as well as safety and security issues related to the samples themselves. The 2014 West Africa Ebola outbreak brought biobanks back to the forefront of debate within the global health security community, compelling the World Health Organization (WHO) to embark on a consultative process to define and guide the development and use of biobanks as repositories for samples collected during epidemics and a research resource. This case study provides an overview of the issues surrounding biobanking in the context of epidemics, particularly in resource-constrained settings.

What Is Biobanking?

The exact definition of a "biobank" varies depending on the context, audience, and application of the facility. However, the core principle, which most definitions have in common, is that a biobank is a managed repository of biological material and its associated information that can be accessed for research and other purposes.[12,13] Biobanks tend to focus on human-derived material, such as tissue, blood, and urine samples, but could also encompass animal samples (particularly for veterinary or zoonotic disease applications) and even plant or other organismal specimens.

As biobanks are often the final destination of samples collected during outbreaks, they are commonly implicated in the broader debate surrounding the transport, sharing, and management of samples, particularly across borders. Many of these issues also apply to samples once deposited in biobanks, when requests are made for later access and use. As such, it is important to consider biobanking as part of a larger set of sample-related activities.

Ethical, Safety, and Security Concerns

The management of samples taken during outbreaks, and the related creation and use of biobanks as a resource for future research, has raised a number of practical, ethical, safety, and security concerns. Particularly in the context of biobanks operating in more economically developed countries, practical concerns relating to data management capacity and interoperability tend to dominate the debate.[14] While important to global governance of biobanks, these issues are less pertinent directly to biobanks in the context of outbreaks, and especially those in less economically developed countries. The greater challenges associated with biosecurity is related to biobanks in resource-poor environments.

Over the last two decades, a major concern related to sample management during outbreaks was the concept of sample sovereignty and the rights retained (or imposed) by the country of origin over access to and use of samples containing infectious disease agents. Historically, biobanks and other repositories of infectious disease samples have been primarily located in more economically developed countries, where most research on development of vaccines, therapeutics, and other countermeasures took place. When outbreaks occurred in less economically developed countries, there was an expectation that samples would be sent out to these research centers and biobanks to facilitate countermeasure development.

In 2007, the Government of Indonesia decided to withhold samples of highly pathogenic H5N1 avian influenza virus from the WHO, citing "sovereignty" over the genetic material under the provisions of the Convention on Biological Diversity (CBD). Their concern stemmed from the use of this material by foreign companies to develop vaccines, which were not being made available to Indonesia at locally reasonable prices, as patents were being taken out on specific strains without necessarily requiring the consent of the country of origin. The ensuing debate highlighted concerns from developing countries over equitable access to the benefits derived from samples taken during outbreaks, which had been shared in good faith with the international community to assist with surveillance and countermeasure development.[15] The debate reared its head once more in 2013, with the emergence of Middle East Respiratory Syndrome (MERS) coronavirus in Saudi Arabia and accusations from the Government of Saudi Arabia that samples of the virus had been sent to Erasmus Medical Center (EMC) in the Netherlands without appropriate clearance.

(continues)

EMC furthermore sought to patent the virus, claiming it was necessary to facilitate pharmaceutical companies using the material for countermeasure development. While EMC claimed it was willing to share the virus freely with all those interested in using it for public health research, there were concerns that the Material Transfer Agreement (MTA) used by EMC actually did include provisions intended to support intellectual property claims on outcomes of any research conducted using the material.[16]

Beyond questions of sovereignty and equity of access, there are safety and security concerns to consider when samples containing extremely dangerous pathogens are kept in research collections and biobanks. To be viable for research, samples need to be kept under strict environmental control and nonfluctuating temperature; conditions which may be challenging or expensive to attain in countries with unreliable electricity grids and frequent blackouts. Curation of the collections also requires staff trained in high-level biosafety procedures, in order to prevent accidental exposure and risk of infection from contact with the samples. Finally, samples containing deadly pathogens pose a security risk, as nefarious actors might seek to acquire the samples as a source of viral material for biological weapons or other nonpeaceful purposes.

These issues were brought into sharp focus by the 2014 West Africa Ebola outbreak. Dozens of organizations were involved in response efforts across Guinea, Liberia, and Sierra Leone, collecting tens of thousands of samples from confirmed, suspected, and probable Ebola patients. Unfortunately, to date, no complete inventory exists for all the clinical and diagnostic samples collected during the outbreak, though all three of the most heavily affected countries have undertaken efforts to catalogue at least those samples that remain within their borders. Although transparency has been low, it is likely that a large number of samples were exported, either to research facilities elsewhere in West Africa or further afield to Europe, China, and the United States. Few organizations have publicly declared how many samples they hold or where they are being maintained; in their defense, some organizations, such as the Public Health Agency of Canada, which operated mobile diagnostic labs in West Africa during the outbreak, explicitly cited safety and security concerns as their reason for not disclosing this information.[17,18] Their laboratories destroyed a large number of clinical samples immediately after diagnosis rather than store them, notably when operating in locations with limited electricity and other infrastructure. Sample sovereignty was also a concern in the context of the Ebola outbreak; in many cases, it is not clear whether MTAs were in place when samples were exported, contributing to the confusion over the total number of extant samples and their location. Samples remaining within Guinea, Sierra Leone, and Liberia have been kept by government facilities as well as the international organizations who collected them, with infrastructure challenges such as interrupted electricity raising concerns over the long-term viability of the samples for future research.

Global Reaction

In recognition of the challenges posed by sample management and storage, and prompted largely by the perceived shortcomings of the global response to Ebola, there has been renewed interest in developing global guidelines for biobanking.[19] In 2015, WHO held two consultations on biobanking, one in Geneva and the other in Sierra Leone, to discuss not only the fate of the remaining Ebola samples but also the concept of establishing national biobanking facilities in the three most affected countries.[17,20,21] This latter sentiment has been echoed in numerous other calls to foster African research resources and capabilities, and thus address, perhaps in a more comprehensive way, some of the past challenges associated with sample sovereignty.[18,22] More broadly, one of the recommendations of the Ebola Interim Assessment Panel—the body that was tasked to review WHO's performance during the 2014 Ebola outbreak—was that WHO should develop guidelines and mechanisms to improve the conduct of research during outbreaks.[23] In response, the WHO embarked on a consultative process on research and development, which resulted in an "R&D Blueprint for Action to Prevent Epidemics"—broadly speaking, a plan of action document outlining critical issues to be addressed. Biobanking is covered under developing norms and standards tailored to an epidemic context, and specifically related to "developing guidance and tools to frame collaborations and exchanges."[24]

Conclusion

Over the previous decades, momentum has increased toward developing a global governance structure for sample management and biobanking specifically, particularly in the context of epidemics. Responding positively to criticism leveled in the wake of the 2014 West Africa Ebola outbreak, the WHO has stepped forward to take a leadership role in this conversation, with the aim of developing tools and guidelines—with the consensus of the global health community—to facilitate equitable, safe, and secure management of samples in the future. However, at the time of writing, few deliverables have been finalized, and consultations remain predominantly at the informal and informational level. The question remains: Will a framework for global governance of biobanks be in place in time for the next pandemic, or will we repeat the lessons observed from H5N1, MERS, and Ebola yet again?

▶ Medical Countermeasures

A key component of public health preparedness is the development, production, and distribution of MCMs. The policies, strategies, and methodologies behind the development and delivery of MCMs have developed over the decades and are now part of what is known as the Public Health Emergency Medical Countermeasures Enterprise (PHEMCE).

As discussed earlier in the text, the Project Bioshield Act was passed in 2004, with the purpose of establishing a market to purchase MCMs to treat exposures to biological, chemical, or radiological agents. A Special Reserve Fund was established, with $5.6 billion to be used over 10 years, to purchase these countermeasures to put into the Strategic National Stockpile (SNS).[25] The federal government, usually through NIH, was able to provide funding for the initial research associated with discovery, and valuation. Drug-development companies were then on their own to move the initial discovery into a tested, safe product—a process that might take up to 10 years, before the government could provide funds again to do final testing and purchase the product. Bioshield also did not provide companies with liability protection if a product was used for emergency purposes, but had not yet completed all final stages of approval by the Food and Drug Administration (FDA). (This problem was addressed by passage of the Public Readiness and Emergency Preparedness (PREP) Act in 2005.) As a result, few companies were willing to invest in the development of products.

The 2006 Pandemic and All-Hazards Preparedness Act (PAHPA) legislation addressed some of the problems in Bioshield, allowing companies to receive payments before delivery of the product, which enables them to move a product through testing with financial support. PAHPA also established the Biomedical Advanced Research and Development Authority (BARDA), which sits in HHS Office of the Assistant Secretary for Preparedness and Response to manage the development of MCMs against CBRN threats, emerging infections, and pandemic influenza.[26(Title IV)] At about the same time, HHS established PHEMCE to coordinate across organizations the planning and execution of developing MCMs (BOX 7-3).

The federal process for PHEMCE starts with DHS, which is tasked with conducting risk and threat assessments and creating a list of agents and conditions. These agents and conditions then become the priorities for the development of MCMs, and HHS directs that countermeasures be produced to counter these threats.

NIH, and NIAID in particular, then fund basic and applied research to address the threat list. When basic science leads to the potential for an MCM, BARDA becomes involved to manage advanced product development. Throughout the drug-development process, FDA provides review and regulatory oversight and eventual approval for licensing. Products are acquired through Project Bioshield, which are then transferred to CDC where the countermeasures are stored and maintained. CDC continues to manage acquisition after the product becomes part of the SNS. If the agent then has to be utilized, CDC is in charge of releasing it from the SNS and HHS is in charge of coordinating deployment and utilization.[2,29]

While BARDA and PHEMCE have guided the MCM development and delivery process in the United States, several international efforts have emerged to guide and accelerate this process. In 2015, in response to the West Africa Ebola outbreak, the WHO began to develop what would become known as the R&D Blueprint for potentially epidemic disease. The purpose of this endeavor was to accelerate the time between the start of an outbreak and the deployment of effective MCMs. The blueprint addressed research and development for diagnostics, vaccines, therapeutics, vector control, and research on epidemiology.[27] To guide this effort, the blueprint prioritizes diseases, and since its development, there have been specific R&D road maps created for both MERS and Zika, as well a coordinated effort to identify new platform technologies.

BOX 7-3 Public Health Emergency Medical Countermeasures Enterprise Strategic Goals

1. Identify, create, develop, manufacture, and procure critical medical countermeasures (MCMs)
2. Establish and communicate clear regulatory pathways to facilitate MCM development and use
3. Develop logistics and operational plans for optimized use of MCMs at all levels of response
4. Address MCM gaps for all sectors of the American civilian population

Data from Assistant Secretary for Preparedness and Response; U.S. Department of Health and Human Services. *The Public Health Emergency Medical Countermeasures Enterprise Review, Transforming the Enterprise to Meet Long-Range National Needs.* August 2010. Available at: https://www.medicalcountermeasures.gov/media/1138/mcmreviewfinalcover-508.pdf. Accessed May 2017.

Following the WHO's R&D Blueprint, a new coalition of states and philanthropic organizations came together and in 2017, formally launched the Coalition for Epidemic Preparedness Innovations (CEPI). CEPI endeavors to provide a new system to try to address some of the barriers to epidemic vaccine development by focusing on moving vaccine candidates through late preclinical studies to larger trials, and to support new technological platforms to rapidly develop vaccines against unknown pathogens.[28]

▶ Stockpiling and Distribution of Medical Countermeasures

In 1999, CDC established what was known as the National Pharmaceutical Stockpile (NPS); it was renamed the Strategic National Stockpile in 2003. The purpose of the SNS is to amass and store large amounts of drugs, vaccines, and medical equipment that can rapidly be deployed to any locality in the country in response to a public health emergency. Once federal officials determine that an emergency exists and that SNS assets should be deployed, an

initial delivery of drugs, antidotes, and supplies can be made to any location in the country within 12 hours. An additional shipment, if necessary, can be available in 24–36 hours. CDC, in collaboration with the rest of the PHEMCE partners, determines what should be in the stockpile and ensures the material has not expired (**FIGURES 7-6** and **7-7**).[30]

▶ Cities Readiness Initiative

When the SNS is deployed, it is the responsibility of the state and local officials to accept the material, store it, and distribute it to the affected population. The Cities Readiness Initiative (CRI) is a federally funded program to help prepare local entities to respond to a public health emergency and to develop distribution plans for getting needed medical supplies and countermeasures to their populations. It was established in 2004 and now funds 72 metropolitan statistical areas, representing 60% of the U.S. population. CDC provides technical assistance to the 72 sites so that they can effectively and efficiently receive items from the SNS, store them, and deliver them. The program is funded through Public Health Emergency Preparedness cooperative agreement[30] (**BOX 7-4**).

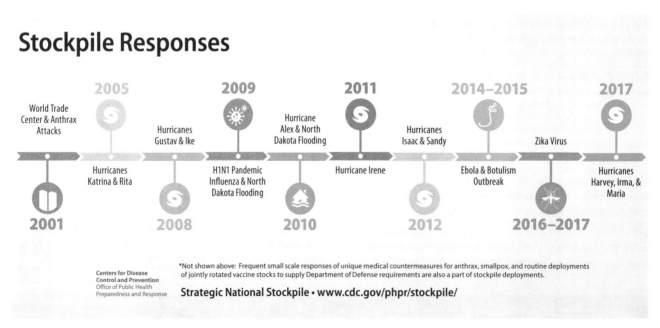

FIGURE 7-6 Examples of when the stockpile has been used since 2001

Reproduced from CDC. *Timeline of Stockpile Responses.* Available at: https://www.cdc.gov/phpr/stockpile/timeline.htm. Accessed May 2017.

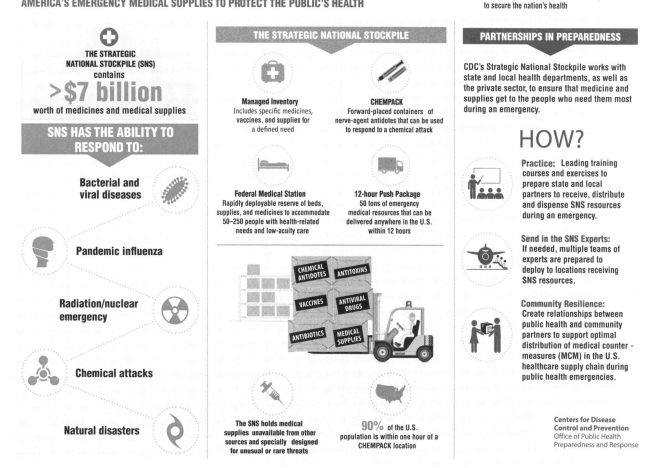

DIVISION OF STRATEGIC NATIONAL STOCKPILE
AMERICA'S EMERGENCY MEDICAL SUPPLIES TO PROTECT THE PUBLIC'S HEALTH

To prepare and support partners and provide the right resources at the right time to secure the nation's health

THE STRATEGIC NATIONAL STOCKPILE (SNS) contains

> $7 billion

worth of medicines and medical supplies

SNS HAS THE ABILITY TO RESPOND TO:

Bacterial and viral diseases

Pandemic influenza

Radiation/nuclear emergency

Chemical attacks

Natural disasters

THE STRATEGIC NATIONAL STOCKPILE

Managed Inventory
Includes specific medicines, vaccines, and supplies for a defined need

CHEMPACK
Forward-placed containers of nerve-agent antidotes that can be used to respond to a chemical attack

Federal Medical Station
Rapidly deployable reserve of beds, supplies, and medicines to accommodate 50–250 people with health-related needs and low-acuity care

12-hour Push Package
50 tons of emergency medical resources that can be delivered anywhere in the U.S. within 12 hours

CHEMICAL ANTIDOTES / ANTITOXINS / VACCINES / ANTIVIRAL DRUGS / ANTIBIOTICS / MEDICAL SUPPLIES

The SNS holds medical supplies unavailable from other sources and specially designed for unusual or rare threats

90% of the U.S. population is within one hour of a CHEMPACK location

PARTNERSHIPS IN PREPAREDNESS

CDC's Strategic National Stockpile works with state and local health departments, as well as the private sector, to ensure that medicine and supplies get to the people who need them most during an emergency.

HOW?

Practice: Leading training courses and exercises to prepare state and local partners to receive, distribute and dispense SNS resources during an emergency.

Send in the SNS Experts: If needed, multiple teams of experts are prepared to deploy to locations receiving SNS resources.

Community Resilience: Create relationships between public health and community partners to support optimal distribution of medical counter-measures (MCM) in the U.S. healthcare supply chain during public health emergencies.

Centers for Disease Control and Prevention
Office of Public Health Preparedness and Response

FIGURE 7-7 CDC Information on the stockpile: What is in it, how it is managed, and how it is used for preparedness and response

Reproduced from CDC. *Overview*. Available at: https://www.cdc.gov/phpr/stockpile/infographic.htm. Accessed May 2017.

MCMs in Response to the 2014–2015 Ebola Outbreak

Several of the federal preparedness laws and regulations of the early 2000s focused on the need to develop and stockpile a ready supply of medical countermeasures (MCMs) to be deployed in the event of a public health emergency. However, many pathogens of concern are relatively rare or occur endemically only in lower-income or resource-constrained countries. As such, there was reluctance from the pharmaceutical and drug-manufacturing industries to commit significant research and development dollars to products that might not have a commercially viable market. The Project Bioshield Act of 2004 sought to change that, by establishing a government-funded market for such countermeasures, and thus incentivizing the development of vaccines and therapeutics that would not otherwise be cost-effective. Subsequent legislation changed how the development of MCMs were funded to better incentivize private-sector companies to remain committed and financially viable during the lengthy process between initial development of a product and final approval by the FDA.

Given the length of time required for a product to come to market, Project Bioshield Act also allowed for HHS to authorize the emergency use of countermeasures even if they had not yet been approved by the FDA. Of course, FDA approval processes are critical for determining safety and efficacy, so the concern was raised about liability—in the event that a non-FDA approved countermeasure, used for a legitimate public health emergency, produced a severe side effect or failed as a treatment. Manufacturers feared that liability in these situations would

(continues)

fall on them, leading to a reticence to even engage in the development of the product. In response, Congress passed the Public Readiness and Emergency Preparedness Act of 2005 (PREP Act, see Chapters 1 and 5) which provides immunity from liability for any claims resulting from the use of an MCM approved for use during a public health emergency.

Starting in late 2013, erupting in 2014, and continuing into 2015, Ebola virus disease spread through Guinea, Sierra Leone, and Liberia, infecting and killing thousands more people than any previous Ebola outbreak. The virus spread to countries outside of West Africa, including the United States, through global travel and the return of infected medical volunteers. The scale of the outbreak prompted several pharmaceutical companies to accelerate research and development of Ebola vaccines and therapeutics; despite such products being incentivized under the Project Bioshield Act, virtually no companies had focused on Ebola virus, and so few countermeasures were at an advanced stage of testing. There was tremendous public fear and pressure mounted on public health and medical officials to do ensure that the U.S. patients with Ebola were given every available treatment, even if experimental. In August 2014, the media widely reported on the remarkable recovery of two American Ebola patients in Liberia, who had been given doses of an experimental drug called ZMapp. It is not clear if and what liability protections were waived for the initial use of this and other, experimental Ebola therapeutics on U.S. patients, though the provision of these treatments were sanctioned under the auspices of FDA's "compassionate use exemption" whereby a patient may receive unapproved treatment outside of clinical trials. However, HHS later issued a PREP Act declaration providing immunity from liability for the manufacturing, administration, and use of Ebola-related vaccines, including several Ebola vaccines under development, and later issuing a declaration for therapeutics such as ZMapp.

This example demonstrates the importance of establishing a legal framework for preparedness to ensure the appropriate and timely use of MCMs in the event of a public health emergency. Having a process in place to protect manufacturers allowed them to move forward with getting potentially life-saving products into a frightened, at-risk population.

Data from US Congress. Global Efforts to Fight Ebola: Hearing Before the Subcommittee on Africa, Global Health, Global Human Rights, and International Organizations. Serial No. 113-239. Washington, DC: USG Publishing Office; 2015. Available at: http://www.gpo.gov/fdsys/pkg/CHRG-113hhrg89811/html/CHRG-113hhrg89811.htm. Accessed June 2017; Department of Health and Human Services Office of the Secretary. Ebola Virus Disease Vaccines: ACTION: Notice of Declaration under the Public Readiness and Emergency Preparedness Act. December 10, 2014. Available at: https://s3.amazonaws.com/public-inspection.federalregister.gov/2014-28856.pdf. Accessed June 2017; Department of Health and Human Services Office of the Secretary. Ebola Virus Disease Therapeutics: ACTION: Notice of Declaration Under the Public Readiness and Emergency Preparedness Act. April 22, 2015. Available at: http://www.gpo.gov/fdsys/pkg/FR-2015-04-22/html /2015-09412.htm. Accessed June 2017.

BOX 7-4 Smallpox Destruction Debate

In 1966, the WHO launched an international campaign to eradicate smallpox (**FIGURE 7-8**). After 11 years, they succeeded, making it one of the most profound public health accomplishments to date. Following eradication, there was a laboratory accident in 1978 that lead to two infections and one fatality. This lab incident led the World Health Assembly to pass Resolution 33.4 in 1980, which urged all countries to destroy their smallpox stocks or transfer them to one of the four designated collaborating centers established by WHO. Three years following Resolution 33.4, CDC in Atlanta, Georgia, and the State Research Centre for Virology and Biotechnology (VECTOR) in the then Union of Soviet Socialists Republics and now the Russia Federation were named the exclusive repositories of the smallpox virus.

Despite naming VECTOR and CDC as the only two repositories of smallpox in the world, evidence was compiled that the virus was not only in multiple countries, including Iran, Iraq, and North Korea, but that it was also potentially being used to develop biological weapons. In addition, inspectors found evidence that the Soviet Union had transferred the smallpox to an offensive biological weapons facility and was using it as part of their offensive biological weapons program. Following the collapse of the Soviet Union, security experts worried that smallpox samples may have left the country. By 1996, the concern about undetected stocks had increased and Resolution 49.10 was adopted by the WHO recommending that all smallpox virus stocks be destroyed by June 30, 1999. However, concerns of a possible bioterrorist attack and the need for more antiviral drugs and vaccines in preparation for such an event led the CDC to reconsider the resolution and to conserve the remaining stocks.

With influence and scientific backing from the National Academies of Science Institute of Medicine (now called the National Academy of Medicine (NAM)), the WHO established a 3-year program (Resolution 52.10) which allowed for applied research with the smallpox virus at the two authorized repositories, for the benefit of public health. At the end of the 3-year research period in 2002, the WHO passed Resolution 55.15, which extended the smallpox research for an indefinite period of time until all research goals and needs had been accomplished.

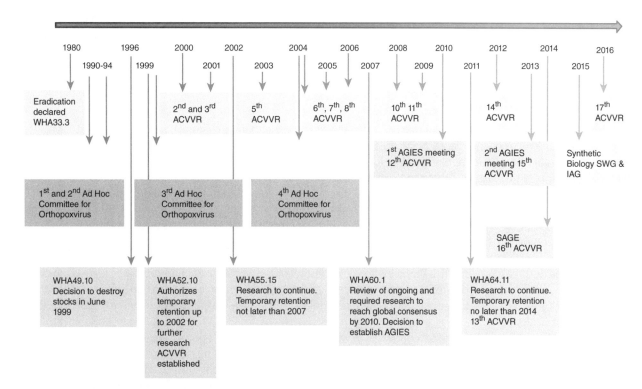

FIGURE 7-8 Smallpox timeline

Reproduced from Khalakdina A, Costa A, Briand S. Smallpox in the post eradication era. *WHO Weekly Epidemiological Record*. May 20, 2016; 91(20), 259. Available at: http://www.who.int/wer/2016/wer9120.pdf.

By 2006, most of the research goals had been fulfilled and, as a result, 46 member states of the WHO drafted a resolution to have the final smallpox stocks in VECTOR and the CDC destroyed by June 30, 2010. However, the United States, Russia, and multiple other countries blocked the resolution. This led to Resolution 60.1 the following year, which claimed the need for a consensus on the issue of the smallpox destruction and recommended a major review in 2010. This review was to provide guidance to the World Health Assembly (WHA) of May 2011, where a final conclusion was planned to be made on the destruction of the smallpox stocks. Instead, the WHA decided in 2011 to postpone the decision until 2014, and in 2014, the decision was postponed again until May 2019.

Retentionists (those in favor of preserving the last two remaining smallpox stocks) claim that the potential for a smallpox outbreak comes more from the threat of unknown stocks or from *de novo* synthesis, and not from the two remaining repositories holding the smallpox virus. They also argue that research is still needed in order to create novel ways to contain the virus in the event there is a bioterrorist attack leading to a smallpox pandemic.

In contrast to these retentionists, those opposed to the saving of the smallpox virus, known as destructionists, believe that an accidental outbreak could cause devastation, leaving the most efficient prevention of this type of incident to be the destruction of the virus. Further, they strongly believe in the "insider threat," which is represented by a scientist with access to the smallpox virus at either of the repositories using that access to bring the virus to outside, dangerous sources.

In the interim, there is still no clear decision on what to do about the samples. Research continues to be approved on public health issues related to smallpox, and the WHO maintains a Smallpox Vaccine Emergency Stockpile, which in 2017 consisted of 33.7 million doses.

Fenner F, Henderson DA, Arita I, et al. *Smallpox and its Eradication*. Geneva: World Health Organization; 1988; Gellman B. *4 Nations Thought To Possess Smallpox: Iraq, N. Korea Named, Two Officials Say*. The Washington Post. November 5, 2002. Available at: http://www.washingtonpost.com/wp-dyn/content/article/2006/06/12/AR2006061200704.html. Accessed May 2017; Mangold T, Goldberg J. *Plague Wars: The Terrifying Reality of Biological Warfare*. New York: St. Martin's Press; 1999; Institute of Medicine, Board on Global Health, Committee on the Assessment of Future Scientific Needs for Live Variola Virus. *Assessment of Future Scientific Needs for Live Variola Virus*. Washington, DC: National Academy Press; 1999; Sixtieth World Health Assembly. *Smallpox Eradication: Destruction of Variola Virus Stocks*; WHA60.1; Agenda Item 12.2. World Health Organization. May 18, 2007; Butler D. *WHO Postpones Decision on Destruction of Smallpox Stocks—Again*. Nature Newsblog. May 28, 2014. Available at: http://blogs.nature.com/news/2014/05/who-postpones-decision-on-destruction-of-smallpox-stocks-again.html. Accessed June 2017; WHO. *WHO Advisory Committee on Variola Virus Research: Report of the Eighteenth Meeting*. November 2–3, 2016. Available at: http://www.who.int/csr/resources/publications/smallpox/18-ACVVR-Final.pdf?ua=1. Accessed June 2017.

🔍 *CASE STUDY: Research Note on Data Integration for Effective Response to Public Health Emergencies*

By Ellie Graeden

Public health emergencies develop over a much more extended timeline than the natural disaster events that have historically been the focus of emergency planning and response in the federal emergency management community. **No-notice** events are those, such as earthquakes, for which some risk information may be available, but predictive analysis is unreliable or unavailable. **Advanced-notice** events include hurricanes and other extreme weather events for which predictive analysis is available and largely reliable. By contrast, biological outbreaks are **delayed-notice** events: the data required to define an event must be collected and analyzed in an ongoing manner with a focus on recognizing outlier events that indicate emergency status (e.g., unusual disease types, clusters of cases above a baseline, or unusual disease transmission patterns; see **FIGURE 7-9**). A single case of most diseases is not a cause for concern, even when recognized; but in another context, it may be the earliest signal of an outbreak or public health emergency. In the case of the 2014 Ebola outbreak in West Africa that grew to the largest recorded, initial cases of hemorrhagic fever, even once confirmed as Ebola, were assumed to reflect seasonal endemic flare-ups. Initial cases of Zika virus in Brazil failed to raise any concern until a pattern of microcephalic births were recognized and a wide-scale effort launched to determine the cause.

Figure 7-12 the timelines show the differing rates at which different event types unfold. **No-notice** events, such as earthquakes, have a rapid, immediate impact. **Advanced-notice** events, such as hurricanes, have a relatively long period of preparation prior to the event, during which the federal emergency response is typically initiated. Most casualties are incurred within hours of landfall. **Delayed-notice** events, such as biological outbreaks, unfold slowly and the federal emergency response is not initiated until the majority of casualties are incurred, long after the onset of the event, despite the need for key response actions very early in the event.

Once an emergency event has occurred and there is sufficient evidence or anticipation of significant loss of life and economic impacts, a federal emergency response is authorized rapidly. However, much of the challenge in responding effectively to public health emergencies is in defining at what point an outbreak or cluster of cases constitutes an emergency. Defining public health emergencies requires the collection of data across state and national borders, analysis by subject matter experts, and communication of the analytical or modeling results to decision makers.

Although decision makers within the federal emergency management community have not traditionally been assumed to play a significant role in public health emergencies, the Federal Emergency Management Agency (FEMA) and other emergency management-focused agencies have been tapped to help coordinate and manage the response

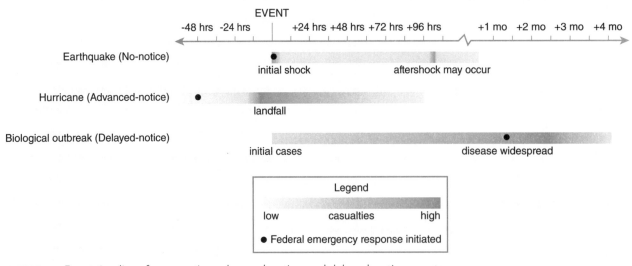

FIGURE 7-9 Event timelines for no-notice, advanced-notice, and delayed-notice events

to a series of large-scale public health emergencies in recent years, including the 2014 Ebola outbreak in West Africa; the 2016 response to Flint, Michigan, water contamination; and the 2016 Zika virus outbreak. With this emerging role, FEMA and the broader federal emergency management community need access to data and modeling about the events, as they unfold, to inform effective response measures and coordinate with the appropriate measures.

The Challenge

Effective response to public health emergencies requires identifying and characterizing the event itself and initiating the response early—even when the scope, scale, and severity of the outbreak are poorly defined. Ongoing data collection and analysis are required to calibrate the scale of these response efforts and determine whether the response measures are sufficient. These data and the corresponding analysis to make the information relevant to decision makers is particularly key for public health emergencies, because management of an event requires high consequence decision-making, including decisions to trigger vaccine development, implementing travel restrictions, or administering prophylactic medical countermeasures (MCMs) to the affected population.

The challenge to effectively initiating these response efforts are twofold: (1) the public health emergency must be recognized and (2) the appropriate response triggered. However, the federal authority to act in response to a public health threat is dependent on declaration of an emergency; public health emergencies are only declared once there is significant loss of life or large-scale disease spread. By the time there is a large enough number of cases to cause either significant loss of life or economic impacts from a public health emergency, it is too late to mount an effective prevention or response effort. Therefore, the trigger for a public health emergency must be based on biosurveillance analysis and predictive epidemiological modeling, and this information must be readily available and relevant to the emergency management decision makers tasked with initiating the response.

Secondly, Emergency Support Function (ESF) #8 (see Chapter 4) is tasked in the National Response Framework as the lead for public health emergencies. Department of Health and Human Services (HHS) is the lead agency for ESF #8, with the Centers for Disease Control and Prevention (CDC) taking the lead role for public health surveillance and ongoing public health efforts both domestically and internationally. HHS Office of the Assistant Secretary for Preparedness and Response (ASPR) is the lead for managing and coordinating an ESF #8 response once a public health emergency is declared. However, ASPR does not have a well-established coordination role within the U.S. federal emergency management community, as is necessary to effectively manage and coordinate a response. Therefore, this role has recently fallen to FEMA, even though the agency is not well positioned to manage or coordinate public health data and, indeed, often does not have ready access to operational information that supports the coordination mission.

Public Health Data and Analysis for Emergency Management

To address the role of the federal emergency management community and better understand the data that are available to help support the emergency management mission for public health emergencies, the Emergency Support Function Leadership Group (ESFLG), a group of senior-level decision makers from across the federal government, tasked the Modeling and Data Working Group with identifying and characterizing the data and models used to inform operational decision-making for public health emergencies. The results of the biological hazard analysis highlighted the current state of data and modeling access and use to the emergency management community in ways that had been suspected previously, but never confirmed.

The data and analysis required to inform emergency management efforts for disease outbreaks include event characterization (e.g., biosurveillance and epidemiological data collection), consequence modeling (e.g., epidemiological modeling to estimate disease spread, casualties, and fatalities), and decision support (e.g., MCMs required, nursing requirements, and hospital bed requirements). The inventory of datasets and models collated by the ESFLG Modeling and Data Working Group (available at: https://gis.fema.gov/Model-and-Data-Inventory/) suggest that there are no widely used sources of event characterization or consequence analysis available to the emergency management community.[31] This finding is confirmed by evidence from 2014 Ebola outbreak and 2016 Zika outbreak during which the federal government's primary source of information were conference calls hosted by ASPR, which were largely a forum for academic exchange with very limited discussion of specific actions or coordination efforts within the federal community.

Based on the results of the working group, the primary source of biosurveillance data, epidemiological analysis, and modeling is the academic community. Even those data collected and analyzed by the CDC, a federal agency with an emergency management mission, are typically only made available once they have been made public through publication in the academic literature. Indeed, this analysis is rarely designed to support the operational emergency management decisions required of those tasked with managing and coordinating the response. While ongoing data collection and analysis is required to calibrate the scale of public health emergency response efforts, these data are, therefore, not typically available to federal emergency managers in a format that is readily applicable to their mission.

(continues)

Three key points should be considered regarding the best path forward for public health emergency response. These begin to address the challenge in managing and coordinating the response to large-scale public health emergencies that require access to event characterization and consequence analysis that inform practical, operationally relevant decision-making. Furthermore, this information needs to be broadly available across the federal government and shared rapidly and smoothly between the agencies tasked with coordinating all aspects of the response.

1. How can biosurveillance data and analysis be more effectively performed and the outputs shared to help identify the event and communicate that information to those leading the response?

   Public health sharing is often limited by privacy issues. However, data sharing methods have been developed for other types of sensitive data. It may be possible to define specific metadata that can be shared or types of analysis and data aggregation that can be performed without putting privacy at risk.

2. How could standardized consequence analysis, performed by subject matter experts, be developed to support emergency management operations?

   Consequence assessments need to be disseminated early and widely during a public health emergency, even when there is uncertainty in what is happening. This information sharing is an essential function of the public health mission and is aligned with the academic culture of many public health organizations. A new understanding is needed to balance the need for accuracy and peer review with the immediate requirements of providing the data needed for effective emergency response.

3. How can the roles of agencies involved in public health emergency response be clarified?

   HHS, ASPR, HHS CDC, FEMA, and DHS have intersecting, overlapping roles in public health response. Improving coordination between the agencies is critical and will depend on better aligning these roles with the practical realities of public health emergency response.

Key Words

Biomedical research
Centers of Excellence
Cities Readiness Initiative
Fort Detrick

High-containment laboratories
Medical countermeasures
National Biodefense Analysis and
   Countermeasures Center

Public health emergency medical
   countermeasures enterprise
Smallpox research and retention
Strategic National Stockpile

Discussion Questions

1. What are the arguments for keeping or destroying the smallpox virus? Which do you agree with and why?

2. Do we need more or fewer BSL-4 facilities?

3. Would you be comfortable with a BSL-4 facility in your neighborhood? Why or why not?

4. Can you think of ways the private sector might assist in the rapid distribution of medical countermeasures?

5. What should the United States have in its stockpile? Should every country have a stockpile?

6. What are the necessary tasks that need to be completed by response agencies during public health emergencies?

7. What constitutes a public health emergency? How would you define a public health emergency? How does the U.S. federal government define a public health emergency?

8. How can concerns about patient privacy be addressed while ensuring that decision makers have access to the data they need?

9. How can the necessary data and modeling results be tailored for use by decision makers who are not public health experts?

References

1. NIH, NIAID. *Biodefense and Related Programs.* Available at: https://www.niaid.nih.gov/research/biodefense. Accessed May 2017.

2. Glowinski IB, Bernstein JB, Kurilla MG. National Institute of Allergy and Infectious Diseases. In: Katz R, Zilinikas R, eds. *Encyclopedia of Bioterrorism Defense.* 2nd ed: Wiley & Sons; 2011.

3. NIH, NIAID. *Biodefense & Strategic Plan.* August 7, 2015. Available at: https://www.niaid.nih.gov/research/biodefense-strategic-plan. Accessed May 2017.

4. NIH, NIAID. Introduction. *The Need for Biosafety Labs.* 2010. Available at: https://www.niaid.nih.gov/research/biosafety-labs-needed. Accessed June 2017.

5. FAS. *BSL-4 Laboratories in the United States.* 2013. Available at: https://fas.org/programs/bio/research.html. Accessed June 2017.

6. NIH, National Institute of Allergy and Infectious Diseases. *Biodefense and Emerging Infectious Diseases Research Infrastructure.* Available at: https://www.niaid.nih.gov/research/biodefense-emerging-infectious-diseases-research-infrastructure. Accessed May 2017.

7. NIH, National Institute of Allergy and Infectious Disease. Biodefense: Introduction to Biodefense Research. Available at: https://www.niaid.nih.gov/research/biodefense-introduction. Accessed May 2017.

8. Fitch JP. National Biodefense Analysis and Countermeasures Center. In: Katz R, Zilinikas R, eds. *Encyclopedia of Bioterrorism Defense.* 2nd ed: Wiley & Sons; 2011.

9. NIH, NIAID. Office of Chief Scientist, Integrated Research Facility (OCSIRF). October 30, 2008. Available at: https://www.niaid.nih.gov/about/chief-scientist-integrated-research-facility. Accessed May 2017.

10. Gottron F, Shea DA. *CRS Report for Congress: Oversight of High-Containment Biological Laboratories: Issues for Congress.* Federation of American Scientists. May 4, 2009. Available at: http://www.fas.org/sgp/crs/terror/R40418.pdf. Accessed May 2017.

11. Takafuji ET. NIAID/NIH Biodefense Research Efforts and Biocontainment Laboratories. *Applied Biosafety.* 2004;9(3):160–163.

12. Shaw DM, Elger BS, Colledge F. What is a Biobank? Differing Definitions among Biobank Stakeholders. *Clinical Genetics.* March 2014;85:223–227.

13. Fransson MN, Rial-Sebbag E, Brochhausen M, et al. Toward a Common Language for Biobanking. *European Journal of Human Genetics.* 2014;23:22–28.

14. Harris JR, Burton P, Knoppers BM, et al. Toward a Roadmap in Global Biobanking for Health. *European Journal of Human Genetics.* 2012;20:1105–1111.

15. Fidler DP. Influenza Virus Samples, International Law, and Global Health Diplomacy. *Emerging Infectious Diseases.* 2008;14(1):88–94.

16. Fidler DP. Who Owns MERS? The Intellectual Property Controversy Surrounding the Latest Pandemic. *Foreign Policy.* 2013. Available at: https://www.foreignaffairs.com/articles/saudi-arabia/2013-06-06/who-owns-mers. Accessed August 30, 2017.

17. WHO Media Center. *WHO Meeting on Survivors of Ebola Virus Disease: Clinical Care, Research, and Biobanking.* August 2015. Available at: http://www.who.int/mediacentre/events/2015/meeting-on-ebola-survivors/en/. Accessed May 2017.

18. Hayden E. Proposed Ebola Biobank would Strengthen African Science. *Nature.* 2015;524:146–147.

19. Chen H, Pang T. A Call for Global Governance of Biobanks. Bulletin of the World Health Organization. 2015;93:113–117. Available at: https://www.ncbi.nlm.nih.gov/pmc/articles/PMC4339960/.

20. WHO. *WHO First Consultation on Ebola Biobanking.* May 2015. Available at: http://www.who.int/medicines/ebola-treatment/1st_consult_ebola_biobank/en/. Accessed May 2017.

21. WHO. *Report on the 2nd WHO Consultation on Biobanking: Focus on West Africa.* 2015. Available at: http://www.who.int/medicines/ebola-treatment/meetings/2nd_who_biobaking-consultation/en/. Accessed May 2017.

22. Ho CWL. After Ebola, Social Justice as a Base for a Biobanking Governance Framework. *Asia-Pacific Biotech News.* 2016. Available at: http://www.asiabiotech.com/20/2002/20020021x.html. Accessed May 2017.

23. WHO. *WHO Secretariat Response to the Report of the Ebola Interim Assessment Panel.* 2015. Available at: http://www.who.int/csr/resources/publications/ebola/who-response-to-ebola-report.pdf. Accessed May 2017.

24. WHO. *Ebola R&D Summit to Develop R&D Plan of Action for Next Global Health Emergency.* 2015. Available at: http://www.who.int/medicines/ebola-treatment/ebola_r-d_summit/en/. Accessed 30th July 2016.

25. Tucker JB. Developing Medical Countermeasures: From BioShield to BARDA. *Drug Development Research.* June 2009;70(4):224–233.

26. Pandemic and All-Hazards Preparedness Act; Public Law No. 109-417.

27. WHO. *An R&D Blueprint for Action to Prevent Epidemic.* WHA A70/10. May 2016. Available at: http://www.who.int/csr/research-and-development/WHO-R_D-Final10.pdf. Accessed May 2017.

28. Coalition for Epidemic Preparedness Innovations. Overview. Available at: http://cepi.net/sites/default/files/CEPI_2pager_27_Apr_17.pdf. Accessed May 2017.

29. HHS. Assistant Secretary for Preparedness and Response. *Public Health Emergency Medical Countermeasures Enterprise (PHEMCE) Review.* August 2010. Available at: https://www.medicalcountermeasures.gov/media/1138/mcmreviewfinalcover-508.pdf. Accessed May 2017.

30. Centers for Disease Control and Prevention. Strategic National Stockpile (SNS). Emergency Preparedness and Response. May 21, 2010. Available at: http://www.bt.cdc.gov/stockpile/. Accessed May 2017.

31. DHS, ESFLG. Model and Data Inventory. 2016. Available at: https://gis.fema.gov/Model-and-Data-Inventory/. Accessed June 2017.

CHAPTER 8

Natural Disasters and Humanitarian Response

LEARNING OBJECTIVES

By the end of this chapter, the reader will be able to:

- Identify the role of federal agencies in responding to the public health implications of natural disasters
- Identify the role of international organizations in providing the humanitarian response to disasters
- Describe the international governance of natural disasters and coordinated humanitarian response

▶ Natural Disasters

It is an absolute certainty that natural disasters will occur all over the world: hurricanes and tsunamis will form, earthquakes will occur near fault lines, active volcanoes will erupt, tornadoes will sweep through regions, snow will fall, fire will spread, and low-lying regions will flood.[1] Some disasters are exacerbated by human actions, such as drought leading to famine or shores becoming contaminated with oil. Public health emergency preparedness is as much about planning for and responding to these types of disasters as it is about responding to terrorist events. In fact, the public health community is much more likely to engage in a response to a natural or humanitarian disaster than to an intentional or accidental one, based on probability of events.

Natural disasters have the potential to impact very large populations. They can lead to morbidity and mortality, disrupt basic services, pose environmental challenges, and completely unhinge a community (BOX 8-1). TABLE 8-1 illustrates the magnitude, as measured in mortality, of major natural disasters and BOX 8-2 describes one particular natural disaster in the U.S.

Public health professionals have long been engaged in disaster response; as long as there have been emergencies, there have been medical and health personnel attending to the needs of populations. In the United States, Centers for Disease Control and Prevention (CDC) started responding officially to international disasters in the 1960s, when an Epidemic Intelligence Service (EIS) team traveled to Nigeria to help maintain public health programs in the midst of a civil war. Over the decades, CDC has developed public health and epidemiologic tools to address the realities of disaster situations and displaced populations. The public health community enters a disaster situation and establishes prevention and control measures, collects critical data to support response, and works to meet the short- and long-term needs of the population.[2,3] Often, the most experienced public health and medical professionals on the ground during an emergency come from the non-governmental organization (NGO) community, which has decades of experience responding to and helping populations recover from disasters. In fact, the American Red Cross, an NGO, has a federal charter to engage in disaster relief, and has specific responsibilities outlined in the National Response Framework based on its recognized expertise in this area.[4] In addition, military assets are utilized during emergencies to get qualified personnel to the event site quickly and, most importantly, provide logistical support, since some disasters require resources only the militaries of the world possess (e.g., the ability to reach isolated populations, bring supplies to remote regions, and establish care and living centers in harsh environments).[5,6]

For most natural disasters and humanitarian emergencies that occur in the United States, Federal Emergency Management Agency (FEMA) is the lead federal agency. FEMA leads an all-of-nation approach, as captured in the National Planning Frameworks. The National Mitigation Framework brings together all segments of society to focus on preparedness and lessen the impact of disasters. FEMA also runs Threat and Hazard Identification and Risk Assessment (THIRA), which is discussed in Chapters 10 and 11.[7]

▶ International Disaster Response

Globally, the number of humanitarian emergencies and disasters have increased at an unprecedented scale. Over 200 million people are affected by natural and technological disasters every year. Approximately,

---

BOX 8-1 Quote Defining Humanitarian Emergency

A humanitarian emergency is an event or series of events that represents a critical threat to the health, safety, security or wellbeing of a community or other large group of people, usually over a wide area.

—Humanitarian Coalition

Reproduced from Humanitarian Coalition. *What Is a Humanitarian Emergency?* Available at: http://humanitariancoalition.ca/media-resources/factsheets/what-is-a-humanitarian-emergency. Accessed June 2017.

TABLE 8-1 Select Major Natural Disasters, 1900–Present

Date	Event	Location	Approximate Death Toll
March 11, 2011	Earthquake/tsunami	Tohoku, Japan	15,800–18,500
January 12, 2010	Earthquake	Port-au-Prince, Haiti	230,000
May 2, 2008	Cyclone	Myanmar	138,000
October 8, 2005	Earthquake	Pakistan	75,000
December 26, 2004	Tsunami (Indian Ocean)	Indonesia, Thailand, Sri Lanka, India, and more	220,000+
July 28, 1976	Earthquake	Tangshan, China	242,000–655,000
November 13, 1970	Cyclone	Bangladesh	500,000
May–August 1931	Yellow River and Yangtze River floods	China	1–3.7 million
May 22, 1927	Earthquake	Xining, China	200,000
September 1, 1923	Earthquake and fires	Tokyo, Japan	143,000
December 16, 1920	Earthquake	Haiyuan, China	200,000

Data from Noji E. *The Public Health Consequences of Disasters.* p 5. New York: Oxford University Press, 1997; CBC News. The World's Worst Natural Disasters: Calamities of the 20th and 21st Centuries. *CBC News.* August 30, 2010. Available at: http://www.cbc.ca/world/story/2008/05/08/f-natural-disasters-history.html?rdr=525. Accessed July 8, 2015; U.S. Agency for International Development, Office of U.S. Foreign Disaster Assistance. *Disaster History: Significant Data on Major Disasters Worldwide, 1900-Present.* August 1993. Available at: http://pdf.usaid.gov/pdf_docs/PNABP986.pdf. Accessed July 8, 2015; Associated Press. Haiti Raises Earthquake Toll to 230,000. *The Washington Post.* February 10, 2010. Available at: http://www.washingtonpost.com/wp-dyn/content /article/2010/02/09/AR2010020904447.html. Accessed July 8, 2015; U.S. Geological Survey. *Magnitude 9.1—Off the West Coast of Northern Sumatra: Summary.* Available at: https://earthquake. usgs.gov/earthquakes/eventpage/official20041226005853450_30#executive. Accessed July 8, 2015.

BOX 8-2 Hurricane Katrina and the Public Health Response

On August 29, 2005, Hurricane Katrina landed on the Gulf Coast of the United States, reaching Mississippi, Louisiana, and Alabama. It came ashore with 115–130 mph winds and brought with it a water surge that in some locations rose as high as 27 feet. The surge pushed 6–12 miles inland and flooded approximately 80% of the city of New Orleans. Some 93,000 square miles were affected, resulting in 1300 fatalities, 2 million displaced persons, 300,000 destroyed homes, and almost $100 billion in property damage.

Katrina was the worst domestic natural disaster in recent history, but the consequences of the event were made worse by a faltering levee system designed by the U.S. Army Corps of Engineers and a failure of government at all levels to properly prepare for and respond to the disaster. First, long-term warnings went unheeded. It was clear that a hurricane of this type would eventually hit the region, yet local and state officials, even after running exercises based on such a scenario, failed to properly prepare. Local and state officials were unable to evacuate all of the citizens, struggled with logistics, and did not make proper preparations for dealing with vulnerable populations, including nursing home residents. The federal government failed to adequately anticipate the needs of the state and local authorities, and the insufficient coordination resulted in a lack of resources and a too-slow response.

The public health and medical response coordinated by the federal government followed the traditional response to a flood or hurricane: focus on sanitation and hygiene, water safety, surveillance and infection control, environmental health, and access to care. Katrina, though, also presented unique challenges, such as the inability of displaced persons to manage chronic disease conditions and access medications, death and illness from dehydration, and mental health problems; all associated with the widespread devastation among those affected.

Almost all offices and branches of the federal Department of Health and Human Services (of which CDC is a part) eventually became involved in the response to Katrina. CDC sent staff to the affected areas, deployed the Strategic National Stockpile (SNS) to provide drugs and medical supplies, and developed public health and occupational health guidance. The Food and Drug Administration issued recommendations for handling drugs that might have been affected by the flood. The National Institutes of Health set up a phone-based medical consultation service for providers in the region. The Substance Abuse and Mental Health Services Administration set up crisis counseling assistance and provided emergency response grants.

In addition, the National Disaster Medical System deployed 50 Disaster Medical Assistance Teams to try to accommodate and treat hurricane victims. Disaster Mortuary Operational Response Teams also deployed to help process bodies. The Department of Defense set up field hospitals at the New Orleans International Airport and aboard naval vessels. The Department of Veterans Affairs evacuated both of its local hospitals—one prior to the storm, one afterward.

Data from The White House. *The Federal Response to Hurricane Katrina: Lessons Learned*. February 2006. pp 5–9. Available at: http://library.stmarytx.edu/acadlib/edocs/katrinawh.pdf. Accessed July 8, 2015; Greenough PG, Kirsch TD. Hurricane Katrina. Public Health Response—Assessing Needs. *The New England Journal of Medicine*. 2005;353(15):1544–1546; Lister SA. *CRS Report for Congress: Hurricane Katrina: The Public Health and Medical Response*. September 21, 2005. Available at: http://fpc.state.gov/documents/organization/54255.pdf. Accessed July 8, 2015.

---

130 million people around the world are in need of humanitarian assistance and more than 65 million people are displaced.[8]

▶ Disaster Risk Reduction

Disaster risk reduction (DRR) is defined as, "the development and application of policies, strategies and practices to reduce vulnerabilities and disaster risks throughout society."[9] It is designed to address the failures that occur when people and communities are not prepared for recurring natural disasters, nor have the resiliency to recover from such events. Since the late 1980s, the international community has been trying to address DRR through a series of international agreements and strategies to engage not just national governments, but also the nongovernmental community and populations that are directly impacted by disasters. In 2005, countries agreed to the Hyogo

Framework for Action 2005–2015, which provided guidance to reduce disaster risk, while aligning with the Millennium Development Goals. Implementation of Hyogo, however, was challenging and highlighted a series of gaps in the agreement, including building resilience at all levels of society.

According to the United Nations, in the 10 years that followed the Hyogo Framework:

Disasters have continued to exact a heavy toll and, as a result, the well-being and safety of persons, communities and countries as a whole have been affected. Over 700 thousand people have lost their lives, over 1.4 million have been injured and approximately 23 million have been made homeless as a result of disasters. Overall, more than 1.5 billion people have been affected by disasters in various ways, with women, children and people in vulnerable situations disproportionately affected. The total

UNISDR
The United Nations Office for Disaster Risk Reduction

www.preventionweb.net/go/sfdrr
www.unisdr.org
isdr@un.org

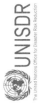

Chart of the Sendai Framework for Disaster Risk Reduction
2015-2030

Scope and purpose

The present framework will apply to the risk of small-scale and large-scale, frequent and infrequent, sudden and slow-onset disasters, caused by natural or manmade hazards as well as related environmental, technological and biological hazards and risks. It aims to guide the multi-hazard management of disaster risk in development at all levels as well as within and across all sectors.

Expected outcome

The substantial reduction of disaster risk and losses in lives, livelihoods and health and in the economic, physical, social, cultural and environmental assets of persons, businesses, communities and countries

Goal

Prevent new and reduce existing disaster risk through the implementation of integrated and inclusive economic, structural, legal, social, health, cultural, educational, environmental, technological, political and institutional measures that prevent and reduce hazard exposure and vulnerability to disaster, increase preparedness for response and recovery, and thus strengthen resilience

Targets

Substantially reduce global disaster mortality by 2030, aiming to lower average per 100,000 global mortality between 2020-2030 compared to 2005-2015	Substantially reduce the number of affected people globally by 2030, aiming to lower the average global figure per 100,000 between 2020-2030 compared to 2005-2015	Reduce direct disaster economic loss in relation to global gross domestic product (GDP) by 2030	Substantially reduce disaster damage to critical infrastructure and disruption of basic services, among them health and educational facilities, including through developing their resilience by 2030	Substantially increase the number of countries with national and local disaster risk reduction strategies by 2020	Substantially enhance international cooperation to developing countries through adequate and sustainable support to complement their national actions for implementation of this framework by 2030	Substantially increase the availability of and access to multi-hazard early warning systems and disaster risk information and assessments to people by 2030

Priorities for Action

There is a need for focused action within and across sectors by States at local, national, regional and global levels in the following four priority areas.

Priority 1
Understanding disaster risk

Priority 2
Strengthening disaster risk governance to manage disaster risk

Priority 3
Investing in disaster risk reduction for resilience

Priority 4
Enhancing disaster preparedness for effective response, and to «Build Back Better» in recovery, rehabilitation and reconstruction

FIGURE 8-1 Sendai Framework for Disaster Risk Reduction 2015–2030

Reproduced from UNISDR. *Chart of the Sendai Framework for Disaster Risk Reduction 2014–2030*. Available at: http://www.preventionweb.net/files/44983_sendaiframeworksimplifiedchart.pdf. Accessed June 2017. ©2017 United Nations. Reprinted with the permission of the United Nations.

economic loss was more than $1.3 trillion. In addition, between 2008 and 2012, 144 million people were displaced by disasters. Disasters, many of which are exacerbated by climate change and which are increasing in frequency and intensity, significantly impede progress towards sustainable development.[10]

To address the shortcomings of Hyogo and move forward with DRR, 185 countries participated in 150 official planning sessions, along with international organizations, NGOs, private sector, and local representatives to agree to the Sendai Framework for Disaster Risk Reduction 2015–2030 (**FIGURE 8-1**). The Sendai Framework includes four priorities for action:

1. Understanding disaster risk
2. Strengthening disaster risk governance to manage disaster risk
3. Investing in disaster risk reduction for resilience
4. Enhancing disaster preparedness for effective response, and "Build Back Better" in recovery, rehabilitation, and reconstruction[10]

This framework fully integrates all levels of society, setting global targets and guiding principles under the four priorities for action.

DRR and risk management are areas that are now being more fully adopted at regional levels, and particularly within the health field. For example, in 1997, the World Health Organization (WHO) Regional Committee for Africa adopted a Regional Strategy for Emergency and Humanitarian Action. In 2011, a new regional strategy on disaster risk management for the health sector was adopted, and with this strategy, a set of tools that included a country capacity assessment, vulnerability risk assessment and mapping, safe health facility index, and recovery framework (**FIGURE 8-2**).[11]

▶ U.N. System

To coordinate activities across all of the United Nations during humanitarian organizations, the United Nations created the Inter-Agency Standing Committee (IASC). This organization, established in 1991, underwent major revisions in 2005 (known as

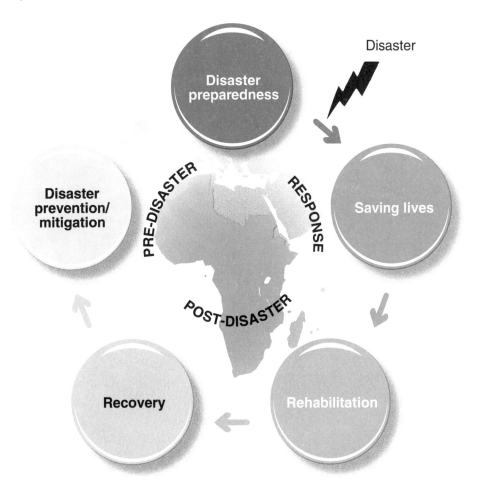

FIGURE 8-2 Disaster risk management cycle

Reproduced from Kalambay K, Manzila TC, Kasolo FC, et al. WHO, African Health Observatory. *Disaster Risk Management: A Strategy for the Health Sector in the African Region.* November 2013. p 5. Available at: http://www.afro.who.int/sites/default/files/2017-06/ahm18.pdf

the Humanitarian Reform Agenda) to rethink how the international community responds to disasters in an effort to be more predictable, accountable, and coordinated.[12] This was followed by another major revision in 2011, known as the Transformative Agenda. This group develops protocols and processes for responding to large-scale disasters that require multiple U.N. agencies. The IASC provides what is known as the cluster approach to large-scale humanitarian emergencies. This cluster approach attempts to clarify the roles and responsibilities across multiple sectors of a response;

there are now 11 different sectors (**FIGURE 8-3**). The WHO leads the health cluster (**TABLE 8-2**).

In order for the cluster system to work, numerous organizations and entities come together. The entire cluster system is coordinated by the U.N. OCHA.[17] An Emergency Relief Coordinator (ERC) oversees the emergency, and is often appointed by a humanitarian coordinator (HC) who assesses if the response is necessary and if so, organized appropriately. The IASC develops the policies and agrees on clear delineation of responsibilities for the humanitarian response.[18]

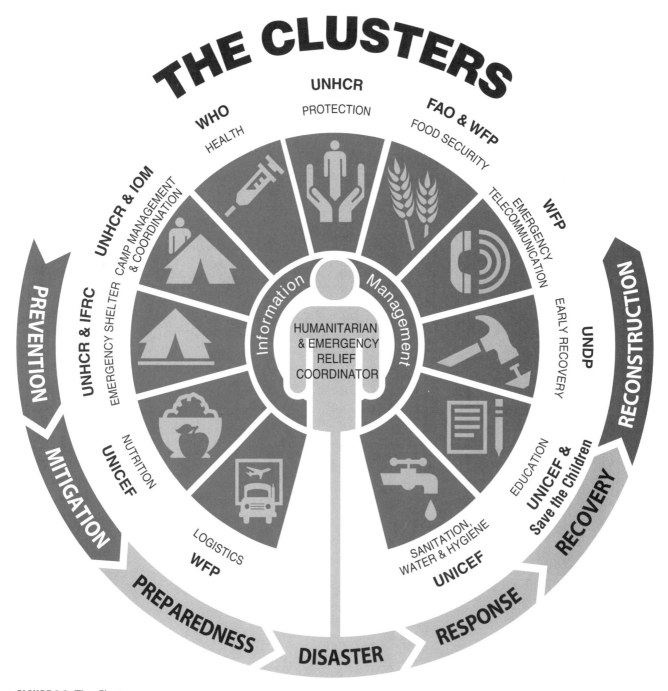

FIGURE 8-3 The Clusters

TABLE 8-2 Global Cluster Leads

Global Clusters	Global Cluster Leads
Camp Coordination/Management	IOM & UNHCR
Early Recovery	UNDP
Education	UNICEF & Save the Children
Emergency Shelter and NFI	IFRC & UNHCR
Emergency Telecommunications	WFP
Food Security	FAO & WFP
Health	WHO
Logistics	WFP
Nutrition	UNICEF
Protection Areas of Responsibility (AoRs): 1. Child Protection 2. Gender-Based Violence 3. Housing Land and Property 4. Mine Action	UNHCR AoRs' respective focal point agencies: 1. UNICEF 2. UNFPA 3. NRC and IRFC 4. UNMAS
Water, Sanitation, and Hygiene	UNICEF

Each cluster also has multiple public and private sector partners

Data from UN OCHA. Global Clusters. *Humanitarian Response*. Available at: https://www.humanitarianresponse.info/en/coordination/clusters/global. Accessed September 9, 2017.

🔍 CASE STUDY: Flooding in Pakistan

In July 2010, monsoon rains caused severe flooding in Pakistan, leaving approximately one-fifth of the country under water and affecting more than 20 million people (**FIGURES 8-4**and **8-5**).[13] The Pakistani government utilized helicopters and ships to move displaced people, but quickly became overwhelmed and looked to the international community for assistance. People were displaced and many were left without any shelter or access to clean water, raising the risk of epidemics. The government was also looking at the long-term consequences, as many livestock drowned, approximately 80% of the harvests were destroyed, and communities would have to be rebuilt.[14,15]

In Pakistan, the response was led by the National Disaster Management Authority (NDMA) and the Provincial and District Disaster Management Authorities (PDMA/DDMA) at the subnational levels. U.N. Office for the Coordination of Humanitarian Affairs (OCHA) coordinated information through ReliefWeb online, and WHO along with the Ministry of Health led the health cluster. NDMA prioritized the food, health shelter, and WASH clusters; and the cluster system was decentralized to the provincial level to address the differing concerns in each region of the country. While the cluster system worked, there were still challenges of fragmentation and delays in funding.[16]

(continues)

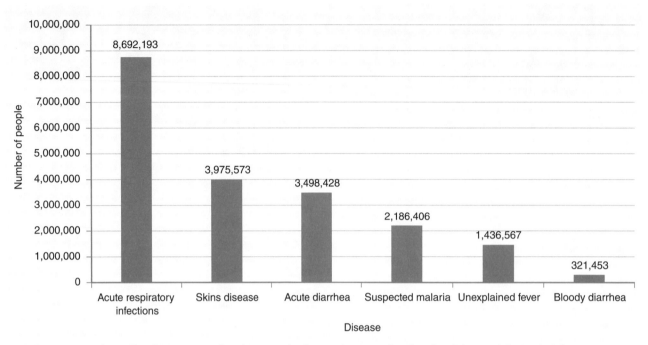

FIGURE 8-4 Number of leading causes of seeking medical consultations after flood in Pakistan July 2010–July 2011

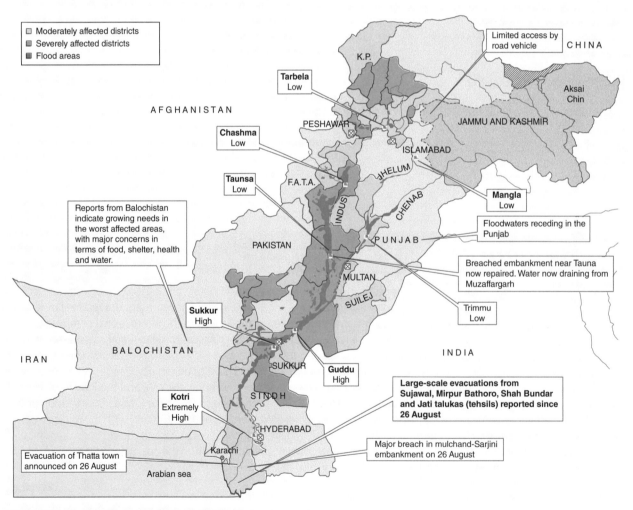

FIGURE 8-5 Flood affected districts in Pakistan

This process has emerged as the best way to coordinate the multitude of entities that must be engaged in a complex humanitarian emergency.

▶ World Health Organization

In 2016, there were approximately 50 countries requiring emergency operations, and WHO monitored over 160 public health events in just that year.[19] Under an Emergency Response Framework (ERF), the WHO clarifies its roles and responsibilities in emergencies, sets out WHO's core commitments, and details the steps that the organization needs to take during emergencies, including event verification and risk assessment. The ERF provides guidance for how to grade an emergency—a process that guides and triggers internal actions. Events range from "ungraded," which are monitored, but do not yet require a response, to grade 3 events in which the WHO or the larger international community must provide a substantial response (**FIGURE 8-6**).

TABLE 8-3 shows the graded events that WHO was working on in 2016. The majority of these events derive from conflict or complex humanitarian crises (40%). Only 16% of the graded events were outbreaks,

11% earthquakes, 11% storm, and the rest (22%) from other types of events. To respond to these events, WHO prioritizes the emergency response, to meet the immediate needs of the population, followed by recovery to build and restore services, and lastly they focus on risk reduction to mitigate risk and reduce vulnerabilities. Per the ERF, the WHO's core commitments to emergency response are as follows:

1. Develop evidence-based health-sector response strategy
2. Ensure disease surveillance and early warning and response systems are in place and functional
3. Provide current information on the health situation
4. Monitor the application of best practices
5. Provide relevant technical experts[20]

To address humanitarian emergencies, WHO uses two systems to bring in relevant technical expertise and expand the health emergencies workforce: Global Outbreak Alert and Response Network (GOARN) and Emergency Medical Teams (EMTs). The Global Outbreak Alert and Response Network is

Ungraded: an event that is being assessed, tracked or monitored by WHO but that requires no WHO response at the time.

Grade 1: a single or multiple country event with minimal public health consequences that requires a minimal WCO response or a minimal international WHO response. Organizational and/or external support required by the WCO is minimal. The provision of support to the WCO is coordinated by a focal point in the regional office.

Grade 2: a single or multiple country event with moderate public health consequences that requires a moderate WCO response and/or moderate international WHO response. Organizational and/or external support required by the WCO is moderate. An Emergency Support Team, run out of the regional office,[6] coordinates the provision of support to the WCO.

Grade 3: a single or multiple country event with substantial public health consequences that requires a substantial WCO response and/or substantial international WHO response. Organizational and/or external support required by the WCO is substantial. An Emergency Support Team, run out of the regional office, coordinates the provision of support to the WCO.

FIGURE 8-6 World Health Organization grade definitions

TABLE 8-3 World Health Organization's List of Acute/Graded Emergencies between January 1–October 1, 2016

Country, Territory, or Area/Emergency	Type of Crisis	Date of Initial Emergency Grading	Date of Revision of Grading	Current Grade
Afghanistan	Earthquake	October 28, 2015		1
Angola	Yellow fever outbreak	February 12, 2016		2
Bangladesh	Tropical cyclone Roanu	May 21, 2016		1
Cameroon	Conflict/civil strife	April 1, 2015	August 18, 2016	2
Central African Republic	Conflict/civil strife	December 13, 2013 (grade 3)	June 3, 2015	2
Democratic People's Republic of Korea	Floods	September 12, 2016		1
Democratic Republic of the Congo	Cholera outbreak	June 23, 2016		2
	Yellow fever outbreak	April 27, 2016		2
	Complex emergency	July 20, 2013		2
Ecuador	Earthquake	April 17, 2016		2
Ethiopia	Impact of El Niño phenomenon	November 18, 2015		2
Fiji	Tropical cyclone Winston	February 24, 2016		1
Guinea	Ebola virus disease outbreak	March 24, 2014	June 1, 2016 (grade end)	Ungraded
Indonesia	Mount Sinabung eruption	May 22, 2016		1
Iraq	Conflict/civil strife	August 12, 2014		3
Kenya	Severe acute respiratory illness outbreak	April 20, 2016		1
Liberia	Ebola virus disease outbreak	July 26, 2014	June 9, 2016 (grade end)	Ungraded
Libya	Conflict/civil strife	August 28, 2014 (grade 1)	December 10, 2015	2
Mali	Conflict/civil strife	February 4, 2013 (grade 2)	October 16, 2015	1
Myanmar	Floods	August 12, 2015		2
Niger	Conflict/civil strife	April 1, 2015	August 18, 2016	2
	Rift Valley fever outbreak	September 26, 2016		2

Nigeria	Complex emergency	April 1, 2015 (grade 2)	August 18, 2016	3
Pakistan	Earthquake	October 28, 2015		1
	Displacement	June 20, 2014		1
Papua New Guinea	Drought related to El Niño/ food insecurity	September 1, 2015	May 31, 2016	1
Philippines	Moro conflict in Mindanao	October 24, 2013		2
	Typhoon Koppu	October 25, 2015		1
Sierra Leone	Ebola virus disease outbreak	July 26, 2014	June 9, 2016 (grade end)	Ungraded
South Sudan	Conflict/civil strife	February 12, 2014	February 12, 2015	3
Sri Lanka	Floods/landslides	May 15, 2016		1
Syrian Arab Republic	Conflict/civil strife	January 3, 2013	August 26, 2015	3
Thailand	Conflict/civil strife	October 19, 2013		1
Ukraine	Conflict/civil strife	February 20, 2013 (grade 1)	February 12, 2015	2
United Republic of Tanzania	Refugee displacement	May 18, 2015 (grade 1)	December 15, 2015	2
	Cholera outbreak	December 15, 2015		2
West Bank and Gaza Strip	Conflict/civil strife	July 13, 2014 (grade 2)	November 10, 2015	1
Yemen	Complex emergency	April 4, 2015 (grade 2)	July 1, 2015	3
Zika virus disease outbreak—globally (75 countries)	Public Health Emergency of International Concern	January 20, 2016		2

a coalition of now over 200 partners around the world. This group expands the reach of the WHO, providing health experts and operational support and contributing to all aspects of preparedness, detection, and response during health emergencies. EMTs are teams of clinicians, logisticians, and others who agree to be part of the global health emergency workforce, and can provide temporary surge capacity to areas in need during crises. As of 2017, over 75 organizations around the world had begun the process of training and quality improvement to be certified for deployment under the WHO.[8]

▶ Sphere Project

The Humanitarian Disaster Response community works with populations at their most vulnerable. In 1997, a group of seasoned humanitarian response professionals founded the Sphere Project, to improve the quality of humanitarian response and hold organizations and individuals accountable to affected populations, donors, and constituents. There were two founding principles for the Sphere Project:

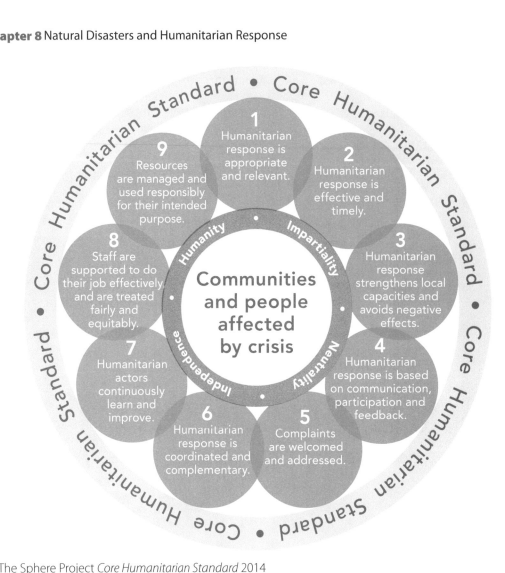

FIGURE 8-7 The Sphere Project *Core Humanitarian Standard* 2014

Reproduced from Core Humanitarian Standard. *Core Humanitarian Standard on Quality and Accountability*. 2014. p 4. Available at: https://corehumanitarianstandard.org/files/files/Core%20
Humanitarian%20Standard%20-%20English.pdf.

■ Those affected by disaster or conflict have a right to life with dignity and, therefore, a right to assistance.

■ All possible steps should be taken to alleviate human suffering arising out of disaster or conflict.[21]

There are nine core humanitarian standards (see **FIGURE 8-7**) and a core text, known as the *Humanitarian Charter and Minimum Standards in Humanitarian Response*, which provide detailed guidance for working with health systems and providing essential health services.[22]

Key Words

Cluster system
Disaster risk reduction
Grading for emergencies

Hurricane Katrina
Natural disasters
Sendai Framework

Sphere Project

Discussion Questions

1. How did the public health community respond to Hurricane Katrina? What lessons can be learned to better prepare for future response efforts?

2. What is the cluster system and do you believe it works? If not, what would make it work better?

3. Why was it important to create the Sphere Project?

4. How can international response to natural disasters be better coordinated?

References

1. Portions of this chapter come from Katz R, Standley, C. Public health preparedness policy. In: Teitelbaum, JB, ed. *Essentials of Health Policy & Law*, 3rd ed. Burlington, MA: Jones & Bartlett Learning; 2017:253–270.

2. Noji E. *The Public Health Consequences of Disasters*. New York: Oxford University Press, 1997.

3. Gregg MB. *The Public Health Consequences of Disasters. CDC Monograph*. Atlanta, GA: Centers for Disease Control and Prevention, 1989.

4. The American National Red Cross. *Our Federal Charter*. Available at: http://www.redcross.org/about-us/history/federal-charter. Accessed June 8, 2017.

5. Wiharta S, Ahmad H, Haine J-Y, et al. *The Effectiveness of Foreign Military Assets in Natural Disaster Response*. Stockholm International Peace Research Institute. 2008. Available at: http://reliefweb.int/sites/reliefweb.int/files/resources/236476AD3257088DC125741000474F20-sipri_mar2008.pdf. Accessed July 8, 2015.

6. VanRooyen M, Leaning J. After the Tsunami—Facing the public health challenges. *The New England Journal of Medicine*. 2005;352(5):435–438.

7. Department of Homeland Security. *National Strategy Recommendations: Future Disaster Preparedness*. September 6, 2013. Available at: https://www.fema.gov/media-library-data/bd125e67fb2bd37f8d609cbd71b835ae/FEMA%20National%20Strategy%20Recommendations%20(V4).pdf. Accessed June 2017.

8. Secretariat; WHO. *Health Workforce Coordination in Emergencies with Health Consequences*. A70/11. April 13, 2017. Available at: http://apps.who.int/gb/ebwha/pdf_files/WHA70/A70_11-en.pdf. Accessed June 2017.

9. Twigg J. Overseas Development Institute. *Disaster Risk Reduction. Good Practice Review*. 2015. Available at: http://goodpracticereview.org/wp-content/uploads/2015/10/GPR-9-web-string-1.pdf. Accessed June 2017.

10. United Nations. *Sendai Framework for Disaster Risk Reduction 2015–2030*. 2015. Available at: http://www.preventionweb.net/files/43291_sendaiframeworkfordrren.pdf. Accessed June 2017.

11. Kalambay K, Manzila TC, Kasolo FC, et al. WHO, African Health Observatory. *Disaster Risk Management: A Strategy for the Health Sector in the African Region*. November 2013. p 5. Available at: https://www.aho.afro.who.int/sites/default/files/ahm/reports/736/ahm-18-01-disaster-risk-management-strategy-health-sector.pdf. Accessed June 2017.

12. UN, OCHA. *How the Cluster System Works*. Cluster Coordination. Available at: https://www.unocha.org/legacy/what-we-do/coordination-tools/cluster-coordination. Accessed June 2017.

13. Gronewold N. Flooding in Pakistan? *Scientific American*. October 12, 2010. Available at: https://www.scientificamerican.com/article/what-caused-the-massive-flooding-in-pakistan/. Accessed June 2017.

14. FAO. *Questions and Answers Pakistan Floods*. August 10, 2010. Available at: http://www.fao.org/fileadmin/user_upload/newsroom/docs/pakistan_qa.pdf. Accessed June 2017.

15. Péchayre M. Feinstein International Center. *Humanitarian Action in Pakistan 2005–2010: Challenges, Principles, and Politics*. January 2011. Available at: http://fic.tufts.edu/assets/pakistan.pdf. Accessed June 2017.

16. Shabir O. A Summary Case Report on the Health Impacts and Response to the Pakistan Floods of 2010. *PLOS Currents Disasters*. April 11, 2013. doi:10.1371/currents.dis.cc7bd532ce252c1b740c39a2a827993f. Available at: http://currents.plos.org/disasters/article/dis-13-0009-a-summary-case-report-on-the-health-impacts-and-response-to-the-pakistan-floods-of-2010/.

17. O'Brien S. UN System Coordination on Outbreaks and Health Emergencies. Statement Presented at: UN General Assembly, November 11, 2016; New York. Available at: https://docs.unocha.org/sites/dms/Documents/StatementonCoordinationonOutbreaksandHealthEmergencies.pdf. Accessed June 2017.

18. OCHA, Humanitarian Response. *Who Does What?* Available at: www.humanitarianresponse.info/en/about-clusters/who-does-what. Accessed June 2017.

19. Director General; WHO. *Health Emergencies: WHO Response in Severe, Large-Scale Emergencies*. A70/9. April 10, 2017. Available at: http://apps.who.int/gb/ebwha/pdf_files/WHA70/A70_9-en.pdf. Accessed June 2017.

20. WHO. *Emergency Response Framework*. 2013. p 19. Available at: http://www.who.int/hac/about/erf_.pdf. Accessed June 2017.

21. The Sphere Project. *What is Sphere? Humanitarian Charter and Minimum Standards in Humanitarian Response*. Available at: http://www.spherehandbook.org/en/what-is-sphere/. Accessed June 2017.

22. The Sphere Project. *The Sphere Handbook*. 2011. Available at: http://www.sphereproject.org/handbook/. Accessed June 2017.

CHAPTER 9

Surveillance and Attribution Investigations

LEARNING OBJECTIVES

By the end of this chapter, the reader will be able to:

- Understand the literature surrounding the differentiation between natural and intentional outbreaks
- Describe an attribution investigation
- Discuss the role of microbial forensics
- Describe how domestic investigations of alleged biological or chemical weapons use are conducted
- Describe how international investigations of alleged biological or chemical weapons use are conducted
- Discuss the roles of the Federal Bureau of Investigation and public health community

▶ Introduction

Detecting and responding to disease outbreaks and public health events are core components of the public health mission. Detection relies upon a comprehensive disease surveillance system, which then allows for the rapid detection, identification, characterization, and containment of biological threats. Once an outbreak has been detected, basic field epidemiology outlines the steps public health professionals need to take next: determine the existence of an outbreak; confirm the diagnosis; define a case; count cases; identify person, place, and time (the who, what, and when of the event); determine who is at risk of becoming ill; develop and test hypothesis regarding exposure; and contain the outbreak to minimize morbidity and mortality in the population. Epidemiologists are trained to conduct these investigations. They know how to determine if an epidemic is taking place, they work with

the public health laboratories to examine specimens, they identify possible and probable cases, they coordinate with the healthcare system to appropriately treat patients, they analyze data to determine causation, and they use all of the resources available to them to contain and mitigate the consequences of the event.

But what happens when a disease outbreak or public health emergency is suspected of being an intentional event? And can public health officials anticipate and plan for such an event?

In this chapter, we first describe the current system for biosurveillance and the tools for detection of potential biological threats and other public health emergencies. We then examine how one begins to differentiate between naturally occurring events and intentional events, and if an event is suspected of being intentional, what steps must be taken to minimize the damages incurred. The investigation can suddenly become much more complicated and involve many new players. We look at some of the work that has been done to build relationships between the organizations that need to work together on these types of investigations (**BOX 9-1**).

Biosurveillance can be defined as any method to detect and monitor a biological incident whether of intentional or natural origin. The 2007 Homeland Security Presidential Directive (HSPD-21) defines biosurveillance as follows:

> The process of active data-gathering with appropriate analysis and interpretation of biosphere data that might relate to disease activity and threats to human or animal health—whether infectious, toxic, metabolic, or otherwise, and regardless of intentional or natural origin—in order to achieve early warning of health threats, early detection of health events, and overall situational awareness of disease activity.[1]

This notion of situational awareness is defined as the basic ability to understand what is going on in a given area. It is the ability to collect and analyze data in order to make appropriately informed predictions and decisions (**BOX 9-2**).

Disease surveillance as a concept has evolved from the observation of individuals suspected of being ill to the current conception of ongoing, systematic collection, analysis, and reporting of health-related data.[2,3] The purpose of these activities is to monitor disease and population health and detect abnormal events. Understanding the baseline health conditions of a population allows decision makers to set priorities, design research programs, and identify short- and long-term public health risks. Being able to detect an abnormality, an unusual health threat, an emerging infectious disease, or any other potential public health emergency allows for a quick and effective response to treat patients, contain the spread of disease, and mitigate the consequences of the event. This last step—response—is essential, as it has been said that *surveillance without response is just documentation of misery.*

There are many different kinds of public health surveillance activities, ranging from periodic surveys to real-time reporting through direct communication from either laboratories or clinicians or warnings from advanced data algorithms designed to pick up unusual syndromes or behaviors. While surveys and surveillance of endemic diseases are essential to the public health community, it is the surveillance of emerging infections, unusual events, and potential public health emergencies which most inform public health preparedness, and are the situations in which rapid detection is essential for saving lives. **FIGURE 9-1**

BOX 9-1 Global Health Security Agenda Action Packages For Real-Time Biosurveillance (Detect 2/3) and Linking Public Health with Law and Multisectoral Rapid Response (Respond 2)

Real-Time Biosurveillance

Desired National Impact: A functioning public health surveillance system capable of identifying potential events of concern for public health and health security, and country and regional capacity to analyze and link data from and between strengthened real-time surveillance systems, including interoperable, interconnected electronic reporting systems. Countries will support the use of interoperable, interconnected systems capable of linking and integrating multisectoral surveillance data and using resulting information to enhance the capacity to quickly detect and respond to developing biological threats. Foundational capacity is necessary for both indicator- (including syndromic) and event-based surveillance, in order to support prevention and control activities and intervention targeting for both established infectious diseases and new and emerging public health threats. Strong surveillance will support the timely recognition of the emergence of relatively rare or previously undescribed pathogens in specific countries.

Public Health with Law and Response Action Package

Desired National Impact: Development and implementation of a memorandum of understanding (MOU) or other similar framework outlining roles, responsibilities, and best practices for sharing relevant information between and among appropriate human and animal health, law enforcement, and defense personnel and validation of the MOU through periodic exercises and simulations. In collaboration with Food and Agriculture Organization (FAO), International Criminal Police Organization (INTERPOL), Organization for Animal Health (OIE), World Health Organization, individual Biological and Toxin Weapons Convention states parties (and where appropriate the Implementation Support Unit), the U.N. Secretary-General's Mechanism (UNSGM) for Investigation of Alleged Use of Chemical and Biological Weapons, and other relevant regional and international organizations as appropriate, countries will develop and implement model systems to conduct and support joint criminal and epidemiological investigations in the event of suspected biological incidents of deliberate origin.

Reproduced from CDC. *Global Health Security Agenda: Action Packages.* Available at: https://www.cdc.gov/globalhealth/security/pdf/ghsa-action-packages_24-september-2014.pdf. Accessed June 2017.

In February 2010, the Centers for Disease Control and Prevention (CDC) released a National Biosurveillance Strategy for Human Health V2.0. Within this strategy, CDC defined biosurveillance as follows:

Biosurveillance in the context of human health is a new term for the science and practice of managing health-related data and information for early warning of threats and hazards, early detection of events, and rapid characterization of the event so that effective actions can be taken to mitigate adverse health effects. It represents a new health information paradigm that seeks to integrate and efficiently manage health-related data and information across a range of information systems toward timely and accurate population health situation awareness.

The scope and function of biosurveillance includes the following:

- All hazards: including biological, chemical, radiological, nuclear and explosives.
- Defined by urgency and potential for multi-jurisdictional interest.
- Urgent notifiable conditions and non-specific and novel health events.
- Ad hoc data gathering, analysis, and application of information.
- Functions: Case Detection, Event Detection, Signal Validation, Event Characterization, Notification and Communication and, Quality Control and Improvement.
- Supports rapid and efficient discharge of responsibilities for the International Health Regulations [IHR (2005)].

Data from CDC. *National Surveillance Strategy for Human Health*. Version 2.0. February 2010. Available at: https://www.hsdl.org/?view&did=690766. Accessed June 2017.

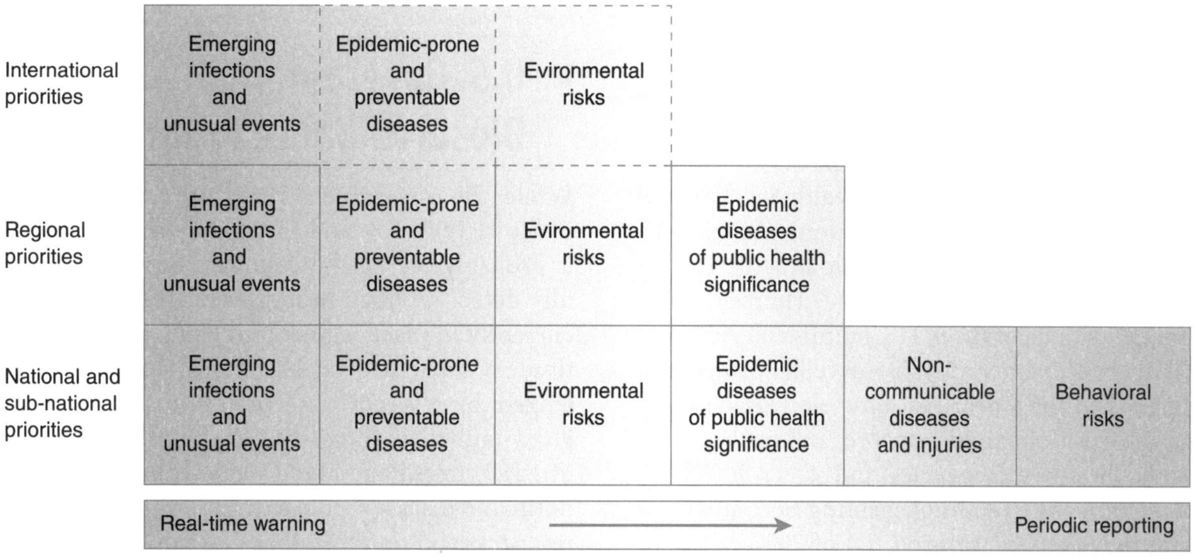

FIGURE 9-1 Public health surveillance targets arrayed by urgency of action and priority

Reproduced from Fischer JE, and Katz R. *The International Health Regulations (2005): Surveillance and Response in an Era of Globalization*. Stimson Center. June 2011. p 16. Available at: https://www.stimson.org/sites/default/files/file-attachments/The_International_Health_Regulations_White_Paper_Final_1.pdf. Accessed November 2017.

shows the range of public health surveillance targets, arranged by priority (from national to international) and urgency of action.[4] While the types of targets vary, effective surveillance for all requires adequate infrastructure, sufficient human capabilities, appropriate tools, and standardized processes.

Surveillance activities themselves involve multiple actors at different levels of government and private sectors. Detection of an unusual disease event may start with an astute clinician, who is able to discern that something is different/unusual/threatening about a particular patient or cluster of patients (be them human or animal) and alerts authorities. Specimen samples must then be transferred in an appropriate manner to a laboratory with the proper equipment and expertise to perform accurate and reliable diagnostic tests. A communication network must then be in place so that data from clinicians and laboratories feeds into a system that allows for effective data analysis. In addition, hospitals may report into this system using discharge data or other markers. Pharmacists and other stores may report prescription and over-the-counter sales of drugs as well as other indicator items, such as toilet paper sales. School or workplace absenteeism may be tracked to provide early indication of illness circulating in a community. Traditional and social media may be monitored for new information, individual citizens reporting disease events, or early trends pointing to unusual behaviors. All of this data may be actively collected by public health officials reaching out to all of the potential data sources, or through passive surveillance relying upon the various actors to report events to authorities.

Regardless of how data are collected, all data must be integrated and analyzed to differentiate between expected levels of morbidity and mortality and indications of an unusual or unexpected event, as well as to validate rumors. The information collected should facilitate action so control measures can be taken. The data alone is not enough; trained public health professionals must analyze the data to determine proper actions.

▶ Policy Directives

The importance of biosurveillance to public health preparedness and national and homeland security has been addressed in a variety of policy directives and legislation over the past decade. There have been calls for an integrated, functional domestic biosurveillance system starting with the Public Health Security and Bioterrorism Preparedness and Response Act of 2002. Further legislation in 2006 (Pandemic and All-Hazards Preparedness Act—PAHPA) and 2007 (Implementing Recommendations of the 9/11 Commission Act) reiterated the need for strong biosurveillance systems. PAHPA called for a near real-time electronic system to enable detection, rapid response, and management of public health emergencies and other infectious disease outbreaks.[5] The Implementing Recommendations of the 9/11 Commission Act of 2007 called for a coordinated, national biosurveillance capability, but the primary focus was on the role the Department of Homeland Security (DHS) should play in providing an integrating center for all surveillance data.[6] And in 2013, the Pandemic and All-Hazards Preparedness Reauthorization Act once again called for better integration of national biosurveillance.[7]

The executive branch has released a series of policy directives and strategies highlighting the importance of disease surveillance and calling for a strong biosurveillance capability. In January 2004, the Bush administration released HSPD 9: Defense of United States Agriculture and Food, which, among other things, directed a series of federal agencies to develop a coordinated surveillance system—primarily for animals, plants, food, and water (**FIGURE 9-2**).[8] HSPD 10: Biodefense for the 21st Century, also released in 2004, reiterates the importance of early detection of a bio event and the importance of an integrated surveillance system.[9] The major directive for surveillance released by the Bush administration, though, was HSPD 21: Public Health and Medical Preparedness, which explicitly calls for a robust, integrated, and comprehensive biosurveillance system as a primary pillar of public health preparedness (**BOX 9-3**). HSPD 21 also focuses on the importance of connecting domestic biosurveillance to global disease surveillance systems, in order to achieve effective early warning and characterization of disease outbreaks.[1]

The Obama administration, building on the recognition of the importance of strong biosurveillance for public health preparedness, released a series of strategies (all discussed in earlier chapters) that speak to the need for a robust, integrated surveillance system. This included National Strategy for Biosurveillance and an accompanying implementation plan.

▶ U.S. Government Biosurveillance Programs

While the government recognizes the importance of biosurveillance, and in practice the United States is probably one of the countries best suited to rapidly detect a public health event, the system that is currently in place is uncoordinated, relies on a multitude of separate data collection systems, and is challenged by the governmental infrastructure which gives individual states the lead and authorities for disease surveillance, and only voluntarily sharing notifiable diseases with federal entities. Most of the resources and responsibilities for public health activities, including disease surveillance, lie at the local and state levels. Federal entities work with these state and local groups to encourage voluntary cooperating and information sharing with the federal level.

There are numerous surveillance programs that are disease or syndrome specific, most of which are operated by Centers for Disease Control and Prevention (CDC). In addition, there is a multitude of surveillance systems designed to capture data on disease events, including laboratory data. In 2010, the U.S. Government Accountability Office (GAO) described a selected set of such federally operated programs, which included more than 60 different programs, operated by the DHS, the Department of Defense (DoD), the Department of the Interior, the

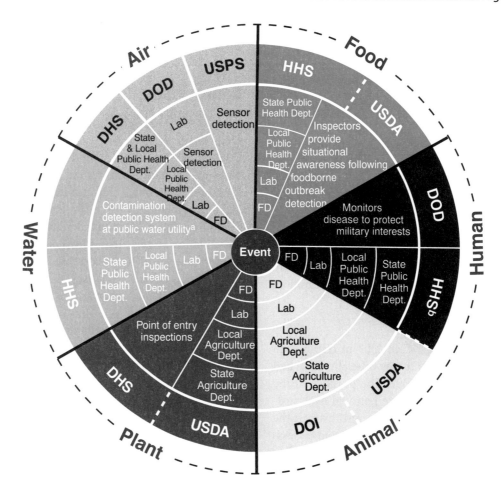

FD   Refers to first detector which could be any of the professionals described in figure 4.
- - -   Indicates coordination between agencies.

FIGURE 9-2 Roles and responsibility for detection across the intergovernmental, cross-domain biosurveillance network

BOX 9-3   HSPD 21: Public Health and Medical Preparedness Call for Robust Biosurveillance Capacity

The United States must develop a nationwide, robust, and integrated biosurveillance capability, with connections to international disease surveillance systems, in order to provide early warning and ongoing characterization of disease outbreaks in near real-time. Surveillance must use multiple modalities and an in-depth architecture. We must enhance clinician awareness and participation and strengthen laboratory diagnostic capabilities and capacity in order to recognize potential threats as early as possible. Integration of biosurveillance elements and other data (including human health, animal health, agricultural, meteorological, environmental, intelligence, and other data) will provide a comprehensive picture of the health of communities and the associated threat environment for incorporation into the national "common operating picture." A central element of biosurveillance must be an epidemiologic surveillance system to monitor human disease activity across populations. That system must be sufficiently enabled to identify specific disease incidence and prevalence in heterogeneous populations and environments and must possess sufficient flexibility to tailor analyses to new syndromes and emerging diseases. State and local government health officials, public and private sector health care institutions, and practicing clinicians must be involved in system design, and the overall system must be constructed with the principal objective of establishing or enhancing the capabilities of State and local government entities.

Environmental Protection Agency (EPA), the Department of Health and Human Services (including CDC and Food and Drug Administration [FDA]), the Department of Agriculture, and the U.S. Postal Service.[10]

Integration Efforts

Given the enormity of the task and the multitude of surveillance systems that currently exist in the country, most experts and policymakers have recognized the need for a means to integrate data collection and analysis in a way that pools all of the available information, rapidly analyzes data, and provides early warning and response to public health emergencies. Several programs have tried to accomplish this (**FIGURE 9-3**); although to date, there are still challenges related to data and systems integration.

BioSense

BioSense was started by CDC in 2003 in response to the 2002 Bioterrorism Act; it was officially launched in 2004 and redesigned in 2007. The purpose of the program is to collect and analyze national near real-time data from a variety of sources, and through the use of advanced algorithms, provide rapid assessments of disease trends. The program collected data on patient complaints from more than 550 acute-care hospitals and 1300 DoD and Veterans Affairs hospitals and clinics. It also collects sales data from over 27,000 pharmacies. In 2010, BioSense was redesigned into BioSense 2.0; but in 2016, it was discontinued in favor

of standardized and integrated software to be shared across CDC and its partners.[11]

National Biosurveillance Integration System

DHS hosts the National Biosurveillance Integration Center (NBIC). This center is designed to integrate and analyze data from human health, animal, plant, food, and environmental monitoring systems to create a single picture of bio-related activities. NBIC relied heavily on Argus, a federally funded but private surveillance system that filters media sources from around the world to collate disease-related information. The program also uses data from ESSENCE, a DoD surveillance program, as well as information from U.S. Fish and Wildlife Services and the EPA. There have been some challenges in implementing the program. Data from all federal agencies has not been readily shared, and when shared, it is often in formats that need to be translated before integrated, and analysis has not always been fully informed. The program is rebuilding and strengthening its capacity.

Biowatch

Biowatch is an environmental monitoring program operated by the DHS, with partners at CDC and EPA. These are environmental "sniffers" designed to detect when a particular biological agent is present in the

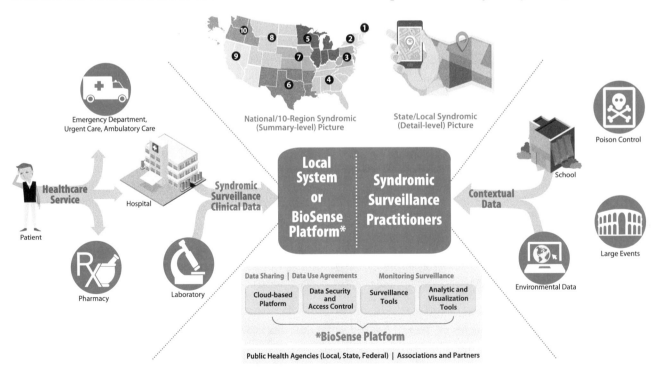

FIGURE 9-3 Public health syndromic surveillance data flow

Reproduced from CDC. *National Syndromic Surveillance Program (NSSP)*. 2016. Available at: https://www.cdc.gov/nssp/overview.html. Accessed June 2017.

environment. These sniffers are currently located in cities throughout the United States.

Global Surveillance

Because a biological threat can emerge anywhere, a weakness in the disease surveillance and response capacity in one part of the world is a potential risk to all nations. Therefore, it is vital that we take a global policy outlook in addition to national efforts, so that we understand the global biosurveillance capacity, identify essential components of effective biosurveillance, and develop policies that will enable nations—particularly in resource-poor environments—to establish systems that will quickly identify and respond to biological threats so that they may be contained prior to global spread.

The United States is committed to this concept through support of the World Health Organization's (WHO's) International Health Regulations (IHR), and the obligations under Article 44 of IHR. Under Article 44 of the IHR, state parties are encouraged to provide technical and financial assistance to help other countries achieve their IHR core capacities, which are necessary capacities to detect, respond to, and contain public health emergencies of international concern.[12] The United States also supports building global disease surveillance capacity through the Global Health Security Agenda and programs like CDC's Global Disease Detection and Response regional centers, the DoD Armed Forces Health Surveillance Branch, U.S. Agency for International Development's (USAID's) Emerging Pandemics Threats program, and a multitude of other engagements through cooperative threat reduction programs at the Departments of State and Defense.

Other agencies, including the Intelligence Community; DHS; the Departments of Commerce, Energy, and the Interior; EPA, and NASA have also been engaged in supporting global disease surveillance efforts. These combined efforts are designed to strengthen national capacities to detect, report, and respond to public health events, particularly public health emergencies. Some programs focus on developing workforce expertise, such as the CDC's Field Epidemiology and Laboratory Training Program (FETP and FELTP). Some of the programs focus on infrastructure development, building laboratories for national and regional use. Several programs work on technological advances that can be utilized in both high- and low-resource environments to enable enhanced surveillance. And some of the programs provide support for pathogen discovery, outbreak investigation, and response and mitigation after the emergence of a public health event.

Global Systems

The U.S. government (USG)–funded activities to promote disease surveillance capacity fit into a larger picture of global surveillance. A robust network of networks exists to support disease surveillance in all parts of the globe. These systems and networks overlap at the national, regional, and global levels, and are designed to be coordinated at the international level by the WHO through the Global Outbreak Alert and Response Network (GOARN). One of the electronic surveillance system utilized by the WHO to detect reports of disease through the media is the Global Public Health Information Network (GPHIN), a system developed by Canada. Other online information sources include less formal systems, such as PROMED (an online community of mostly health professionals sharing data about disease emergence) and HealthMap (visually depicts events around the world). There are regional versions of this listserve as well, which also feed into the WHO. In addition to online sources, the WHO receives reports of disease emergence from ministries of health, WHO regional and national offices, laboratory networks, nongovernmental organizations (particularly those entities working on the ground in remote regions), militaries, and other entities within the U.N. system.[13]

Overall, there are a multitude of surveillance systems around the world, all designed to detect and report the emergence of a public health emergency as rapidly as possible to enable a timely response that will prevent morbidity and mortality. These systems range in effectiveness, and some parts of the world are better equipped than others in this arena. There appears, however, to be a strong commitment at the national and global policy levels to build stronger surveillance systems, and we should expect great strides in the next few years to strengthen our domestic capabilities and build a comprehensive global system.

When Epidemiology and Law Enforcement Come Together

Once a public health event has been identified through surveillance systems, teams must begin the epidemiologic investigation to determine the causative agent of an outbreak and enact appropriate measures to mitigate the consequences. If, however, there is a suspicion that the disease event was not naturally occurring, this process becomes complicated by the need to not only identify the causative agent, but also the bad actor, and do so in a way that maintains evidentiary standards so that findings can be someday used to prosecute wrongdoers. Law enforcement will also become engaged to protect public safety.

Because of this need to work together, a new area has emerged called Crim-Epi. This is a joint effort led by the CDC and Federal Bureau of Investigation (FBI) to train law enforcement and public health officials to work together to build relationships, share information, conduct joint threat assessments, and work together during outbreak investigations. CDC and FBI are now engaged with communities around the world to conduct Crim-Epi trainings and enhance multisectoral cooperation in response to potentially deliberate events (**FIGURES 9-4** and **9-5**).[14]

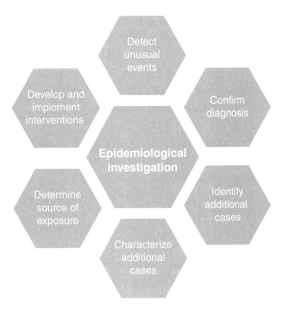

FIGURE 9-4 Elements of an epidemiological investigation

Reproduced from US Department of Justice, FBI, CDC. *Benefits of Joint Criminal–Epidemiological Investigations.* Available at: http://www.nwhrn.org/media/Crim-Epi-Flyer.pdf. Accessed June 2017.

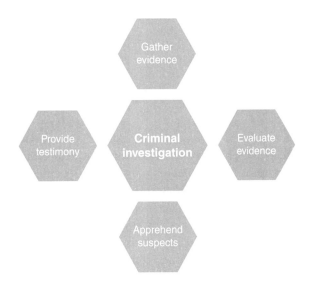

FIGURE 9-5 Elements of a criminal investigation

Reproduced from US Department of Justice, FBI, CDC. *Benefits of Joint Criminal–Epidemiological Investigations.* Available at: http://www.nwhrn.org/media/Crim-Epi-Flyer.pdf. Accessed June 2017.

▶ Differentiating Between Natural and Intentional Events

One of the ways in which biological agents can be effective weapons is through plausible deniability—they can be extremely difficult to detect. In fact, it can be almost impossible to differentiate between a naturally occurring disease and an intentional event. Of course, this is not always the case. A cluster of smallpox cases outside of the designated smallpox repository laboratories would automatically be considered an intentional event, as smallpox is no longer circulating naturally. A large explosion releasing a visible cloud of agents resulting in population morbidity and mortality would most certainly be investigated as an intentional event. Other outbreaks, though, are more complicated. Several researchers have tried to identify and characterize the epidemiology of an intentional event, to provide clues that something might not be of natural origin.[15–17] Their collective findings include the following:

- Intentional events are more likely to have a point source. This means that individuals are exposed to the agent during one time period, so that infected individuals begin to show symptoms at about the same time. The epi curve for a point source event usually has a sharp rise in cases at one time, with most cases developing within a short-time period (**FIGURE 9-6**).
- An intentional event may involve a larger than expected number of cases.
- The disease may be more severe than expected from a naturally occurring event.
- There may be unusual routes of exposure (e.g., airborne as opposed to gastrointestinal).
- The disease may be unusual for a given geographical area.
- The outbreak may involve an unusual strain or variant of an agent.
- There may be distinctly higher attack rates in individuals exposed to the agent during specific times or in specific areas.
- Simultaneous morbidity and mortality in animals may signal an airborne release of an agent.
- There may be corroborating intelligence information suggesting intent by an actor to use biological agents.

Regardless of whether the event is naturally occurring or intentional (or even accidental), it will still start with detection through surveillance mechanisms,

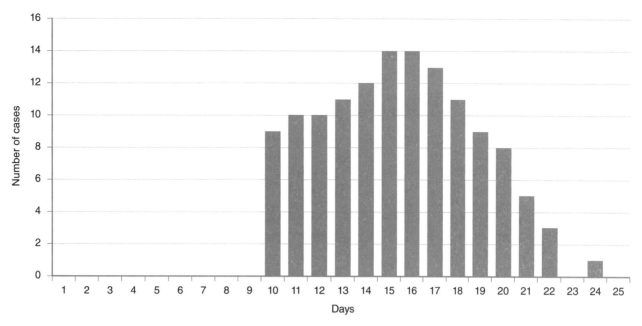

FIGURE 9-6 Point source Epi-Curve

followed by an investigation. The public health community will need to detect, identify, and characterize the event and respond through treatment and containment. If the event is not naturally occurring, there will also need to be an attribution assessment to determine the source of the agent and the perpetrator(s) of the attack.

▶ Attribution Assessments

While the public health community is responsible for detecting, identifying, and responding to an intentional use event to safeguard population health, law enforcement officials and policymakers are responsible for determining and verifying the origin or source, sponsorship, delivery, and responsible party associated with an intentional use event. The task of answering "Who did it?" is called an attribution assessment. This assessment may be used for a variety of purposes ranging from criminal prosecution of individuals to diplomatic actions against nations. The strength of the evidence necessary for the attribution assessment, however, may vary depending on the intended use; strong evidence may be used in a court of law, while weaker evidence may be used to spark diplomatic actions.

In order to make an attribution assessment, investigators need to link the agent used in an event to a source and a specified perpetrator. They need to identify if a crime occurred, and if so, what exactly happened, when, and why. They need to determine what evidence is necessary to answer

these questions.[18] Depending on the evidence and the event, microbial forensics may need to be used. Microbial forensics is the application of both forensic science and molecular epidemiology to problems involving biological agents.[19] It employs themes and concepts from these disciplines to determine the molecular identity of the agent, if it can be linked to a source, and if so, how precisely it can be linked. Depending on the availability of source data, microbial forensics may provide useful data that can be used during a criminal prosecution, or possibly an investigative lead that can assist in the larger attribution investigation.

▶ Domestic Investigations of Suspected Biological Weapons Use

The first indication that a potential intentional use event has occurred will likely come from the local public health surveillance systems. That event is then reported to state and possibly federal authorities, while at the same time, public health officials begin to investigate the event. At the first indication that the event may be intentional, law enforcement personnel become involved. Law enforcement personnel then engage in the process of evidence collection, ensuring chain of custody of evidence is maintained so that it can be introduced at trials, delivering biological samples to specific laboratories in the Laboratory Response Network (LRN) to ensure proper

🔍 *CASE STUDY: Amerithrax*

In the weeks following the 9/11 attacks, several letters containing anthrax were mailed to news outlets and U.S. senators. The letters contained white powder as well as a cursory note. The letter sent to Senator Leahy read, "YOU CAN NOT STOP US. WE HAVE THIS ANTHRAX. YOU DIE NOW. ARE YOU AFRAID? DEATH TO AMERICA. DEATH TO ISRAEL. ALLAH IS GREAT."[20] The letters led to 22 cases of anthrax, 5 deaths, large-scale decontamination efforts, and what amounted to a 7-year investigation by the Federal Bureau of Investigation and the U.S. Postal Service inspectors.

Massive amounts of evidence were collected during the investigation, but investigators were limited by the scientific methods available to them. Over the course of the investigation, new methods in microbial forensics were developed to eventually trace the anthrax sent in the letters to a single spore-batch of anthrax. The final determination of the perpetrator required a combination of traditional law enforcement methods with new methods of scientific analysis.

In the end, the investigation led to Dr. Bruce Ivins, an employee at U.S. Army Medical Research Institute of Infectious Diseases (USAMRIID) at Fort Detrick, Maryland. Dr. Ivins committed suicide in July 2008 before he could formally be indicted.

AMERITHRAX by the Numbers:

- At least 5 letters sent in September and October 2001.
- 22 cases of anthrax.
- 5 dead from anthrax.
- Another 31 tested positive for exposure but did not become ill.
- 10,000 "at-risk" individuals underwent antibiotic prophylaxis.
- 35 postal facilities and mailrooms contaminated.
- Anthrax detected in 7 buildings on Capitol Hill.
- In October–December 2001, the LRN tested more than 120,000 clinical and environmental samples.
- 7-year investigation.

- 600,000 investigator work hours.
- 10,000 witness interviews.
- 80 searchers.
- 6000 items of potential evidence.
- 5730 samples collected from 60 sites.
- Cooperation from 29 government, university, and commercial labs.
- Amerithrax task force staffed by 25–30 full-time investigators.
- 5750 grand jury subpoenas.
- 1000 possible suspects.
- 1 perpetrator, never tried for the crime.[20]

analysis, obtaining original documents when appropriate, and taking witness statements regarding the event.

▶ International Investigations of Suspected Biological Weapons Use

International investigations of suspected deliberate use events, like those in the domestic arena, often will start with a local public health system detecting that something out of the ordinary in kind or scope has happened. In some cases, these first reports may come from nongovernmental organizations, particularly if the reports are from refugee camps or remote populations. The event is then reported to the national level authorities and, depending on the type of event, it may be reported to either the WHO or the United Nations.

Under the IHR, states parties must notify the WHO of any event that may constitute a Public Health Emergency of International Concern

(PHEIC). These include events that are unusual or unexpected in nature, including those of unknown causes or sources. In the case of an intentional (or suspected intentional) use event, the state would notify the WHO. Under Article VII of the Biological and Toxin Weapons Convention, states parties are obligated to assist nations that have been victim of a violation of the treaty—a deliberate use of a biological agent.

When a country suspects that there has been an intentional use of biological or chemical weapons, the country can make a request to the U.N. Secretary-General to formally investigate the allegations (Article VI of the Biological Weapons Convention, see **BOX 9-4**). The U.N. General Assembly and the Security Council established a mandate through multiple resolutions (including Resolution 620 in 1988, and 42/37C) for the Secretary-General to carry on biological or chemical weapons use investigations. This mandate is known as the U.N. Secretary-General's Mechanism (UNSGM) for Investigation of Alleged Use of Chemical and Biological Weapons (CW and BW). This applies to both BW and CW events, but the United Nations has an agreement to partner with the

---

BOX 9-4 Article VI of the Biological Weapons Convention

Article VI

(1)   Any State Party to this Convention which finds that any other State Party is acting in breach of obligations deriving from the provisions of the Convention may lodge a complaint with the Security Council of the United Nations. Such a complaint should include all possible evidence confirming its validity, as well as a request for its consideration by the Security Council.

(2)   Each State Party to this Convention undertakes to cooperate in carrying out any investigation which the Security Council may initiate, in accordance with the provisions of the Charter of the United Nations, on the basis of the complaint received by the Council. The Security Council shall inform the States Parties to the Convention of the results of the investigation.

Reproduced from U.S. Department of State. *Text of the Biological Weapons Convention.* March 26, 1975. Available at: https://www.state.gov/t/isn/bw/c48738.htm. Accessed June 2017.

Organization for the Prohibition of Chemical Weapons (OPCW) to investigate CWs events.

The Secretary-General's Mechanism allows any member state to submit a report of alleged use to the Secretary-General. The Secretary-General can then decide to launch an investigation utilizing a team of qualified experts, provided by the member states. The investigation, however, can only operate in countries that have provided express permission. The mechanism was used a dozen times starting in the early 1980s, with the last investigations occurring in 1992 before again being invoked for chemical weapons allegations in Syria over a decade later.[21]

One of the challenges of the Secretary-General's Mechanism was that it is difficult to get experts on the ground to conduct an investigation in a timely fashion. Thus, attempts to determine the facts of a case are complicated by time delays and inability to access evidence. In 2010, the United Nations signed a MOU with the WHO that will allow the WHO to share information and resources, including data collected during its own investigations, with the U.N. fact-finding teams.[22] Several additional MOUs with International Organizations are currently in process.

In addition to the UNSGM, the GOARN, and the other international organizations involved in alleged use investigations, there are many national and regional entities that would/could become involved in investigations, each bringing their own expertise to the situation. The North Atlantic Treaty Organization (NATO), for example, has a Multinational Chemical, Biological, Radiological and Nuclear (CBRN) Defense Battalion that can provide response teams, laboratory assets, and logistical support, while investigating allegations of biological or chemical weapons use in NATO countries. The European Union Center for Disease Prevention and Control (ECDC) has a unit for responding to outbreaks and other health threats of unknown origin. Interpol and Europol both support law enforcement officials in the field, providing a resource for national level law enforcement efforts in response to an alleged intentional use event.[23] Finally, in most cases, outbreak investigations and alleged use investigations will be led by the national entity. Depending on the resources available to that country, there may be assistance from the any of the previously mentioned organizations.

🔍 CASE STUDY: Investigating Chemical Weapons Use in Syria

Syrian President Bashar Al-Assad's family has held power for more than 40 years. But in March 2011, demonstrator launched a series of protest against the leader, eventually leading to a civil war by the mid-2012.[24–26] Allegations of chemical weapons use came almost immediately after the start of armed conflict. By the mid-2013, there had been 12 separate chemical weapons events reported in Syria by the media, with accusations of use by both the Syrian government and the opposition forces.[27–33] The U.N. Independent International Commission of Inquiry on the Syrian Arab Republic stated in June 2013 that "there are reasonable grounds to believe that chemical agents have been used as weapons."[34]

By March 2013, both the Syrian government and the opposition forces called for independent fact-finding investigations through the UNSGM for Investigation of Alleged Use of Chemical and Biological Weapons. The investigation was officially launched by the Secretary-General on March 21, 2013.[35]

(continues)

Invoking the UNSGM marked the first time the mechanism had been used in over a decade. During this period, the Chemical Weapons Convention (CWC) had entered into force and with it the establishment of the OPCW. The purpose of the OPCW was to implement the CWC, assist with the destruction of existing chemical weapons stockpiles, and conduct challenge inspections to ensure that member states were not maintaining offensive chemical weapons programs. In 2000, OPCW established an agreement with the United Nations to "agree to cooperate closely within their respective mandates and to consult on matters of mutual interest and concern."[36] Additionally, a corresponding 2011 MOU between World Health Organization (WHO) and the U.N. states that the WHO will "provide technical support in assessing the public health, clinical, and event-specific health aspects of an alleged use."[37] So when UNSGM was invoked in March 2013, the United Nations requested that OPCW support the investigation into alleged chemical weapons use in Syria, and asked the WHO to work in partnership with the OPCW on the investigative team.[38]

After several months of investigations, the OPCW–WHO fact-finding mission delivered a final report to the Secretary-General in December 2013.[39] The report found that chemical weapons had, in fact, been used in Syria on multiple occasions.

The U.N. Security Council condemned the use of chemical weapons in Syria (Resolutions 2118 and 2209) and adopted a resolution in 2015 (Resolution 2235) to establish the OPCW–UN Joint Investigative Mechanisms (known as the JIM [Joint Investigative Mechanisms]) to identify the perpetrators, organizers, and sponsors of Syrian chemical weapons use events. Multiple reports were issued by the JIM, including conclusions that there was sufficient information to determine that both the Syrian Armed Forces and the Islamic State in Iraq and the Levant were responsible for chemical weapons attacks.

▶ Conclusions

It is evident that responding to public health emergencies to protect population health is complicated. Responding to public health emergencies with the goal of protecting population health as well as determining if the event was intentional, and if so, finding who committed the crime in a manner that will provide strong enough evidence to bring a perpetrator to justice or influence foreign policy decisions are even more complicated. Many entities need to become involved, not all of which have the same goals, but many of which need to use the same data. Collaboration between law enforcement, security, and public health entities greatly strengthens the ability of all sectors to do their jobs well.

Key Words

Amerithrax
Attribution assessment
Biosurveillance
Crim-Epi

Global Outbreak Alert and Response Network
Outbreak investigation
Microbial forensics
Surveillance

U.N. Secretary-General's Mechanism for Investigation of Alleged Use of Chemical and Biological Weapons

Discussion Questions

1. If you could design a biosurveillance system from scratch, what information would you want to collect and how? How would that information then be relayed to decision makers?
2. What are some of the successes and challenges of the current disease surveillance system in the United States?
3. Describe how countries' disease surveillance is interrelated. Who should be supporting global disease surveillance capacity building?
4. If faced with a suspicious disease outbreak, what questions would you ask to begin to determine if the event was natural, intentional, or accidental?
5. What organizations would you work with to make the above determination?
6. What could/should be improved to make accurate and timely attribution assessments?
7. What kind of cooperation do you think would be necessary to have a complete international investigation of an alleged biological or chemical weapons use event?

References

1. The White House. *Homeland Security Presidential Directive /HSPD-21*. October 2007. Available at: https://georgewbush-whitehouse.archives.gov/news/releases/2007/10/20071018-10.html. Accessed June 2017.
2. Raska K. National and International Surveillance of Communicable Disease. *WHO Chronicle*. September 1996;20(9):315–321.
3. Thacker SB, Berkelman RL. Public Health and Surveillance in the United States. *Epidemiologic Reviews* 1988;10:164–190.
4. Fischer JE, Katz R. *The International Health Regulations (2005): Surveillance and Response in an Era of Globalization*. Stimson Center. June 2011. p 16. Available at: https://www.stimson.org/sites/default/files/file-attachments/The_International_Health_Regulations_White_Paper_Final_1.pdf. Accessed November 2017.
5. Pandemic and All-Hazards Preparedness Act, P. L. 109-417 p 202. 2006.
6. Implementing Recommendations of the 9/11 Commission Act of 2007, P. L. 110-53 pp 1101–1102.
7. Pandemic and All-Hazards Preparedness Reauthorization Act (PAHPRA), P. L. 113-5. 2013.
8. The White House. *Homeland Security Presidential Directive /HSPD-9*. January 30, 2004. Available at: https://www.gpo.gov/fdsys/pkg/PPP-2004-book1/pdf/PPP-2004-book1-doc-pg173.pdf. Accessed June 2017.
9. The White House. *Homeland Security Presidential Directive 10: Biodefense for the 21ˢᵗ Century*. Federation of American Scientists. April 28, 2004. Available at: https://fas.org/irp/offdocs/nspd/hspd-10.html. Accessed June 2017.
10. GAO. *Biosurveillance: Efforts to Develop a National Biosurveillance Capability Need a National Strategy and a Designated Leader*. GAO-10-645. June 2010. Available at: http://www.gao.gov/assets/310/306362.pdf. Accessed June 2017.
11. CDC. *BioSense 2.0. National Syndromic Surveillance Program (NSSP)*. 2016. Available at: https://www.cdc.gov/nssp/biosense/biosense20.html. Accessed June 2017.
12. WHO. *Article 44 Collaboration and Assistance. Revision of the International Health Regulations*. WHA58.3. 2005. p 35. Available at: http://www.who.int/csr/ihr/WHA58-en.pdf. Accessed June 2017.
13. Grein TW, Kamara KB, Rodier G, et al. Rumors of Disease in the Global Village: Outbreak Verification. *Emerging Infectious Disease*. 2000;6(2):97–102.
14. US Department of Justice, FBI, CDC. *Benefits of Joint Criminal-Epidemiological Investigations*. Available at: http://www.nwhrn.org/media/Crim-Epi-Flyer.pdf. Accessed June 2017.
15. Pavlin JA. Epidemiology of Bioterrorism. *Emerging Infectious Diseases*. July–August 1999;5(4):528–530.
16. Khan AS, Morse S, Lillibridge S. Public-Health Preparedness for Biological Terrorism in the USA. *The Lancet*. September 2000;356(9236):1179–1182.
17. Dembek ZF, Kortepeter MG, Pavlin JA. Discernment between Deliberate and Natural Infectious Disease Outbreaks. *Epidemiology and Infection*. April 2007;135(3):353–371.
18. Bahr E. Attribution of Biological Weapons Use. In: Katz R, Zilinikas R, eds. *Encyclopedia of Bioterrorism Defense*, 2nd ed. Wiley and Sons, New York; 2011.
19. Budowle B, Burans JP, Breeze RG, et al. Microbial Forensics. In: Budowle B, Schutzer SE, Breeze RG, eds. *Microbial Forensics*. Cambridge, MA: Elsevier Academic Press; 2005.
20. U.S. Department of Justice. *Amerithrax Investigative Summary*. U.S. Department of Justice. February 19, 2010. Available at: http://www.justice.gov/amerithrax/docs/amx-investigative-summary.pdf. Accessed December 10, 2010.
21. Smidovich N. *The Secretary-General's Investigations of Alleged Use of Chemical, Biological or Toxin Weapons*. The United Nations Office at Geneva. August 25, 2010. Available at: http:// www.unog.ch/80256EDD006B8954/(httpAssets)/68C1707BD779563BC125778B0046B251/$file/2_UNODA_SGM_Mechanism_BWC.pdf. Accessed June 2017.
22. Implementation Support Unit. *The Role of International Organizations in the Provision of Assistance and Coordination in the Case of Alleged Use of Biological or Toxin Weapons*. Geneva: Meeting of the States Parties to the Convention on the Prohibition of the Development, Production and Stockpiling of Bacteriological (Biological) and Toxin Weapons and on Their Destruction. August 5, 2010. Available at: http://repository.un.org/handle/11176/290574. Accessed June 2017.
23. Commission of the European Communities. *Bridging Security and Health: Towards the Identification of Good Practices in the Response to CBRN Incidents and the Security of CBR Substances*. 2009. Available at: http://ec.europa.eu/health/ph_threats/com/preparedness/docs/bridging_en.pdf. Accessed June 2017.
24. Amos D. *In Syria, Opposition Stages Massive Protests*. NPR. July 15, 2011. Available at: http://n.pr/oKyu3R. Accessed June 2017.
25. Mid-East Unrest: Syrian Protests in Damascus and Aleppo. *BBC*. March 15, 2011. Available at: http://bbc.in/18kMa1N. Accessed June 2017.
26. UN Official Calls Syria Conflict 'Civil War.' *Al Jazeera*. June 13, 2012. Available at: http://www.aljazeera.com/news/middleeast/2012/06/201261222721181345.html. Accessed June 2017.
27. McDonnell PJ. At Least Three Allegations of Chemical Use in Syria. *Los Angeles Times*. April 28, 2013. Available at: http://www.latimes.com/news/world/worldnow/la-fg-wn-chemical-syria-20130428,0,4685355.story. Accessed June 2017.
28. Zeiger A, Winer S. Syrian Rebels Claim Recent Alleged Chemical Attack Not the First. *The Times of Israel*. December 25, 2012. Available at: http://toi.sr/Tp9O6s. Accessed June 2017.
29. Holmes O, Solomon E. Alleged Chemical Attack Kills 25 in Northern Syria. *Reuters*. March 19, 2013. Available at: http://reut.rs/WAJrtL. Accessed June 2017.
30. Syria Chemical Weapons Allegations. *BBC*. October 31, 2013. Available at: http://bbc.in/12HmdCL. Accessed June 2017.
31. Remy JP. Chemical Warfare in Syria. *Le Monde*. May 27, 2013. Available at: http://www.lemonde.fr/proche-orient/article/2013/05/27/chemical-war-in-syria_3417708_3218.html. Accessed June 2017.
32. Lynch C. Britain Refers More Claims of Syrian Chemical Weapons Use to U.N. *The Washington Post*. May 29, 2013. Available at: http://wapo.st/Zf894d. Accessed June 2017.
33. Syrian Rebels: Dozens Hurt in Chemical Weapons Attack in Damascus. *The Times of Israel*. May 18, 2013. Available at: http://toi.sr/11M7X0a. Accessed June 2017.

34. UN Human Rights Council. *Report of the Independent International Commission of Inquiry on the Syrian Arab Republic.* June 4, 2013. Available at: http://www.ohchr .org/Documents/HRBodies/HRCouncil/CoISyria/A-HRC -23-58_en.pdf. Accessed June 2017.

35. UN News Centre. *UN Chief Announces Independent Probe into Allegations of Chemical Attack in Syria.* March 21, 2013. Available at: http://www.un.org/apps/news/story.asp? NewsID=44450. Accessed June 2017.

36. UN. *Agreement Concerning the Relationship between the United Nations and the Organization for the Prohibition of Chemical Weapons.* June 18, 2001. Available at: http://www.un.org /documents/ga/docs/55/a55988.pdf. Accessed June 2017.

37. UN. *Memorandum of Understanding between the World Health Organization and the United Nations Concerning WHO's Support to the Secretary-General's Mechanism for Investigation of the Alleged Use of Chemical, Biological or Toxic Weapons.* January 31, 2011. Available at: https://unoda -web.s3-accelerate.amazonaws.com/wp-content/uploads /assets/WMD/Secretary-General_Mechanism/UN_WHO _MOU_2011.pdf. Accessed June 2017.

38. OPCW. *Statement by the Chairperson of the Executive Council Following the Council Meeting on 27 March 2013.* March 27, 2013. Available at: http://www.opcw.org/fileadmin/OPCW /PDF/Statement_EC_Chair_27_March.pdf. Accessed June 2017.

39. UN, General Assembly Security Council. *Identical Letters Dated 13 December 2013 from the Secretary-General Addressed to the President of the General Assembly and the President of the Security Council.* December 13, 2013. Available at: http:// undocs.org/A/68/663. Accessed June 2017.

PART V

Practical Applications and Operations

CHAPTER 10

The Preparedness Cycle

LEARNING OBJECTIVES

By the end of this chapter, the reader will be able to:

- Describe the preparedness cycle
- Explain the six-step planning process

▶ Introduction

Preparedness can be defined as a state of being ready. It can take shape in many forms, such as planning for an incident or event. An event is something we typically prepare for, such as the State of the Union address, and an incident is something that happens, such as the bombing of the World Trade Center that happened in 1993. Each of these examples is something we can prepare for, but an event is something that we are actively engaged in at the time. For example, in the event of a State of the Union event, the U.S. Secret Service conducts hundreds of investigations into threats and actively takes steps to prevent them from happening. Steps taken by the U.S. Secret Service to prepare can include adding extra security, including extra physical presence, and extra screening of participants using metal detectors and explosive-sniffing dogs. In the event of an incident, we prepare by planning any contingency, such as a truck filled with explosives being parked in an underground parking deck, providing the right equipment and organization to the incident or event, from training police and security personnel on what to look for to conducting exercise to ensure everyone knows their jobs, and evaluating these exercises to see what went right and what went wrong.

In each of these instances, we can take an active role in preparing; it just may be that our response time is delayed based on whether we were actively engaged at the time of the event or incident.

▶ The Preparedness Cycle

The U.S. government developed what is called the preparedness cycle to actively prepare us for any event or incident (**FIGURE 10-1**). The Federal Emergency Management Agency (FEMA) developed what is called the National Preparedness Goal. The purpose of the National Preparedness Goal is for the whole community to be prepared for all types of disasters and emergencies.[1] The goal simply states, "A secure and resilient nation with the capabilities required across the whole community to prevent, protect against, mitigate, respond to, and recover from the threats and hazards that pose the greatest risk."[1(p1)] Risks and hazards can include natural disasters such as tornadoes, hurricanes, floods, disease outbreaks, and chemical spills; and man-made disasters such as terrorist attacks and cyber-attacks.

In the world of public health, all disasters have a health component. Let us explore a cyber-attack for health effects. While the health effects of a

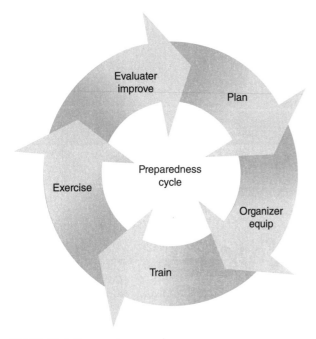

FIGURE 10-1 Preparedness cycle

Reproduced from Department of Homeland Security, FEMA. *Developing and Maintaining Emergency Operations Plans*. 2010. pp 1–4 Available at: https://www.fema.gov/media-library-data/20130726-1828-25045-0014/cpg_101_comprehensive _preparedness_guide_developing_and_maintaining_emergency_operations_plans_2010.pdf. Accessed May 2017.

cyber-attack may not seem obvious, let us think about an attack itself. If terrorists or a nation-state conduct a cyber-attack on our power grid, the first-order effects would be obvious, such as loss of power. If the attack were particularly devastating and long lasting, the grid could go down for an extended period of time. If the power were out long enough, backup generators at hospitals would eventually run out of fuel. Almost all fuel stations require electricity to pump fuel from underground storage tanks. If we were unable to refuel generators because we were unable to get fuel out of the ground, we would begin to lose patients that require electricity to power their life-saving equipment, such as respirators. Thus, a cyber-attack could have devastating health effects.

Homeland Security Presidential Directive 5 (HSPD 5), the National Incident Management System (NIMS), says that the federal government is to work with state, local, territorial, and tribal partners, as well as private industry and nongovernmental sectors, to conduct planning to prevent, prepare for, respond to, and recover from natural and man-made disasters. Included in this is planning for specific events, such as the aforementioned State of the Union address, the inauguration of a new president, or large athletic events such as the Super Bowl. HSPD 5 also sets forth the directive that the federal government develop a National Response Plan (NRP). The NRP was eventually replaced by the National Response Framework.

Taking preparedness one step further, HSPD 8 outlines a National Preparedness System. HSPD 8 is a companion to HSPD 5, in that it develops a system of preparedness activities as part of the NIMS. In particular, it does the following:

- Directs the federal government to work with its partners to develop a National Preparedness Goal
- Allows for federal preparedness assistance to partners
- Streamlines procedures for developing and adopting appropriate equipment for first responders
- Establishes training and exercise procedures to standardize program delivery
- Directs the heads of federal departments and agencies to conduct preparedness activates
- Establishes national citizen preparedness programs, such as the Community Emergency Response Teams (CERT)

As part of federal assistance to partners, the Secretary of Health and Human Services (HHS) is named as a partner to state, local, territorial, and tribal governments. Part of this assistance is the administration of the Public Health Emergency Preparedness (PHEP) cooperative agreement. The PHEP cooperative agreement outlines preparedness activities for its recipients, and in exchange for their participation, HHS provides funds for use in developing preparedness programs. Programs include planning, training, exercising, equipping first responders, and preparing health departments for disasters.[2,3]

The Planning Process

The preparedness cycle is arranged as a cycle for a reason; the cycle never ends. That being said, the usual starting point is planning. Planning can be defined as the process of making a plan for something, such as how you will handle an emergency. We conduct planning in our everyday lives. Think about when you get up in the morning and get ready for work. Many of us watch television or listen to the radio to find out what traffic is like before we leave for work. If traffic is bad on our normal route to work, we often decide to take an alternate route. You wouldn't get in your car and start driving and take random roads to see if it gets you to work. If you took a wrong turn you could end up in another state. In order to know the right way to go, more than likely you have either driven the route you are going to take or you have looked up the route on a mapping program or website. You have done your homework! This is all part of the planning process. Planning can be a long process, but often the process is what gives us the information we need in order to make informed decisions. Also, we do not conduct the planning process alone. All parties that can or could be affected by the plan should be invited to be part of the planning process.

Community Preparedness Guide 101 (CPG 101) was published in July 2013. CPG 101 outlines the planning process to be followed by all partners. The goal of CPG 101 is to allow the integration of all community planning efforts into the overall federal response plans. CPG 101 lays out the process in six steps (**FIGURE 10-2**).

Step 1 of the planning process begins with identifying the core planning team. The core planning team is made up of emergency management professionals as well as all sectors that have a stake in the plan. One group that should always be involved is public health. As discussed previously in the cyber-attack example, there is a health component to all disasters. Some more groups that should be included as appropriate include law enforcement, fire services, emergency medical services, hospitals and healthcare facilities, public works and utilities, education, agriculture, animal control, social services, military, private industry, as well as civic, social, and faith-based organizations. Each of these groups brings a unique perspective to the planning process. Let us take education for example. What would education bring to the table in a disaster? If a public health department were to have a mass vaccination campaign during a disaster response, such as a pandemic influenza, schools could be used as a location for those clinics. Schools offer a lot of space, an abundance of parking, and a definite path for traffic to follow when arriving and departing the school grounds. Schools are easy to secure, so security forces could be kept to a minimum by keeping doors locked and funneling foot traffic a certain way. Without the education sector, schools would not be able to be used effectively. Part of the planning process is to identify resources available during a disaster response. By bringing in all sectors of government and private organizations during the planning process, we can get a good idea of what is available for use during a response. Remember, you can have as many people as you want during a response, but without resources such as equipment, money, etc., you will not be able to do anything during the response.

The approach taken by the planning team once they are assembled is to think about the entire community. This can mean looking at every corner of society within your community. For example, if we were planning a communications campaign to let the community know about an upcoming mass vaccination clinic at the local school, there are many things to consider. We can advertise by radio, television, or newspaper, website, social media, etc. But what about those without access to those things, or those who do not speak English. Every community should be aware of what types of languages are prevalent within their community. If there is a prevalent Spanish-speaking community, then while conducting planning for the mass vaccination clinic, some thought needs to go into how we advertise in Spanish. Maybe there is a community leader within the Spanish-speaking community

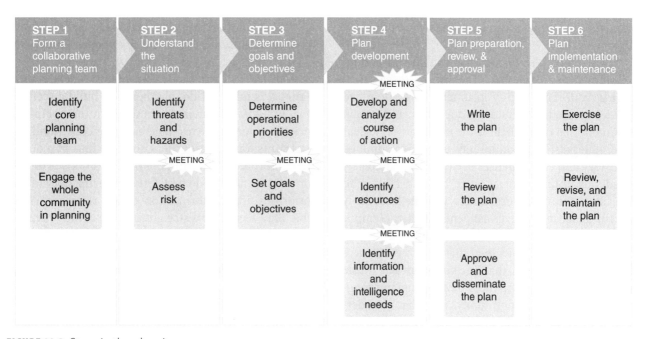

FIGURE 10-2 Steps in the planning process

who can assist with the communications campaign. Without considering a whole community approach to planning, certain parts of the population could be forgotten.

Step 2 of the planning process is to know the situation. This can be explained as knowing what kinds of threats and hazards the community is facing as well as assessing the risk, this is often referred to as a Threat and Hazard Identification and Risk Assessment (THIRA). It is impossible to effectively plan unless you know what you are planning for. This step includes a lot of research, including looking at what has happened in the past to your community. Has the community faced tornados, hurricanes, earthquakes, ice storms, or flooding? Is your community located near a railroad track that has shipments of hazardous materials or waste? Does the interstate system in your area service nuclear waste shipments? Is your city a symbolic location for extremists? For example, New York City is often referred to as the symbol of freedom to the rest of the world, thus making it the target of multiple terrorist attacks. While this may be a planning factor for New York City, it may not be a concern for Lebanon, Missouri. What is the disease burden in the area? Is there a large immigrant population that could inadvertently import a communicable disease?

Understanding these questions helps us realize what kinds of hazards and threats your community faces. Once we know the threats and hazards, we need to figure out the risk associated with each of the threats and hazards. When determining risk, we look at two things: the probability of the event happening and the effect the event would have on the community. Often, the events that are more probable have the least hazardous effect.

For example, let us say that you live in a rural community in Oklahoma. The list of threats and hazards your community planners have identified includes severe thunderstorms, tornados, and a train derailment that could include the transport of nuclear waste materials. The community planners examined the history and consequences of each event and determined that thunderstorms were the most likely to occur and that a train derailment was the least likely to occur (since it has never happened in their community). The planners then looked at the consequences of each event and determined that the consequences of a train derailment that included nuclear waste materials could have the most devastating and long-term effects on the community, and that thunderstorms would have the least effect on the community. While thunderstorms can have effects, such as lightning that causes fires or flash flooding, the potential

consequences of the train derailment could be loss of life, loss of productive farmland, or loss of a transportation route for products coming through the area as well as products coming into the community for use by the community.

Community planners then looked at the probability of each event. It was determined that severe thunderstorms happen quite often in the community. This was followed by tornados, which average around one or two a year. A train derailment has only happened once in the area, and it was 126 years ago, but the trains that come through the area now carry nuclear waste material. So the question facing planners now is which of the threats and hazards should they plan for first?

At this point, you could graph the results and where the probability and the effect line meet, this is what your priority of planning should be. This may not be the most probable event or the most devastating, but it should be the event that could happen more times than naught, and the event that would still have some pretty devastating effects on the community. For our example here, the community planners determined that tornados were the biggest and most likely threat to the community. The community decided to make planning for a tornado the highest priority. This is not a scientific process, therefore the results of the process may not be clean and pretty. The community planners could decide that they fear the train derailment more and decide to plan for it first. That is up to the leaders of the community and the planning team. For the rest of the chapter, we use the tornado scenario as our example.

Step 3 of the planning process is to determine our goals and objectives. Community planners have used THIRA and determined that the tornado was the biggest threat to their small community in Oklahoma. From this information, planners will build a scenario that will force planners to think about the operations priorities during the response as well as constraints and restraints for the response. Using the idea of a devastating tornado, let us think of the operations priorities or what we need to do first. One of the first operational priorities after a tornado is debris removal. While this may seem like a straightforward effort, there are many things to think about when planning for debris removal. Obviously, there have to be trucks, bulldozers, and a location to dump the debris. While planning, a point to consider is that debris may contain hazardous materials, which could be in the form of asbestos, lead-based paint products, Freon from refrigerators, or household hazardous waste such as paint thinners, motor oil, fuel products, etc. Each of these items has a requirement for disposal. The situation this forces is that debris must be removed from the area in order to free up the flow of transportation through the affected area, but it must be sorted in order for proper disposal.

Now let us think about the workers removing debris. As we have said before, every disaster has a health component; the workers removing debris may be faced with sharp, rusted objects. Are they all current on their tetanus vaccinations? Do the community planners need to consider providing tetanus vaccinations to responders?

We have identified some of the resources, now let us look at constraints and restraints. A constraint is something that must be done, and a restraint is something that is preventing something from happening. A constraint to the recovery of the community is the removal of debris. Debris must be removed in order for the community to begin recovery. A restraint to debris removal is the issue of hazardous materials and waste removal from the debris for proper disposal. Planners use the scenario to determine the specific resources needed to respond to the emergency as well as determine specific constraints and restraints to the response.

Step 4 of the planning process is to develop the plan itself. During this step, we develop courses of action and analyze them, identify the resources needed to put the plan into action, and identify the information and intelligence needs. The first action in developing the actual plan is to develop a detailed timeline within the scenario. Following the example of the tornado, what would be Step 1? Would it be a notification from the National Weather Service to the community emergency operations center (EOC)? Would the EOC then start notifying law enforcement, fire services, and public health that a tornado is on the way? Would public health leaders start notifying shelter locations that they may need to be put into service? As we develop the detailed timeline, we need to also identify specific decision points. Who needs to make the decision as well as the consequences of those decisions? Let us look at the decision to activate shelter locations to begin setting up for possible occupants. Who makes that decision? Is it the mayor, the director of emergency management, or the director of public health? What if the shelters end up not being used? Who is paying for all of this? One point to remember about responding to emergencies, everything costs money. Cost is always a factor and could determine which actions are taken and which one are delayed. While this is a reality that no one wants to consider, community planners must take into account the cost of future actions and determine if their planned activities can truly be paid for.

Once community planners have identified decision points, they must identify specific actions to take. Specifically, what is the action to be taken, who is responsible for the action, when should it happen, how long should it take and how much do they actually have to perform that action, what has to happen before that action can be taken, and what resources are needed to accomplish that action? Let us go back to the need for the mass vaccination clinic for tetanus shots for responders. We can break it down by saying the specific action is a vaccination clinic. The public health department will be responsible for the clinic. The clinic should happen as soon as possible to allow for protection of responders. The clinic needs to determine how many responders need to be vaccinated and then determine the throughput of the clinic based on the amount of healthcare works available for the clinic, the location of the clinic, and the available resources (such as the amount of vaccinations available). Some of the steps that need to be taken before the clinic include setting up the clinic itself, advertising for the clinic time and location, and obtaining the right amount of vaccinations. Resources include screeners, nurses, a location for the clinic, needles, vaccination vials, handouts about the vaccination, etc.

Next, we determine which course of action we will take. This can be done by comparing the costs and benefits of each action and determining which action is the best for the overall mission, goals, and objectives for the response. Once the course of action is selected, it is analyzed again to determine the resources needed to complete that course of action. This analysis is done to determine the resource needs without limitations; this estimate is a best-case scenario.

Finally, we look at the information and intelligence needs for our plan up to this point. At this point, we begin to look at the end state of the response. Will the actions move us closer to that? What are the failure points of the plan so far? What would cause us to fail? For example, failure of the vaccination clinic could happen because we are unable to obtain enough vaccine for all the responders. We also look for what we have forgotten in the plan as well as inconsistencies. We also look to see if the plan messes with jurisdictions around us and the next high level of government. In our example of a small rural community in Oklahoma, we would want to make sure that our plans are consistent and complimentary to our neighboring local communities, the county the community resides in, the State of Oklahoma's plans, as well as specific federal plans.

Step 5 of the planning process is to prepare the plan for presentation, review it, and seek approval.

This is the part of the process where a lot of the actual writing takes place. The plan has practically written itself as a result of the previous steps, but here is where it is put into a specific format. CPG 101 has a format that can be followed that matches the steps of the planning process. Some hints for plan writing are the following: keep the language simple and easily understandable, avoid using jargon (words that only certain people will understand) and try not to use acronyms unless you explain them first, use an active voice, and provide detail. After reading the plan, the reader should be able to understand what to do in the case of an emergency.

After the plan has been prepared, it is time to review it using a set of filters. Review the plan for adequacy (Is it large enough in scope to cover the mission?), feasibility (Can we actually do it?), acceptability (Is the plan something that people would be able to accept as an appropriate solution?), completeness (Have we left anything out?), and compliance (Are we in compliance with applicable policies, regulations, and laws?). CPG 101 contains a long list of questions that can be consulted when asking the above questions about the plan.

Once the plan has been prepared and reviewed, the next part of Step 5 is to seek approval for the plan and disseminate the plan. The planning team leaders should arrange a briefing with the approving authority and seek their approval. In this particular case, a verbal approval is not adequate. Anyone picking up the plan to it put into action needs to see that they are operating with approval from the elected officials in the community. In many cases, the city or county has an ordinance that indemnify the responder from legal responsibility, but often the plans outline what actions the responder is responsible for during the response. Disseminating the plan can be done in a few different ways: it could be put on a website, printed and given out, or placed in an easily accessible location.

Step 6 is plan implementation. Plan implementation is actually part of the preparedness cycle. Training and exercising the plan allows us to determine if the plan is going to do what we want it to do in a simulated emergency environment. Training can be accomplished by conducting seminars and workshops with the goal of either training the specifics of the plan or using the plan as a basis for suborganizations to develop standard operating procedures based on the identified actions within the plan. For example, if the public health department was identified as the responsible party in the plan for setting up shelters, then the public health department would come up with its own standard operating procedure for setting up a shelter. Exercising is covered in depth as capacity building

in Chapter 13. But when we refer to exercises, we are talking about using a hypothetical scenario to test our actions against a specific plan, policy, or procedure. This can be accomplished by conducting a tabletop exercise where members of an organizations sit around a table and talk about what they would do according to the plan, all the way to actually setting up a mass vaccination clinic in what is referred to as a full-scale exercise (FSE). As we evaluate the results of the training and exercises, we can determine if the plan needs to be changed or simply updated. For example, if the plan stated that the EOC would notify public health officials in the event of a tornado to begin preparing shelters and during the exercise, the EOC was not able to reach certain officials, the plan will need to be updated with the right contact information.

The last section of the preparedness cycle for us to discuss is organizing and equipping responders. Organizing will be covered in-depth in Chapter 11, but for the purpose of the preparedness cycle, we are looking at how we organize responders and how we equip them to handle the response to a specific disaster or emergency. Organizing can mean that as part of the planning process, we look at how we put certain activities together with the right type of responder. For example, if we care conducting a mass vaccination clinic, do we organize as "Clinic Team 1" or do we separate medical staff from security staff and from janitorial staff? In Step 4 of the planning process, we said that the process will identify resources needed to complete the mission. As we look at that resource, we need to consider what is currently on hand to assist responders in accomplishing their tasks. If the responder needs an item that is not currently available, using the plan can be a great justification for the purchase of that item.

As you can see, the preparedness cycle covers a lot of ground. The cycle never ends as we continually plan, organize, equip, train, exercise, and evaluate our actions. The basis for all of the preparedness cycle activities is the plan. Developing the plan will inform all other actions within the preparedness cycle.[4]

▶ Conclusions

The preparedness cycle as described in national emergency management literature is what guides us through the process of preparing to respond to an emergency. As part of that cycle, planning allows us to ask important questions about what types of threats and hazards the community faces and develop a plan for responding to those threats and hazards. These are the first real steps in building a preparedness and response program. In the next chapter, we look at some practical applications of emergency management principals.

Key Words

Planning process
Preparedness cycle
Threat and Hazard Identification and Risk Assessment

Discussion Questions

1. Describe the steps of the planning process?
2. Why is the THIRA the basis for the planning process?
3. How many parts of the preparedness cycle are there?
4. Briefly explain the parts of the preparedness cycle.

References

1. Department of Homeland Security. *National Preparedness Goal.* September 2015. p 1. Available at: https://www.fema.gov/media-library-data/1443799615171-2aae90be55041740f97e8532fc680d40/National_Preparedness_Goal_2nd_Edition.pdf. Accessed May 2017.
2. Department of Homeland Security. *Homeland Security Presidential Directive 5.* February 28, 2003. Available at: https://www.dhs.gov/sites/default/files/publications/Homeland%20Security%20Presidential%20Directive%205.pdf. Accessed April 2017.
3. Department of Homeland Security. *Homeland Security esidential Directive 8.* December 17, 2003. Available at: https://www.gpo.gov/fdsys/pkg/PPP-2003-book2/pdf/PPP-2003-book2-doc-pg1745.pdf. Accessed April 2017.
4. *Comprehensive Preparedness Guide (CPG) 101: Developing and Maintaining Emergency Operations Plans*, Version 2.0. November 2010. Available at: https://www.fema.gov/media-library-data/20130726-1828-25045-0014/cpg_101_comprehensive_preparedness_guide_developing_and_maintaining_emergency_operations_plans_2010.pdf. Accessed May 2017.

CHAPTER 11

Practical Applications of Public Health Emergency Management

LEARNING OBJECTIVES

By the end of this chapter, the reader will be able to:

- Describe the Incident Command System
- Explain the principals of the Incident Command System
- Explain the steps of the Threat and Hazard Identification and Risk Assessment process

▶ Introduction

So far in the text, we have explored many different things to help us prepare for a disaster. Whether it is legislation that tells us our authorities during a disaster, the role of numerous organizations during a disaster, as well as the national and international response infrastructures, each of these have a role in getting us ready for a disaster. In the previous chapter, we explored the idea of the preparedness cycle and how it can be used to ready us for a disaster. Whether it is through planning, organizing and equipping ourselves, training, exercising our plans, policies and procedures, or evaluating our progress and performance, each of these areas is nothing without putting them into practice. This chapter explores some practical ways of placing these ideas into practice.

▶ The Incident Command System

In the 1970s, California faced a series of devastating wild fires. In 1970, during a 13-day period of fighting fires, 16 lives were lost, 700 structures were destroyed by fire, and over 500,000 acres were burned. The overall cost was over $18 million per day.[1] As you can imagine, these types of losses were unsustainable. It was identified during the aftermath of the fires that communications and organization of firefighters were not handled properly, resulting in the inability to work effectively in putting out the fires. In using what would later become part of the preparedness cycle, evaluation of actions and the incorporation of lessons learned led authorities at the national and state levels to develop a system of organizing and communicating during such disasters. By working together, national and state authorities developed a system called Firefighting Resources of California Organized for Potential Emergencies (FIRESCOPE).[1] FIRESCOPE was a series of command and control protocols that revolved around the idea that each person had a specific job, each person reported to a specific supervisor, and planning, operating, and communicating during a disaster would be done using a common language. No longer would each responding organization work on their own. They would become part of the bigger response that would serve specific objectives all toward the overall goal of solving the problem. These principals would later become the Incident Command System (ICS).

ICS is a standardized system that can be used in any type of disaster, enables a coordinated response among various jurisdictions and municipalities, establishes a common planning process and management of resources, and allows for integration into a common organizational structure. It can be used in any type of event: a natural disaster, a terrorist attack, a disease outbreak, or a preplanned event.

An incident is something that happens that requires us to respond. An event is something that we plan for in advance, such as the State of the Union address. An incident happens and we react versus an event is planned and executed according to the plan. If something happens during the event, it can then become an incident.

Why do we use ICS? ICS helps us with accountability, both personal and resource accountabilities. Personal accountability is supported by having a clear chain of command and a clear role and set of responsibilities for each position. Without ICS, we will not have clear communications. Clear communications mean that we are operating on the same radio channel, have clear lines of reporting information, a central repository for response information, and a clear communications plan. Communications plans lay out who will speak for the response (typically the Public Information Office), what type of information they will communicate to the public, and how that information will be communicated to the public. ICS also gives us a standardized process for planning. Planning develops a course of action that can be agreed upon by all involved and gives the response a clear path toward achieving its objectives. It also allows us to seamlessly include responders into our organization during a response. If everyone is using ICS, then a responder can report to a supervisor and will know what is going on and what their role will be, because each position

has a specific title, role, and responsibility and each structure will be the same. Some of the benefits of ICS include a system that looks out for the safety and welfare of assigned responders, achievement of response objectives that helps us reach the overall goal of the response, and helps effectively manage resources. Some of the features of ICS include the standardization of common terms, establishment of a chain of command with a system of how to transfer command, a dedicated planning and organizational structure, comprehensive resource management, information flow, and an accountability system.

▶ Incident Command System Structure

The basic ICS structure contains a command group and a general staff group (**FIGURE 11-1**). The command group is made up of the incident commander, the deputy incident commander, the public information officer (PIO), the liaison officer, and the safety officer. The incident commander's role is to manage all ICS functions, until that responsibility is transferred to someone else. The incident commander can also delegate his/her authority as needed. Specifically, the incident commander is responsible for the safety of all responders, providing information to partners (both internal and external) and establishing liaisons with other organizations responding to the incident.[2] The deputy incident commander can also serve as the incident manager in his/her absence or when the incident commander needs a rest.

The PIO advises the incident commander on how to give information to the public or to the media. If someone needs to represent the response, either the incident commander or the PIO would conduct the briefing. The incident commander will approve of all materials that are to be released by the response or briefed to the public or media. The safety officer provides advice to the incident commander on the safety of responders and works with others within the ICS structure to make sure responders are briefed on safety concerns and actions taken to mitigate those hazards. The liaison officer serves as a conduit of information between agencies or organizations supporting the response. If the incident is health focused, such as pandemic influenza, more than likely the Centers for Disease Control and Prevention would be in charge, at the national level. Liaison officers from all other U.S. government agencies that are supporting the response will work to provide a two-way flow of information between agencies to better inform

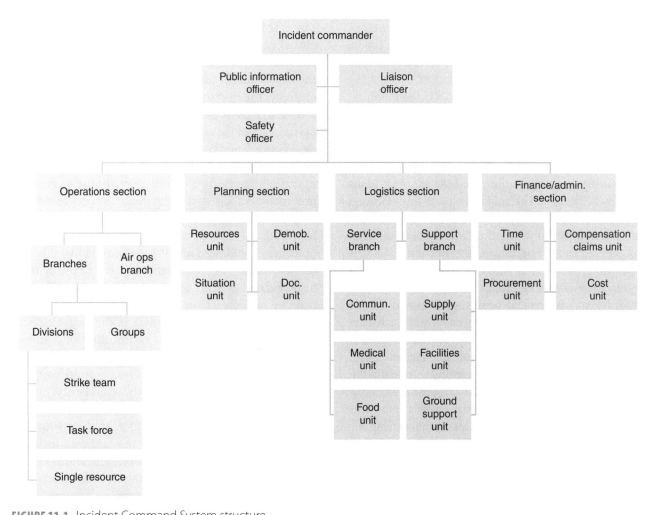

FIGURE 11-1 Incident Command System structure

the response and the decision makers as they weigh options and decisions.

The General Staff of the ICS is made up of the Operations Section, Planning Section, Logistics Section, and the Administrative/Finance Section. Even though the general staff section is made up of these four areas, it does not mean all of them will be used. For example, in a small incident, it may be that there is no need for an Administrative/Finance Section. If the section is not needed, it simply will not be activated. If the need arises for an administrative/finance role, then a person can be appointed to be the Administrative/Finance Section chief. Each of the sections can be expanded to have branches, divisions or groups, units, or single resources. If the Operations Section expands to multiple branches, it does not mean the Planning Section must expand to the same level. The idea behind ICS is that the system is expandable or contractible based on the needs of the response.

The Operations Section is responsible for directing and coordinating all of the actual operations within the response. This could be firefighting operations,

aeromedical evacuations, or providing vaccinations in a mass vaccination clinic. Usually, the Operations Section is the first section activated and to have assets assigned to the response. It usually has the most assets. For example, the Operations Section could have multiple groups assigned to different divisions across the entire response area, whereas the Administrative/ Finance Section may only have one or two people to track all financial transactions. Based on the geographical area of operations, there may be numerous staging areas for assets to get ready for response operations and multiple base camps allowing somewhere responders can rest and relax prior to reporting to a staging area to deploy to a response location. One of the features of ICS is span of control. Span of control means that there are usually three to seven persons working for one supervisor. Any more than seven and the duties of the supervisor become more difficult to execute. The optimal number for supervision in the ICS is five direct reports per supervisor. If there are more than seven direct reports, then they can be broken down into strike teams, task forces, groups, etc.

This will allow for better supervision and accountability of personnel and resources. These personnel can be organized by location into divisions or resource type into groups.

The next major section in the ICS is the Planning Section. The major activities of the Planning Section are collecting, evaluating, and displaying incident intelligence and information; preparing and documenting the Incident Action Plan (IAP); tracking resources; maintaining documentation; and developing plans for demobilization. The major units of the Planning Section are the Resources Unit, the Situation Unit, the Demobilization Unit, the Documentation Unit, and the Technical Specialists. The Resources Unit is responsible for making sure everyone who is part of the response is checked in, accounted for during the response, and is tracked until they are ready to go home. Not only does the Resource Unit track personnel, but they also track all equipment during the response. The Situation Unit collects, analyzes, and displays information for the response. Information can be weather maps, maps of the response area, logistical information such as resource levels, etc. This information can assist response leadership during the decision-making process. The Demobilization Unit makes sure that all assets assigned to the response are sent home when they are no longer needed. Demobilization planning begins as soon as the response begins. When an objective of the response is met, then the Demobilization Unit begins assessing whether resources can be sent home. This process continues until all resources have been sent home. The Documentation Unit collects, maintains, and stores all documentation related to the response. This can be IAPs, receipts for purchases, records of reimbursement, etc. These documents will help write the story of what happened during the response once it is over. This process aides in the development of the after action report that will tell us what went right, what went wrong, and what needs to be improved upon the next time we do a response. Technical Specialists are assigned to the Planning Section as needed. They are subject matter experts that can provide information and technical assistance to the planners for the response.

One of the major responsibilities of the Planning Section is the development of the IAP. The IAP outlines the objectives for the response during the operational period, the resources assigned to the response, the leadership of the response to include the ICS structure, the communications plan, safety plans, maps, and any other information that can assist during the operational period. The operational period is defined as the time frame for which the operations can take place. This can be a 12-hour period, 24 hours, 1 week, etc. This does not mean the entire response will be completed within that time period; it just means that the objectives for that time period have been met. For example, the overall goal of a response may be to stop a wild fire from spreading. For the first operational period, one of the objectives may be to set up the Incident Command Post and assign firefighters to specific divisions to begin firefighting operations. The second operational period objectives may consist of creating firebreaks to assist in slowing down the progress of the fire. Operational periods will continue until the fire is put out. At the end of each operational period, the objectives are viewed and it is determined whether or not the objectives have been met, whether they need to be carried over to the next operational period, or whether new objectives have to be developed.

The next section of the ICS is the Logistics Section. The Logistics Section is responsible for communications, medical support to responders, food for the responders, supplies, facilities, ground support, and maintaining support for the emergency operations center and Incident Command Post. Communications in this instance is different than what the PIO does. Communications in this instance includes radios, frequencies, and other communications equipment such as Wi-Fi devices, computers, fax machines, etc. In today's electronic environment, you are probably wondering why a fax machine is listed. Certain documents are still required to be faxed according to Federal Emergency Management Agency. This assists in maintaining tight document control and does not allow for electronic manipulation of documents after they have been created, signed, and assigned for action. The units within the Logistics Section are divided into two branches: the Service Branch and the Support Branch. The Services Branch provides services for the responders, such as communications, medical services, and food. The Support Branch provides support to the responder, such as ordering supplies, running response facilities, or acquiring facilities needed for the response; and the Ground Support Branch can move resources from one area to another, as well as maintain the response vehicles. This is an important part of the response because vehicles such as bulldozers require strict maintenance protocols that measure in hours used. Once a vehicle or resource reaches its required maintenance hours, it must be pulled from service and cannot return until it has undergone required maintenance.

The last section of the ICS is the Administrative/Financial Section, commonly referred to as the Admin/Finance Section. The overall responsibilities of the Admin/Finance Section include recording personnel time, maintaining contracts, compensation and claims, and conducting overall cost analysis for the incident. While these may not seem like the type of things we do during a response, no response can take place without financial management. Every action in a response costs money. Without financial resources, the response would quickly grind to a halt. Therefore, careful analysis of courses of action during a response must include financial aspects of the action. For example, just because a course of action sounds like a good idea, if it costs too much money, it could be deemed unfit and therefore an alternative course of action must be developed. If there are not enough financial resources available, the Admin/Finance Section can work with leadership and different levels of government to secure those resources. The four major units in the Admin/Finance Section include the Compensation/Claims Unit, Cost Unit, Procurement Unit, and Time Unit. The Compensation/Claims Unit provides compensation for damaged property during a response and processes claims for compensation. The Cost Unit tracks the costs associated with the response and also provides valuable assistance during course of action development, as to which course of action is more economically feasible. The Procurement Unit is responsible for purchasing items needed for the response as well as conducting contracting operations. The Time Unit records times for the response, including time for individuals as well as time for equipment usage. This will allow for proper calculations for things like overtime as well as assisting in the scheduling and costing of required maintenance for equipment.

As you can see, ICS can be a very large organization when it is fully expanded. As was stated before, the beauty of the system is that each section and unit is only activated when needed, which allows for a very flexible and manageable response organization. Sometimes, a person can fill more than one role. All

that is needed for an ICS to be activated is an incident commander. From there, the incident commander can expand the structure as needed, bringing in personnel to fill roles when it becomes necessary. One of the planning methods to predetermine what kind of ICS structure will be needed during a response, it conducts what is called a Threat and Hazard Identification and Risk Assessment (THIRA) process. This process lets us determine what types of threats and hazards our community faces and what type of risk is associated with each one. Once we determine the risk, we can develop a plan for responding to that threat or hazard, which in turn allows us to plan the type of response necessary.

▶ Threat and Hazard Identification and Risk Assessment

The first step in the THIRA process is to identify the threats and hazards of concern to your community (**FIGURE 11-2**). When we consider the threats and hazards a community faces, we look at three categories: natural, technological, and human-caused. Natural threats and hazards can include earthquakes, drought, tornados, tsunamis, severe winter weather, and pandemics, to name a few. Technological threats and hazards can include airplane crashes, dam failures, prolonged power failures, train derailments, mine accidents, and hazardous materials releases. Human-caused disasters can include a biological, chemical, radiological or nuclear attack; bombings; cyber-attacks; electrical grid sabotage, and school/workplace violence. In order to determine which of these threats and hazards a community could face, we can look to history as a guiding tool.[3] For example, in Chapter 10, we used a rural community in Oklahoma's

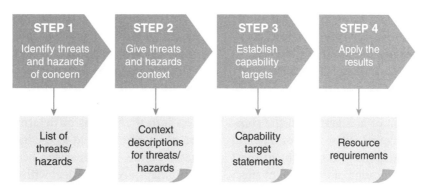

FIGURE 11-2 Threat and Hazard Identification and Risk Assessment steps

Reproduced from Department of Homeland Security. *Threat and Hazard Identification and Risk Assessment Guide, Comprehensive Preparedness Guide (CPG) 201*. August 2013. p 2. Available at: https://www.fema.gov/media-library-data/8ca0a9e54dc8b037a55b402b2a2 69e94/CPG201_htirag_2nd_edition.pdf. Accessed April 2017.

history of tornados as a hazard the community faced. Looking into the history of the community could also show us that multiple train derailments have occurred over time. We can also look at what is currently happening in our community to determine threats and hazards. If the community is in close proximity to an interstate, then we could do a survey of what types of things are being transported via the interstate near or in our community. For example, while conducting our survey, it is determined that nuclear waste material from a nuclear power plant in a neighboring state is transported by trucks using the interstate bordering the community. This could pose multiple threats and hazards from a traffic accident to hijacking of the shipment. All community partners should be involved in the determination of threats and hazards. No threat or hazard should be ignored, because as we saw in an example in Chapter 10, all incidents and hazards can have a health effect. As public health planners, we can find ourselves involved in planning for numerous threats and hazards.

In order for planners to determine the threats and hazards of a community, there are two factors that must be look at: the likelihood of the incident and the significance of the threat or hazard effect. In likelihood, we need to determine the chance that the specific threat or hazard would occur. We can look at historical patterns, such as when tornados typically happen, when a train derailment took place, or how often a truck carrying hazardous materials goes through our community. Once we determine the likelihood, we can determine the significance of that threat or hazard. We have to answer questions such as if the truck carrying nuclear waste material were to crash and spill its contents, what would the effect be? Planners should look at the worst-case scenario, not only looking at their community for examples, but also looking at any type of disaster resulting from the threat or hazard. Some caution should be used when determining effect, as the effects from a nuclear waste spill in New York City would not be of the magnitude of a spill in rural Oklahoma. The types of effects could be the same, but the magnitude could be different.

Once the list of threats or hazards has been determined, each one must be given context. In order to do that, certain questions can be asked: How would the timing of the incident or accident affect the community's ability to manage it? What time of day and what season would be most likely to have the greatest impacts? How would the location of the incident affect the community's ability to manage it? Which locations would be most likely to have the greatest impacts: populated areas, coastal zones, industrial areas, or

residential areas? What conditions or circumstances would make the threat or hazard of particular concern? Multiple events happening at the same time? For example, if we determined that transportation of nuclear waste through the community via the interstate was a threat, we must look at where an accident could occur. Would it make a difference if it occurred on the east side of town, the west side of town, or the middle of the community; if it happened during rush hour, in the middle of the night, or during the middle of the day; or if the accident area was near the retirement community, near a school, or near the industrial park. All of these help us determine the context of the threat, which also helps us determine the potential effects on the community should they happen.

Once we determine the threats and hazards and put them into context, then we can determine what capabilities our community must have in order to respond to those threats or hazards. If it is determined that transportation of nuclear waste through the community is a threat, we can determine what types of response capabilities would be needed to respond to that type of incident or accident. Do we need specialized hazardous materials teams, specialized resources at the hospital, or specialized resources at the community morgue to deal with contaminated casualties? Once we determine the answer to those types of questions, we can determine what we need to do to either develop that capability or further develop the capability we already have to deal with the threat or hazard. Planners must also determine the time frame for which a response would be acceptable. For example, if we determined that the threat from a nuclear waste spill would be greatest if it were to happen during rush hour, near the school district, planners must determine if immediate action is required or if the community can wait for assets from another area to be called. If the rural community is outside a major city, could the community rely upon assets from the major metropolitan area for response or must the community have the capability to deal with the incident on their own while they wait for additional assets as needed?

Once we have determined the capability needed in order to deal with the threat or hazard, planners must apply the results. Applying the results leads planners into the process of determining what resources are needed to respond to the incident or accident. As stated before, resources can be personnel, money, or equipment needed to deal with the effects of the incident or accident. Back to our tornado example from before, some of the equipment resources needed to deal with the aftermath of a tornado could include bulldozers and dump trucks to remove debris. In order to determine the amount of bulldozers and dump trucks needed, planners should make an estimate in the amount of debris that could result from the tornado. Once the amount of debris is estimated, then the load capacity of trucks can be determined, and the overall estimate of the debris totals can be divided by the load capacity of the truck to determine the amount of trucks. This number then can be reduced by determining how long one truck can operate before it must rest. This will help planners determine how long it would take for debris removal to occur. While this may seem like a long process, proper planning requires us to determine these things prior to an incident or accident to properly determine how long the debris removal will last and how many resources are needed to make it happen.

Now, how do we apply all of this information to public health? Let us go back to the tornado example. It was determined through the THIRA process that tornados were a threat to the community and must be planned for. One of the effects of a tornado can be standing water. As was seen during the response to the tornado that devastated Joplin, Missouri, in 2011, standing water became a problem the days after the tornado. One of the public health consequences of standing water can be mosquitoes. Mosquitoes breed in standing water and in today's environments of West Nile Virus and Zika, standing water needs to be eliminated. If it cannot be eliminated, then it must be treated. If it cannot be treated, fogging operations should be conducted. The local health department should organize itself by using the ICS. Part of the Operations Section could be a unit dedicated to fogging operations. The Fogging Operations Unit will work with Logistics Section and Admin/Finance Section to procure the necessary chemicals and equipment for prolonged fogging operations. The unit will also work with the Planning Section to determine the best areas and street routing for foggers in the potentially affected area. Once fogging operations have been completed, the unit will work with Logistics Section and Admin/Finance Section to conduct maintenance on the equipment, determine replacement of the fogging chemicals, and determine how much the operations actually cost to recoup the cost of fogging operations.

▶ Conclusions

The ICS and the THRIA process are two foundations for the application of emergency management principles. ICS allows us to organize for any incident or event, while the THIRA process lets us determine which hazards are the most dangerous for the community and lets community planners determine which of those hazards should be prioritized in the planning process. In the next chapter, we discuss how to use ICS and the THIRA process to help develop an emergency operations center.

Key Words

Incident Command System
Threat and Hazard Identification and Risk Assessment

Discussion Questions

1. What are the main features of ICS?
2. Why was ICS created?
3. Briefly describe the THRIA process.

References

1. FEMA. *NIMS and the Incident Command System.* 2004. Available at: https://www.fema.gov/txt/nims/nims_ics _position_paper.txt. Accessed May 2017.
2. FEMA. *ICS 100.B Course.* October 2013. Available at: https:// training.fema.gov/is/coursematerials.aspx?code=IS-100.b. Accessed April 2017.
3. Department of Homeland Security. *Threat and Hazard Identification and Risk Assessment Guide, Comprehensive Preparedness Guide (CPG) 201.* August 2013. Available at: https://www.fema.gov/media-library-data/8ca0a9e54dc8b 037a55b402b2a269e94/CPG201_htirag_2nd_edition.pdf. Accessed April 2017.

CHAPTER 12

Developing a Public Health Emergency Operations Center

LEARNING OBJECTIVES

By the end of this chapter, the reader will be able to:

- Define the term "emergency operations center"
- Explain the basic steps of developing an emergency operations center

▶ Introduction

An emergency operations center (EOC) has been defined by Federal Emergency Management Agency (FEMA) as a central command and control facility responsible for carrying out the principals of emergency preparedness and emergency management, or disaster management functions at a strategic level during an emergency.[1] A public health emergency operations center (PHEOC) integrates traditional public health services and functions into an emergency management model.[2] Using an emergency management model that is centered on prevention, preparedness, mitigation, response, and recovery, we can apply those to all of the public health services and functions.

Day-to-day operations of a local public health department typically center around providing public health services such as wellness screenings, vaccinations, and environmental health services, to mention just a few. Let us take environmental health services for example. Environmental health services can include restaurant inspections, ground water well services, and pest control.

In May 2011, the city of Joplin, Missouri, was hit by a devastating tornado. The tornado damaged a large portion of the city and left essential city services in ruin. As part of the response to any disaster, organizations descend on the affected area to provide aid and services. Sometimes, these volunteers can do more harm than good. For example, many church and civic groups decided to bring cooked food to responders working in the area. While this may seem like a good idea, unregulated and uninspected food can be, and often is, the cause of illness among responders. There is a fine line between accepting help and putting responders at risk by allowing these groups to provide uninspected food. To counter this, environmental health inspectors from the health department in Joplin reached out to these groups and set up an inspection protocol. Food had to be prepared in the area and could not be prepared off-site and brought in to be served. While this may seem like an over burdensome process, it ensured that food was prepared properly and responders who received the food were not put at undo risk from improperly prepared and served food. You have to remember that civic-minded groups only wanted to help, so many of them jumped at the chance to work with the health department to ensure food was properly prepared and served. Each organization that participated with the inspection program received a sheet of paper certifying that their preparations and serving techniques were within acceptable guidelines. Each group would display the sign and responders were briefed that if they approached a food service area that did not display the sign, then they were not permitted to eat at that location. This simple system prevented many illnesses that most likely would have been attributed to ill prepared and served food.

▶ Emergency Operations Center Development

As you can see, there are many areas of activity during a response; environmental health food inspections being just one of them. In order to track all of these services, as well as plan the next actions of the response, coordinate with other responding agencies, and leverage resources during a response, a central location for all of these activities are needed. A PHEOC is needed to do all those things during a disaster.

One of the most common questions is what is an EOC and why do we need one? As stated earlier in the chapter, an EOC is a physical location from which the coordination of information and resources take place in order to support incident management activities. It is the structure, not the people. The people make up the Incident Command System (ICS) or Incident Management System (IMS). In the world of public health, incident command principals have been used to create an IMS that better fits the philosophy of public health operations. An EOC is a place where the IMS can be used to support decision makers in the accomplishment of their task and provides the capability to receive, analyze, display, and monitor incident information. It provides a central location where the identification, organization, collaboration, and coordination of resources can be accomplished, as well as a location for communications, collaboration, and coordination of public health assets during an incident or event.

The EOC is responsible for the strategic or operational overview of the incident. This should not be confused with the Incident Command Post, where tactical decisions are made and operations are coordinated. The EOC provides the next level up of organization and decision-making. Common functions at this level include information analysis, decision-making, continuity of the organization, and determining courses of action for the agency. In most PHEOCs,

there is one person in charge, and that is the incident manager. A PHEOC organizes itself via the IMS structure, which provides a management structure that results in better and more efficient decision-making and use of resources. It is designed for incidents that may involve multiple agencies and should be able to expand or contract (one of the principals of the ICS).

When developing an EOC, planners and developers should answer questions such as what is the mission of the EOC, what will the communications processes of the EOC be, what is the organizational approach of the EOC staff, what will the design of the EOC look like, and are there any specific design considerations that must be taken into account. To define the EOC's mission, planners need to answer the following questions: What will the EOC do? What functions will the EOC perform? How will the EOC be staffed? Under what conditions will the EOC operate? For example, if a community health department were to use the Threat and Hazard Identification and Risk Assessment (THIRA) process (as discussed in the previous chapter) and it was determined that an EOC capability was needed in order to effectively respond to public health threats, the planners would need to ask what the EOC will do during a response to one of those threats. In the case of a mass vaccination campaign that would be run from multiple locations, the EOC could serve as a coordination center for the leverage of personnel and resources during the campaign. Functions of the EOC could include resource tracking and coordination at the health department level. The EOC could also serve as a coordination center for public health leadership to gather, review pectinate data and information to make decisions, and recommend courses of action to make the campaign more efficient in its services. The EOC staffing model should include the IMS. As described before, IMS is modeled after the principals of ICS and therefore allows for easy expansion and contraction of the system as needed. Conditions under which the EOC will operate include what types of shifts will be used (8-hour vs 12-hour), will the EOC operate on the weekends or at night, or where the EOC will conduct virtual operations during a holiday weekend. Sometimes during a prolonged response lasting months at a time, IMS leadership may choose to let everyone be on call and send them home for the weekend. This allows response personnel to have some much-needed downtime but allows for a quick return should the situation change. Other things that can be used to determine the mission of the EOC include relevant municipal codes and laws, regulations, policies, and protocols.

When determining communications, planners should answer the following questions: Who will the

EOC communicate with? What will be communicated by the EOC (as compared to what will be communicated by the ICS team at the scene if there is such a structure)? How often will communications occur? Are there redundant or alternative communications techniques available? Examples of communications during a mass vaccination campaign can include directions to the nearest clinic, information about clinic hours, and information about paperwork that can be found online and needs to be filled out prior to arriving at a clinic.

Planners will also need to determine what types of reports will be generated during EOC operations. Some of the common reports include situation reports (SITREPs), Incident Action Plans (IAP), Health Alert Network (HAN) notifications, and Epidemic Information Exchange (EPI-X) notifications. Planners will also need to determine who those reports will go to once they have been generated. Typically, local health departments will coordinate and report information to counties or districts, then to the state, and then to the federal government. Planners must also remember that information should flow back to the local area once consolidated reports are generated or received. This allows the local level the ability to see the big picture.

Once we have determined the mission of the EOC and the staffing structure, we can develop the facility design. Things to consider when developing the overall design include the location of the EOC, the size, floor layout, what types of technology will be necessary, and how to protect the facility against certain threats such as earthquakes and tornados. The location of the EOC should be close to the health department or the agency it serves. It should be available for use at a moment's notice, and it should be accessible to all employees that are assigned to serve in the EOC. The EOC should be big enough to accommodate all of the response personnel that could be assigned, as well as any other agency that may send representatives. The layout of the EOC should have a floor space where workstations can be set up or used by responders. It should also consider rest areas, bathrooms, a kitchen, showers, meeting spaces, and offices for senior leaders. When considering the daily use of the EOC, planners should think about daily use, such as having a staff that is dedicated to answer phones and inquiries, as well as watch over the news and other intelligence sources, 24 hours a day. Will the space be used as a meeting space? Or will the space only be used during an emergency or an exercise/drill? Planners must also consider the amount and different types of technology that will be used in the EOC. Will the EOC need to be designed to accommodate things such as large projection walls, or will a current space (such as an executive conference room) be used? Once those questions can be answered, they need to be passed through the threats and vulnerabilities filter, asking questions as follows: What do we do if the power is disrupted? What about a physical attack on the facility? Does the facility have, or will we need to acquire, fire suppression? What do we do in the case of severe weather, such as severe winter storms or tornados?

▶ Framework for a Public Health Emergency Operations Centre

As you can see, there are many factors that go into developing an EOC. There are numerous documents and guides to assist in the process. One of those is from the World Health Organization (WHO). The *Framework for a Public Health Emergency Operations Centre*, published in November 2015, is a guide for the international public health community on the development of an EOC. In the United States, most of the emergency management guidance comes from FEMA. For the international audience, there is no global emergency management entity; therefore, health-related emergency management generally falls under the purview of WHO. Since most of the international community looks to WHO to set standards and give guidance, WHO stepped forward to develop guiding documents on the application of emergency management principals to international public health. One result from that effort was the development of the framework.

The framework is laid out into 10 sections, with 9 annexes. The primary sections of the framework lay out planning guidance for establishing the legal authority for a PHEOC. This is an important step for determining what can be legally done during an emergency. Developing an overall Emergency Response Plan is also part of the initial process. Developers of the PHEOC must know what the plan is for a response in order to design a facility that will support response operations. Developers must also consider what would happen if the facility was compromised and leadership had to move to a new location as part of a Continuity of Operations (COOP) Plan. The next section of the framework covers management of health emergencies, covering topics like planning an operational considerations, elements of an emergency management program, the IMS, and event- or hazard-specific response and management plans. For example, if the country was facing a threat from an Ebola outbreak, who would be the incident manager and what would the IMS look like? It is recommended by WHO and other public health emergency management (PHEM) leaders that a viral hemorrhagic fever expert, or more specifically an Ebola virus expert, be the incident manager.

The next section of the framework is about implementing a PHEOC. The section starts with defining the objectives of the PHEOC and what will the EOC do. This is followed by determining the essential functions of the PHEOC, the operations structure of the PHEOC (IMS), role and responsibilities of the PHEOC staff and the IMS, and core components of the PHEOC—such as plans and procedures, the physical structure, and human resources. Section 7 of the framework covers developing a training and exercise program that continuously prepares staff to operate in a PHEOC environment, as well as a general emergency environment. Lessons learned from training and exercise program execution can be measured using a monitoring and evaluation program (section 8 of the framework). Section 9 of the framework covers costing, funding, and sustaining a PHEOC. Maintaining a PHEOC can consist of normal computer replacement schedules, replacing items that were used during a response or an exercise, as well as the need to remodel or expand the PHEOC as the need arises. Section 10 of the framework contains checklists for planning and implementing a PHEOC. The annexes of the framework contain examples of things like concept of operations plans, infrastructure requirements, and minimum data sets for PHEOCs, knowledge, skills and abilities for PHEOC staff, as well as a checklist for planning and implementing a PHEOC.[2]

▶ Public Health Emergency Operations Center Network

The *Framework for a Public Health Emergency Operations Centre* contains all the needed information to get a program started. As was stated before, money is the limiting factor. Developing an EOC costs money and sometimes a country that wants to develop an EOC does not have an abundance of money. To assist in that area, the WHO developed the Public Health Emergency Operations Center Network (EOC-NET). WHO established EOC-NET in 2012 to help identify and promote best practices and standards for EOCs as well as provide support for EOC capacity building in WHO member states. The objectives of EOC-NET include the following:

- To support states parties in building their PHEOC capacity, as part of their national response framework

- To share expertise, lessons, and experiences in building, evaluating, exercising, and utilizing EOC for public health emergency response
- To identify key needs of information and communications technologies, and explore or test possible solutions
- To identify minimum data sets and standards related to public health EOCs
- To develop and make available common procedures and protocols for public health EOCs, and promote best practices
- To develop mechanisms and tools to support necessary information gathering and sharing among relevant PHEOCs during health operations
- To develop and implement EOC training programs

Member states can join EOC-NET and will have access to other member states that are in the network. Members can share lessons learned and products that have been developed that can greatly assist other member states.[3]

▶ Public Health Emergency Preparedness Cooperative Agreement

Domestically, the Centers for Disease Control and Prevention (CDC) have been administering the Public Health Emergency Preparedness (PHEP) cooperative agreement since 2002. The cooperative agreement provides funding to state, local, tribal, and territorial partner health departments to assist them in strengthening their ability to prepare for and respond to public health threats. Since its inception, the cooperative agreement has given out more than $11 billion to partners. The idea behind the cooperative agreement is that partners receive funding in exchange for concentrating efforts on an agreed path. For example, one of the goals of the national preparedness program is that organizations conduct exercises to test their readiness and to make sure that plans, policies, and procedures are correct. The PHEP cooperative agreement asks partners to conduct exercises in exchange for funding programs.

One of the documents produced by the CDC to assist state, local, tribal, and territorial partners in achieving the capabilities to effectively prepare for and respond to public health threats is the *Public Health Preparedness Capabilities: National Standards for State and Local Planning*. This document lays out 15 public health capabilities that state, local, tribal, and territorial partners can use to assist in the development of plans, policies, and procedures to prepare for and respond to public health threats. Some of the capabilities include Medical Countermeasure Dispensing, Emergency Operations Coordination, Medical Surge, Public Health Surveillance and Epidemiological Investigation, and Responder Safety and Health, to name a few. Each capability lists certain functions that must be performed in order to say that the organization is fully capable of executing the capability. Let us use the Emergency Operations Coordination capability as an example. The goal of the Emergency Operations Coordination capability, as listed in the document, is the ability to direct and support an event or incident with public health or medical implications by establishing a standardized, scalable system of oversight, organization, and supervision consistent with jurisdictional standards and practices and with the National Incident Management System (NIMS). As you can see, the capabilities work hand in hand with NIMS and other guiding documents within the national emergency management framework. The *Public Health Preparedness Capabilities* are meant to apply emergency management principals to public health situations and the result is a PHEM program.

In the Emergency Operations Coordination capability, there are five functions:

1. Conduct preliminary assessment to determine the need for public activation
2. Activate public health response operations
3. Develop incident response strategy
4. Manage and sustain the public health response
5. Demobilize and evaluate public health emergency operations

Each function contains a series of tasks that must be accomplished in order to complete the function. For example, Function 1 of Emergency Operations Coordination is to conduct a preliminary assessment to determine the need for public activation. Task 3 of Function 1 is to define incident command and emergency management structure for the public health event or incident. Each function also has performance measures that will allow for measurement of action to see whether or not the function has been completed. Sometimes, the performance measure has a time limit, such as the performance measure for Function 2—activate public health response operations. The performance measure says that the time for pre-identified staff covering activated public health agency incident management lead roles (or equivalent lead roles) to report for immediate duty, performance target: 60 minutes or less. When determining whether or not the organization can meet the target time, a drill or

exercise can be conducted to test the actions of organization to determine if the organization has the capability to conduct Emergency Operations Coordination.

As was mentioned in Chapter 4, the National Preparedness Goal mentions five mission areas:

1. Prevention
2. Protection
3. Mitigation
4. Response
5. Recovery

The core capabilities of the national emergency management level are organized into the mission areas. The FEMA core capabilities work in the same manner as the PHEP capabilities. They are targets for an organization (such as a public health department or county emergency management agency) or jurisdiction (county, city, state, etc.) to meet in order to perform specific functions during an emergency. Some of the core capabilities can be applied to all of the mission areas, such as Planning, Public Information and Warning, and Operational Coordination. Some of them are specific to the mission area, such as Forensics and Attribution are listed in the Prevention Mission Area, Intelligence and Information Sharing is listed in the Prevention and Protection Mission Area, Community Resilience is listed in the Mitigation Mission Area, and Fatality Management Services is listed in the Response Mission Area.

Sticking with the EOC theme, let us look at the core capability of Operational Coordination. The overall objective of Operational Coordination is to establish and maintain a unified and coordinated operational structure and process that appropriately integrates all critical stakeholders, and supports the execution of core capabilities. The Operational Coordination has seven targets, one of which (Target #4) says to mobilize all critical resources and establish command, control, and coordination structures within the affected community. As you can see, Target #4 is very similar to Function 2 of the PHEP capability Emergency Operations Coordination. In fact, Emergency Operations Coordination is just an amplification of the Operational Coordination core capability. The core capability outlines the national goal; it is broad and is meant to apply to more than one type of organization or jurisdiction. The PHEP capabilities are meant to apply specifically to public health organizations. This allows for application to specific public health circumstances.

Before the development of the PHEP capabilities, it was sometimes difficult to apply emergency management principals to public health operations because there was a different mind-set. Public health operations have traditionally been closer to traditional health operations in a clinic or hospital. Most public health leadership comes in the form of medical doctors or epidemiologists, and have not been trained in emergency management. In today's public health, traditional emergency management is being applied to public health operations in the form of PHEM. Public health has applied the principals of emergency management in things such as using the ICS principals in developing the IMS, substituting command for management. The idea is that public health's greatest product is information and recommendations. For example, during the Japan earthquake and radiation disaster, doctors and public health workers were having a hard time equating the potential radiation in the atmosphere to something the public was more familiar with. In order to assist public health professionals, the CDC developed a series of equivalencies that showed what a specific level of radiation might look like. One of the most used examples was an X-ray equivalency. The public messaging contained references, such as "the amount of radiation in the atmosphere is equivalent to 5 X-rays received over a 2 year period." This allowed people the ability to compare what they were seeing with what they knew. While it was/is not an exact science, being able to show the public what something means and then provide information about it is something the CDC can do. Using an IMS allows the CDC to follow a system that allows for the dissemination of information during an emergency. Having a public information officer or a Joint Information Center (JIC) allows the agency the ability to reach into its large organization, use the appropriate subject matter expert, and draft the message alongside communications experts in a way that the public will understand. Using the JIC, the agency can directly disseminate the information to the media or to state, local, tribal, and territorial partners, as well as the international community.[4]

▶ Conclusions

In this chapter, we have covered a lot of ground, both in domestic and international programs. We have reviewed international guidance on the development of an EOC and the network of EOCs around the world that provide lessons learned and good practices to its members. We have covered the PHEP cooperative agreement and its associated public health preparedness capabilities, as well as the national core capabilities. The key point is that we operate in a system that is coordinated from the local level, through the state, through the national, and onto the international level. As each level does its part, it supports the larger picture of response operations around the world. Look no further than the Ebola virus outbreak in West Africa in 2014–2015. While most would consider an Ebola virus outbreak something that will only affect Africa, we saw that because of today's ability to travel worldwide, the United States had to deal with Ebola patients in local hospitals. This makes things like an isolated outbreak a potential worldwide pandemic a real possibility, but working through a preparedness and response system allows us to be ready when that time comes.[5]

Key Words

Emergency operations center
Public health emergency
    operations center
Public health emergency
    operations center network

Public health emergency
    preparedness
Public health emergency
    preparedness cooperative
    agreement

Public health preparedness
    capabilities

Discussion Questions

1. What is an emergency operations center?
2. Describe the public health preparedness capabilities?
3. Name the five National Preparedness Goals.
4. What are the objectives for EOC-NET?

References

1. FEMA. *NIMS Resource Management: Instructor Guide.* August 2010. Available at: https://training.fema.gov/emiweb /is/is703a/instructor%20guide/preparing%20to%20train .pdf. Accessed June 2017.

2. WHO. *Framework for a Public Health Emergency Operations Centre.* November 2015. Available at: http://apps.who .int/iris/bitstream/10665/196135/1/9789241565134_eng .pdf?ua=1. Accessed June 2017.

3. WHO. *Public Health Operations Center Network (EOC-NET).* 2012. Available at: http://www.who.int/ihr/eoc_net /en/. Accessed May 2017.

4. CDC. *Public Health Emergency Preparedness Cooperative Agreement.* 2017. Available at: https://www.cdc.gov/phpr /readiness/phep.htm. Accessed May 2017.

5. CDC. *Public Health Preparedness Capabilities: National Standards for State and Local Planning.* March 2011. Available at: https://www.cdc.gov/phpr/readiness/capabilities.htm. Accessed May 2017.

CHAPTER 13

Links to Exercises and Capacity Building

▶ Introduction

Exercises can and will enable a public health organization a way to test their plans, policies, and procedures prior to an incident or event (as we learned in Chapter 10). Working through the planning process, we can use exercises to validate our planning assumptions and verify that we can do what we say we can do. At this point, we should all understand that an exercise is not a substitute for a real response. Exercises work within a specific parameter of events that is controlled and can be stopped at any time if we feel that we are in physical danger.

Exercises can also prepare us for incidents that have nothing to do with the exercise. For example, in April 2009, the Centers for Disease Control and Prevention (CDC) participated in a Department of Health and Human Services (DHHS) department-wide hurricane exercise. The goal of the exercise was to foster coordination within the department during the disaster and allow each organization within the department

a scenario where they could exercise their response protocols, all using a common scenario. This exercise happened to be a hurricane response, but what the CDC didn't know was there was a larger natural disaster looming in the not so distant future.

Also in April 2009, the world faced the largest pandemic influenza in many years. H1N1 was just emerging as a world-wide pandemic and it was coming fast. Having just come out of a large full-scale exercise, the CDC was able to begin work right away on H1N1 as a national priority. What would normally take days for the agency to spin up for a response, only took hours because all of the major pieces and parts of the agency were ready due to participation in the exercise. This exercise was also special because it had incorporated members of the agency that don't normally participate in a disaster exercise, such as child and maternal health practitioners. As the largest pandemic in years, all of the parts of the CDC became engaged in the response.

A lot was learned from the exercise as well as the response to H1N1. One of those lessons learned was the need to develop capacity in the agency in different areas to respond to incidents and events. Areas that were not normally involved in a response needed to be trained and prepared to serve a role in the Incident Management System, deploy as part of the response, or take on the work of others that were participating in the response. Fast forward a few years, and the CDC would again be faced with a world-wide response: Ebola.

The preparedness cycle contains sections on training, exercising, and evaluating and improving (as we discussed in Chapter 10). In this chapter, we explore those three topics and apply them to public health as part of a Public Health Emergency Management (PHEM) program.

▶ Training Development Process

Up until this point in the preparedness cycle, we have discussed planning and organizing and equipping. We have learned how to develop a plan and to determine the right organization for our response and what types of resources may be needed for a response. The next step in the process is to conduct training on those topics. A plan is no good if it is kept on the shelf. It needs to be read and people need to be trained on its contents. To develop training, there are many different methods, including one followed by the U.S. military and the Federal Emergency Management Agency. This process outlines five different phases of development:

- Phase 1—Analysis
- Phase 2—Design
- Phase 3—Development
- Phase 4—Implementation
- Phase 5—Evaluation and control

Phase 1, analysis, is where training developers look at the item that needs to be trained. It could be a new job performance step; a plan, policy, or procedure; or a new position in the Incident Management System. Training developers will break down the job, task, or plan into its basic parts and look at how it works, how the task is designed, and how best to measure the tasks associated with the plan, policy, procedure, or job. Once that is complete, training developers will look at different options on how best to design the training and then will select the best option for training delivery—also called an instructional setting. This could be an online educational tutorial, traditional classroom settings, or a mixture of the two.

Once the analysis is complete, the next phase is design. This is where the objectives for the training are developed. One of the ways that objectives are developed is using the SMART acronym (**FIGURE 13-1**). SMART has several different meanings, but some of the most common meanings are Simple, Measurable, Achievable, Realistic, and Task Oriented. Some additional meanings include Time Sensitive instead of Task Oriented, Attainable instead of Achievable, and Relevant instead of Realistic. Whichever way you decided to define SMART, the idea is that each objective that is developed fits within a pattern to allow for measurement and evaluations. Objectives that are developed without a way

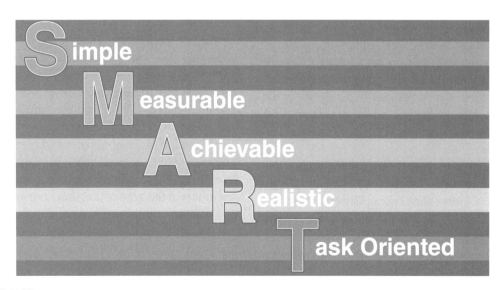

FIGURE 13-1 SMART
Reproduced from DHS. *Homeland Security Exercise and Evaluation Program (HSEEP)* Training Course. Slide 10.

to measure them do not allow for a corrective action process that leads to the ability to fix something that was proved to be broken during training or exercising. Once the objectives are set, training developers develop the tests. While this may seem like putting the cart before the horse, this typically has to do with online or distance-learning environments. If you add in storyboarding, which is just what it sounds like, putting the story step by step on a board, it allows programmers a way forward in designing the software or programming for the training. At this point, training developers are also determining what types of knowledge, skills, and abilities the students should have in order to best comprehend the training, as well as determining the overall sequence and structure of the training.

Phase 3 of the training development process is called development. As one could guess based on the name of the phase, this is where training developers develop the content of the training. This would include developing special learning activities, such as hands-on learning sessions, or in a virtual training world, where the student may be asked to complete a learning exercise as part of the learning process. In this phase, developers will determine the instructional management plan and delivery of training. For example, one block of instruction could be 50 minutes long, require 2 specific handouts, and could be followed by a check on learning and a 10-minute break. Developers will also review any existing materials, such as operating instructions supplied by the manufacturer, for inclusion into the overall training product. Then the fun begins, actually developing the instructional materials, as well as how the instructional materials will be evaluated or validated.

Phase 4 of the process is implementation. This is where instructors use the materials that were developed and teach the course of instruction. This could also mean placing students in front of a computer and letting them use the instructional materials online, or via a CD-ROM, or other delivery method. Instructional materials may also include operating instructions for equipment and may include a period of time where learners can practice those skills using real equipment or training equipment. For example, training to learn how to put on personal protective equipment may only use training equipment and may not allow for the use of actual response equipment due to cost or a limited supply of real-world response equipment.

The last phase, Phase 5, is evaluation and control. This is where training developers will go through a series of evaluations, both internal and external, to determine whether or not the product meets expectations. Internal evaluations are when developers who are part of the development process evaluate the product, and external evaluation is when outside developers are brought in to look at the product for an external perspective. Once those evaluations are complete, the training materials can be revised and once approved are available for widespread use and dissemination.[1]

While this may seem like a long process, it does provide a product that is tested and appropriate for the materials being taught. The most common practice when developing training is when a supervisor or leader tells you to give training on a certain topic, such as the new Continuity of Operations (COOP) plan. What typically happens is someone takes the plan and does a copy/paste into a PowerPoint presentation, then stands up in front of an audience and reads each slide, and says that training was conducted. But let us ask the question, was the training effective? Without a training development process that analyzes, designs, develops, implements, and evaluates training, have we really done the best we can do?

▶ Exercise Development Process

Following along with the preparedness cycle, the next step is to exercise the plan, policy, or procedure. Exercises can provide validation for a plan without having to do an actual response. Exercises also allow us to test sections of the plan, policy, or procedure without having to do the entire process. For example, if we were exercising our ability to operate an emergency operations center (EOC), one of the first steps in that process is activating the leadership and organizational structure of the EOC. If exercise planners just want to exercise the activation protocols, then they would design a drill that would allow them to exercise just the activation protocol.

The Homeland Security Exercise and Evaluation Program (generally known as HSEEP) was first published in 2007 (**FIGURE 13-2**). It is part of the National Exercise Program (NEP). The NEP provides opportunities to periodically train and exercise, identify key policy issues, and refine key incident management processes. The program allows for all levels of government and organizations to participate in a program that can benefit all. For example, the Top Officials (TOPOFF) exercise in 2007 centered on a series of radiological dispersion devices in multiple states and territories. This scenario allowed for multiple levels of government to respond, from cities to counties, state, and federal partners. Exercises such as this allow for a diverse set of

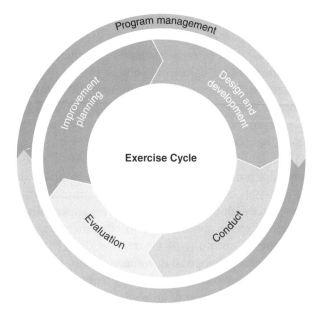

FIGURE 13-2 Homeland Security Exercise and Evaluation Program

Reproduced from Department of Homeland Security. *Homeland Security Exercise and Evaluation Program (HSEEP)*. April 2013. pp 1–2. Available at: https://preptoolkit.fema.gov/documents/1269813/1269861/HSEEP_Revision_Apr13_Final.pdf /65bc7843-1d10-47b7-bc0d-45118a4d21da. Accessed May 2017.

objectives and allow players to determine their level of involvement in advance of the exercise.

HSEEP is designed on the idea of capabilities-based planning. This means that you determine what type of capability you would like to test, then design the exercise around that capability. For example, if our health department decided it wanted to test the Emergency Operations Coordination capability, it would design an exercise that would put us into a position to execute that capability. HSEEP provides a capabilities-based program that provides a standardized methodology and consistent terminology for designing, developing, conducting, and evaluating an exercise. As with all national emergency management program documents, HSEEP sets out to fit into the national doctrine. It provides tools and resources to help build a self-sustaining program, and includes an exercise cycle and different types of exercise activities in varying degrees of complexity.

The exercise process is also designed around a cycle, just as exercising is part of the preparedness cycle. There are five phases of the exercise cycle:

- Phase 1—Establishing the foundation
- Phase 2—Design and development
- Phase 3—Conduct
- Phase 4—Evaluation
- Phase 5—Improvement planning

In order to establish the foundation, exercise planners must complete a series of tasks. The first task is to review the current plan, policy, or procedure that is going to be tested or validated by the exercise. Exercises are designed to be a validation tool, not a tool by which we create a plan, policy, or procedure. The next task is to conduct a specific exercise needs assessment. This task just simply asks "why" we need to conduct an exercise. It could be that the exercise has been mandated by law, such as the exercise requirements in the Radiological Emergency Preparedness program, or it could have been part of an agreement like the Public Health Emergency Preparedness (PHEP) cooperative agreement. Either way, sometimes we have to do an exercise as part of a bigger program. Once planners have determined the why, planners then can determine what capability they want to exercise. Sticking with the EOC idea, planners could determine that they need to exercise the Emergency Operations Coordination PHEP capability. Once the capability has been determined, planners can determine the scope of the exercise; how many people, what organizations, what jurisdictions, etc. Next is the selection of the type of exercise. HSEEP consists of seminars, workshops, tabletop exercises, games, drills, functional exercises, and full-scale exercises. Seminars, workshops, tabletop exercise, and games are discussion-based exercises. This type of exercise does not require as much planning, but it can be a powerful tool as the first step in validating a plan, policy, or procedure. Drills, functional exercises, and full-scale exercises require more planning than a discussion exercise, but they also are as close to a real response as possible. Functional exercises can be designed to only exercise a part of the full operations, typically called a function, and do not require as much planning as full-scale exercises. These exercises are called operations-based exercises. Planners will look at the needs of the exercise, determine the capability, figure out who will be involved in the exercise, set the type of exercise, and then look at how much the exercise will cost. Sometimes, planners are faced with the reality that just because they want to do a big exercise, they are limited by the amount of money that is available for the exercise. Developing a long-term exercise program can help alleviate that problem, as allowing for a 3–5-year plan gives planners the ability to budget for a progressively tougher exercise schedule. After all of that, planners can develop a clear purpose statement for the exercise and then announce that an exercise will take place.

The group of people assigned to develop the exercise is called the exercise planning team. This team is charged with designing, developing, conducting, and evaluating the exercise. It determines exercise objectives, create the scenarios, and develops all exercise documentation. It distributes all the pre-exercise materials, such as the *Situation Manual* for discussion-based exercises like the tabletop exercise. The exercise planning team is organized using the Incident Command System/Incident Management System structure. There is a lead, an operations section, a planning section, a logistics section, an admin/finance section, and a safety officer, as well as a public information officer as needed.

In Phase 2, design and development, the exercise planning team develops the exercise objectives. As was discussed previously, objectives should be developed via the SMART method. Once the objectives have been developed, planners can develop the scenario. Planning the exercise will consist of a series of planning meetings that will assist in the development of exercise documentation, a control simulation system as needed, an evaluation system, and help prepare facilities and logistics.

Phase 3 is the actual conduct of the exercise. This phase will vary based on the type of the exercise. For example, setting up for a tabletop exercise will not be as expansive as setting up for a full-scale exercise. With the increase in complexity comes the increase in setup time, as well as cost. Setting up for a tabletop exercise can consist of setting up the tables and chairs in a configuration that will foster open discussion. If audiovisual products are being used, each participant should be able to see the presentation or video. If the exercise calls for breakout sessions, then the areas should be set up prior to the exercise. This could include making sure that there are writing utensils, easels with pad of paper and markers, and a clock to keep track of the time. Presentations for a tabletop exercise should contain an overview of the exercise, such as the purpose, objectives, and specific instructions; a relevant historical context for the exercise; and the questions to be discussed during the exercise. Facilitation of the exercise is extremely important. Planners need to appoint someone as a facilitator that can keep the participants engaged. Tabletop exercises can quickly get out of hand without the guidance of a skilled facilitator. Once the exercise is complete, the facilitator can lead the participants in a wrap-up that can cover things such as what went right, what went wrong, and what needs to be improved upon in the plan, policy, or procedure that was being exercise. Logistical considerations for a discussion-based exercise include the location of bathrooms, meals or light refreshments, name tags, a sign in area, and

what to do if there is a real-world emergency that would require an evacuation of the facility, like a fire or earthquake.

In an operations-based exercise, players need to be oriented to the scenario as well as the location for which exercise actions are to take place. Players will also be oriented to the type of evaluation that is to take place. If evaluators are using exercise evaluation guides based on operating instructions for a piece of equipment, players should be aware of that. If players will receive messages as part of exercise play, they should be briefed on the procedure for receiving those messages. Most importantly, players should be briefed on the procedures they should follow if there is a real-world emergency during the exercise, such as an accident.

Phase 4 of the process is evaluation. To most exercise planners, evaluation of the exercise is the most important part of the process. If you do not evaluate the exercise, why conduct an exercise. Think back to what was discussed previously, the main purpose of an exercise is to validate a plan, policy, or procedure. In order for planners to determine if the plan, policy, or procedure is valid, evaluators look at how the procedure was accomplished as part of the overall plan. In order to determine if a policy is valid, actions must be observed to make sure the policy covers all the pertinent areas and if the policy addresses specific roles and responsibilities. The evaluation process starts with the objectives. Planners develop procedures to look at the actions of the players to determine if they are in line with the published plans, policies, and procedures. Observers and evaluators then collect their data and conduct an exercise debrief with the players and other observers and evaluators. This is commonly referred to as a "hot wash." This is conducted right after the completion of the exercise in order to gather all pertinent information while the exercise and player actions are still fresh on the minds of all personnel involved. After all the data and information is gathered, an after action report (AAR) can be generated. The AAR lists all of the key observations from the exercise, such as what went right, what went wrong, and what needs to be improved upon.

Phase 5 of the process is called improvement planning. Besides the evaluation, improvement planning is probably the second most important part of the process. This process identifies the improvements to be implemented, finalizes the after action report and improvement plan (AAR/IP), assigns items to the appropriate party, establishes a schedule for completion, determines who is responsible for the improvements, and monitors or tracks progress of implementation (**BOX 13-1**).

Evaluation and improvement processes typically follow an eight-step process:

1. Plan and organize the evaluation
2. Observe the exercise and collect data
3. Analyze the data
4. Develop the draft AAR
5. Conduct an after action conference
6. Identify improvements to be implemented
7. Finalize the AAR/IP
8. Track implementation of the improvement plan

The major product of the improvement planning phase is the improvement plan. The improvement plan is completed as part of the after action conference. This is where all major parties involved in the exercise sit down and discuss what happened and ways that the problems that were identified in the exercise can be fixed. Once the solutions are determined, responsible parties are assigned and a timetable for improvements is established. All of these items are put into a matrix called the improvement plan. As part of overall program management, these items are entered into a database that can be used to track progress of the improvements. This could be something as simple as correcting a procedure or writing a new procedure to accurately capture what has been done, or it can be as complicated as developing an entirely new plan that is needed to fill a gap that was identified as part of the exercise. Each corrective action should be assigned a point of contact for tracking the progress of the corrective action. A timeline is established for progress checks, and periodic reports of progress are done until the corrective action is completed.

The last part of the process is to start the process all over again. This sounds kind of strange, but think back to the reason for an exercise (validating a plan, policy, or procedure) and this will all make sense. If the result of the exercise is an evaluation that leads to an improvement plan, which in turn leads to a corrective action program, the end result of all this effort is a validated plan, policy, or procedure. Often the result of an exercise is that a plan, policy, or procedure needs to be revised. Once that plan, policy, or procedure is revised, the process starts all over again. We must then train on the changes, exercise the modifications, then evaluate whether those modifications were correct, and then the plan is complete.[2]

Conclusions

As was shown in the preparedness cycle, exercising, evaluating, and improvement planning has a prominent place in preparedness. In the absence of a real-world response scenario, exercises provide planners a real opportunity to test their plans, policies, and procedures in a simulated response environment. While simulations often cannot recreate the stress and confusion of a real response, they can offer an opportunity for players to conduct operations in the environment that is the closest thing to real situations. Looking back at the TOPOFF exercise in 2007 that was mentioned at the beginning of the chapter, this exercise dealt with the response to multiple radiological dispersion devices. While no one would actually explode a radiological dispersion devise just for an exercise, planners can take steps to make it as realistic as possible. Real radiation sources can be used (in small quantities) to make detection equipment display readings of real radiation. Real debris can be brought in to show what a collapsed building would look like, and players can be brought in and made up to look like real casualties, adding to the realism of the exercise. Real decontamination showers can be set up, and players can process through the systems to get a real idea of what it takes to operate a decontamination line. Players in personal protective equipment can get a real idea of what it is like to be in Level A fully encapsulated suits for hours at a time. While exercises cannot simulate a real event, they can be used as a powerful tool to show us what it will be like during a real response. They give us an opportunity to put all of our training and planning into operation, without having to respond to a real disaster.

Key Words

After action report and improvement plan
Exercise cycle

Exercise program
Homeland Security Exercise and Evaluation Program

Preparedness cycle
SMART objectives
Training development cycle

Discussion Questions

1. What is the purpose of an exercise?
2. What does the acronym SMART stand for?
3. Describe the eight steps of the evaluation and improvement planning process.
4. Describe the five phases of the exercise cycle.
5. What are the five phases of the training development cycle?

References

1. FEMA. Responder Training Development Center National Training and Education Division. May 2017. Available at: https://www.firstrespondertraining.gov/rtdc/state/. Accessed June 2017.
2. DHS. *Homeland Security Exercise and Evaluation Program (HSEEP)*. Vol II. February 2007. Available at: https://www.hsdl.org/?view&did=470612. Accessed June 2017.

CHAPTER 14

Case Studies in Public Health Response Operations

By the end of this chapter, the reader will be able to:

- Describe recent public health response operations

▶ Introduction

In Part V of this text, we have explored the combination of public health preparedness and emergency management (EM). We have covered the Incident Command System (ICS), the preparedness cycle, the Threat and Hazard Identification and Risk Assessment Process, emergency operations centers (EOCs), and how to develop capacity through training, exercising, and evaluating. In this chapter, we review a few case studies about public health preparedness and EM in action.

The first case study, Public Health Emergency Management in Guinea—Before and After the 2014 Ebola Outbreak, is about the application of public health

EM principles during the Ebola crisis in Guinea. As discussed in Chapter 10, planning can better prepare an organization for a public health emergency. As you read the case study about the application of public health EM in Guinea, please pay particular attention to how the planning process was used to help manage the incident.

The second case study, Risk Communications in a Time of Zika—Conducting Community Assessments during Public Health Emergencies, examines the process of gathering data from the community during a response. This case study also describes the use of the ICS to organize the teams doing the assessments. While this may not seem like a traditional use of ICS, it does show the flexibility of ICS as described in Chapter 11.

🔍 *CASE STUDY: Public Health Emergency Management in Guinea— Before and After the 2014 Ebola Outbreak*

By Claire Standley

In 2016, Guinea was declared free from Ebola virus, having been the origin of the worst Ebola outbreak in history. Along with Liberia and Sierra Leone, Guinea was also one of the three countries most heavily impacted by the disease. The magnitude of the outbreak was compounded through the weak health systems in the affected countries, which have since led to significant international and multilateral efforts to build public health capacity in the region. One of the major areas of investment has been public health emergency management (EM) systems and structures, including emergency operations centers (EOCs) as a critical tool for rapidly and effectively responding to potential public health emergencies. The value of EOCs was recognized as early as the revised International Health Regulations (IHR) (2005), but has since further become enshrined as a core action package under the Global Health Security Agenda (GHSA), and forms one of the U.S. Centers for Disease Control and Prevention (CDC) "core four" areas for capacity building as part of the U.S. government's international commitment to GHSA. This case study uses the framework of EM to examine Guinea's health system before, during, and after the Ebola outbreak, and to highlight the evolution of EM as a tool and approach to public health preparedness and response.

Emergency Management in Guinea Pre-Ebola

Emergency management was not a widely recognized concept in the public health sphere in Guinea prior to the Ebola outbreak. Efforts to establish capabilities for public health preparedness and response were largely centered around implementation of IHR (2005) and the Integrated Disease Surveillance and Response (IDSR) framework. However, as of self-reporting to World Health Organization (WHO) in 2014, Guinea had only met 63% and 64% of the required indicators for the preparedness and response IHR core capacities, respectively, and a mere 22% for the zoonotic disease specific hazard.[1] The Ministry of Health did not possess an EOC. In 2011, Guinea developed a national implementation guide for IDSR, based on the revised technical guidelines produced by CDC and WHO-AFRO in 2010, which aligned IDSR to IHR (2005) at an operational level.[2] However, the guide was not extensively adapted to Guinea's specific health context or needs, and was exclusively implemented by the human health sector with no multisectoral input. The guide also provided little scope or direction for detection and reporting of diseases of unusual or unknown etiology, and the general lack of resources for surveillance activities, combined with Guinea's centralized government structure, resulted in limited education and awareness on IDSR in peripheral parts of the health system. All of these factors proved critical when Ebola emerged in late 2013.

Perhaps the only example of a specific, multisectoral public health preparedness and response planning document from the pre-Ebola era is the Avian Influenza Preparedness and Response Plan from 2006.[3] Funded by the World Bank as part of their global efforts to combat the emergence and spread of highly pathogenic H5N1 avian influenza, the document was developed jointly between the Ministry of Agriculture, Livestock, Water and Forests as well as the Ministry of Health, and with technical assistance from a number of other international and assistance organizations including the Food and Agriculture Organization (FAO), the World Organization for Animal Health (OIE), and U.S. Agency for International Development (USAID). The document provides a risk analysis for the introduction and transmission of avian influenza in Guinea and outlines a number of specific objectives for improved surveillance, diagnostics, case management, coordination between sectors, social mobilization and education, and research priorities. While well-conceived and an important step, the document unfortunately mostly fell short of achieving effective capacity building for zoonotic disease control, largely due to lack of sustained funding after the end of the project. Reorganization of government ministries, which included the separation of the Ministry of Agriculture, Livestock, Water and Forests into three entities, with the Ministry of Livestock now responsible for domestic animal health and veterinary services, but the Ministry of Livestock overseeing wildlife was a further challenge to ongoing coordination. Finally, Guinea never detected any avian influenza cases and only performed a handful of simulations (which ended in 2007), limiting the opportunities for exercising the plan and maintaining robust capabilities.

Outside of the health sphere, EM approaches are largely focused on natural disasters and disaster risk reduction, starting initially in 1990 from the formation of the National Guinean Committee for the International Decade on Prevention of National Hazards and leading to several legislative acts related to disaster management in the 1990s. These efforts are, on paper, multisectoral, with numerous government agencies implicated, though in practice technical ministries such as the Ministry of Health usually have little operational awareness of these acts. The National Service for Humanitarian Action (SENAH), an agency of the Ministry of Territorial Administration and Decentralization, is the lead agency for responses with humanitarian implication; their coordination with health authorities is usually focused at the level of the affected community.

Developments During the Outbreak: 2014–2016

The events that led to the emergence and spread of the outbreak have been well characterized.[4,5] The index case is thought to be a young boy from a rural village in Guéckédou Prefecture, in the remote southeastern forest region of Guinea, who was originally exposed to the virus via contact with a bat. He became ill and spread the disease to several family members, who in turn passed the disease on to healthcare workers at the prefectural hospital. Additional members of the extended family moved the virus further afield. By the beginning of February 2014, a case had been transported to the capital city, Conakry, but the etiology of the disease was still unknown. Although local health workers reported the cases to prefectural authorities at the end of January 2014 and a small investigation was conducted (though Ebola was not identified as the causative agent; in fact, cholera was suspected at the time), the process of investigation, assessment, and confirmation were woefully slow. Indeed, from the very beginning, outside entities were intrinsically and extensively involved in the response effort, starting from the initial investigation of the outbreak by Médecins Sans Frontières in January 2014, and continued to play a major role throughout the outbreak.

The Guinean Ebola response was overseen by the Ebola Coordination Cell (Cellule de Coordination de la riposte contre la maladie à virus Ebola, or CNLEB), created in September 2014 by presidential decree. The structure of the CNLEB was formed of a coordinator and a deputy (both Ministry of Health officials) overseeing a number of technical and operational sections and covering surveillance, case management, communication, security, logistics, etc. Execution of several of these operational areas were delegated to different international or nongovernmental organizations (NGO). For example, WHO was the entity in charge of conducting surveillance and epidemiological functions, including contact tracing and collating data for daily situation reports. The Red Cross was responsible for transport of patients to Ebola treatment units as well as safe and dignified burials. The World Food Program (WFP) played a major role in coordinating logistics. U.N. Children's Fund (UNICEF) was the lead for social mobilization and awareness-raising.

Many agencies and organizations also provided direct support to the CNLEB during the response, through provision of technical, financial, and material assistance. The U.S. CDC (e.g., via funding from the CDC Foundation) renovated several floors of an existing Ministry of Health building into an EOC, to house the CNLEB and affiliated response entities. Concurrently, USAID's Office of Foreign Disaster Assistance (OFDA) provided funding to the International Organization for Migration (IOM) to renovate structures in 28 prefectural and communal health departments to serve as local-level EOCs. CDC partnered with the Public Health Agency of Canada (PHAC) to embed EM experts within the national EOC and provide support and training to members of the CNLEB, mainly on basic managerial and administrative functions such as meeting management, information management, and communications. Finally, CDC and OFDA combined efforts and brought together IOM with George Washington University, to develop and implement a training program on basic EM concepts, targeting prefectural and communal health officials, as a first step toward operationalizing the local-level EOCs.[6] In June 2015, the French government launched its PREPARE project, which included an effort to train multidisciplinary rapid response teams in each of Guinea's eight administrative regions.

In December 2015, Guinea was declared free from Ebola virus for the first time. Success in stemming the number of cases was largely due to extensive social mobilization relating to reporting new cases and community deaths, education on preventing transmission, large-scale contact tracing (including across borders, in coordination with authorities in Sierra Leone and Liberia), and concerted efforts to limit transmission in communities through efforts such as safe and dignified burials. Technological advances, such as the development and deployment of rapid diagnostic tests for point of care testing, and the very promising vaccine candidate trial in Guinea during the latter stages of the outbreak, also likely contributed significantly. In addition to the thousands of Guinean professionals and volunteers, the response involved a vast number of external actors, including international organizations, foreign bilateral donors, foundations, and NGOs.

Sustaining Zero Cases: The Aftermath of the Outbreak

As early as April 2015, the World Bank had begun assisting the three most heavily affected countries with the development of economic recovery plans, acknowledging the severe financial toll the outbreak would take in terms of lost trade and tourism, not to mention the tragic loss of human capital.[7] However, starting from December 2015, Guinea entered "Phase III" of the response, which focused on enhanced surveillance and preparedness for new cases. This included initial plans for future capacity building, with a strong emphasis on the base of the health "pyramid," through strengthening community and prefectural level surveillance, diagnostics, and response efforts. In addition, many of the efforts initiated during the outbreak, which had been intended to focus on the response itself, had been delayed during the height of the crisis, and so were continued during this post-response phase of operations as support for Phase III.

The end of active transmission also emphasized the social recovery that would be needed in the aftermath of the outbreak. In some cases, these efforts coincided with the concern of disease reemergence—for example, survivor monitoring. It had been observed during the outbreak that the Ebola virus can persist for weeks or even months in apparently recovered individuals, and can remain capable of transmitting the disease, meaning that the large numbers of recovered Ebola patients could serve as reservoirs for the virus and be a risk for new cases. Moreover, these survivors

(continues)

faced social stigma and continuing health problems, requiring psychosocial and medical support, and assistance with reintegration into their communities. The SA-CEINT endeavor was launched in 2016 to monitor survivors and offer frequent testing of key bodily fluids, such as semen, blood, and breast milk, in an effort to prevent new cases. Despite these efforts, in February 2016, a new case emerged in Koropara, again in southeastern forest region of Guinea. Despite the CNLEB's vigilance and the continued presence of many of the key response partners, it took the Ministry of Health almost 3 weeks to confirm the cases and report the flare up to WHO.[8]

Preventing Future Infectious Disease Emergencies

Throughout the outbreak and its aftermath, a key concern of the Guinean government has been to ensure that a public health emergency of the scale and scope of the 2014–2016 Ebola epidemic never occurs again. Working with partners, a number of efforts are now underway to better understand the epidemiological dynamics of Ebola, in order to prevent future spillover events. For example, several groups, including USAID's PREDICT program and the Institut de recherche pour le développement (IRD), are surveying wild and domestic animal populations to identify possible reservoir species for the virus. As mentioned previously, another outcome of the outbreak was to rapidly develop and test new technological tools to support response efforts. Results from the vaccine trial in Guinea have been extremely positive, with data from over 5000 vaccinated individuals demonstrating protection from the virus even after possible exposure, adding a powerful new tool to the arsenal for preventing, or at least mitigating, future outbreaks.[9]

With respect specifically to EM, CDC is continuing to support EM training and capacity building in Guinea, in collaboration with IOM, PHAC, and other partners. The national public health EOC has now been placed under the jurisdiction of a new Ministry of Health–affiliated agency, the National Health Security Agency (Agence National de Securité Sanitaire, or ANSS), which will be the lead for outbreak preparedness and response efforts. An EOC manager has been appointed, staff are being trained, and efforts are underway to develop key systems and documents to support future activities, such as a concept of operations (CONOPs), strategic plan, and standard operation procedures (SOPs).

Learning lessons from the past is also a key facet of EM. In addition to the numerous global review processes related to the outbreak as a whole (and WHO's role in particular), there have also been initiatives at the national level in Guinea related to reviewing performance during the outbreak. After the flare-up in Koropara in February–March 2016, a number of stakeholders led by CNLEB, including U.N. Development Programme (UNDP), IOM, WHO, and CDC, planned an after-action review process to determine the causes and consequences of the delayed response, focusing on identifying opportunities for future improvement. More generally, the Ministry of Health has recognized the urgent need to review and update many of the key documents related to disease control; a new National Plan for Health System Development (Plan National de Développement Sanitaire) was released in 2015, for implementation through 2024. In addition, the national IDSR guide is being updated to take into account the developments and enhanced capacity put into place as a result of the Ebola crisis. Crucially, these efforts are not being carried out solely by the Ministry of Health. Another outcome of the outbreak has been a far greater awareness of the importance, and impact, of multisectoral approaches to preparedness and response, even when dealing with a public health emergency. The ANSS, for example, will be guided by an administrative council comprised of representatives from at least six different ministries, as well as the offices of the president and prime minister. These developments suggest that a more holistic, and integrated, approach to infectious disease control is being established, and hopefully sustained even once the funds associated with the Ebola outbreak are no longer available.

Conclusion

Prior to the Ebola outbreak, EM was not widely understood in Guinea, let alone practiced, and was entirely absent as an approach within the health sector. The Ebola outbreak highlighted the benefits of including EM principles, as well as infrastructure such as EOCs, as part of the response effort. Guinea has benefitted from numerous internationally funded efforts to build EM capacity during and after the Ebola outbreak, and is now embarking on expanding and sustaining those capabilities within an explicitly multisectoral framework.

Discussion Questions

1. To what extent does this case study reflect the four distinct stages of the emergency management cycle (preparedness, response, recovery, and mitigation)? Can you provide at least one example of each stage? Are there overlaps between any of the stages?

2. Guinea's experience with emergency management was largely shaped by external actors and international assistance, and was catalyzed by the Ebola outbreak. Compare and contrast this experience with the U.S. domestic experience with developing public health preparedness and response systems. (*Hint: Think about 2001 as a catalyst year for U.S. infectious disease preparedness and response.*)

🔍 CASE STUDY: Risk Communications in a Time of Zika—Conducting Community Assessments during Public Health Emergencies

By Malaya Fletcher and Ami Patel

Introduction

Emerging infectious diseases have a history of causing emotional, societal, and healthcare impact, as evidenced by recent epidemics such as HIV/AIDS, H1N1, and Ebola. To help minimize these impacts and promote disease prevention, public health agencies play a critical role in developing and disseminating health information to the public, at-risk populations, and the healthcare community. To be effective, health information must be accurate, informative, timely, accessible, and direct, among other elements. The creation of effective messages can be particularly challenging during an emerging epidemic due to rapidly changing situations and a paucity of information. Other challenges with developing such information include the need to convey technical material to lay audiences, keep pace with rapidly changing information, and address evolving rumors. Public health agencies frequently have limited methods and resources to contend with these challenges, identify target populations, and reach these populations.

The emergence of Zika virus in the Americas in 2015 compelled public health authorities to rapidly develop and convey competent, comprehensive, and transparent health messages to promote evidence-based knowledge without fostering fear. Such information helps minimize false claims and stigma. The Zika virus is primarily spread through bites from infected *Aedes aegypti* mosquitoes. Zika can also be spread sexually, from mother-to-child during pregnancy, and through blood transfusions and organ donations. Infection with Zika typically causes mild or no symptoms, but can potentially cause Guillain–Barré syndrome and neurologic complications in adults. Infections in pregnant women can lead to microcephaly and other birth defects in the unborn baby. It is these associated adverse outcomes and impact on fetuses that prompted the creation of robust health information campaigns to raise awareness of Zika and associated methods of prevention.

Facts of the Case and Background

In February 2015, the Philadelphia Department of Public Health (PDPH) activated its Incident Command Structure (ICS) to address the growing epidemic of Zika in the United States. Representatives within the ICS included epidemiologists, disease surveillance investigators, public information officers, preparedness planners, clinicians, and mosquito control technicians from within the Divisions of Disease Control, Maternal Child and Family Health, and Environmental Health Services, in addition to the Health Commissioner's Office. Core members of the ICS met monthly to discuss program-specific and department-wide Zika activities and identify key health communication needs for Philadelphia residents and at-risk populations.

Philadelphia is located in a region with the potential for limited local mosquito-borne transmission of Zika. The city has an endemic population of *Aedes albopictus* and projections have included Philadelphia as an area where *A. aegypti* may be reintroduced.[10] Populations identified to be most at risk for Zika included travelers, pregnant women, and women of childbearing age. Philadelphia is a densely populated city with a large Hispanic/Latino population that has close ties to Zika-affected countries. According to 2010 census estimates, 12% of the 1.5 million residents of Philadelphia are Hispanic or Latino. Travel to and migration from Zika-affected countries occurs frequently through the Philadelphia International Airport and other transportation centers in the region with many residents visiting family and friends in their birth country.

Pregnant women and women of childbearing age may also acquire Zika through sexual transmission from an infected partner who traveled to a Zika-affected area. Each year, about 22,000–24,000 live births occur in Philadelphia, and among the 2015 birth cohort, 12% of infants had a parent native to a Zika-affected area. Nearly 50% of these parents were born in Puerto Rico or the Dominican Republic. Further complicating the potential for acquiring sexually transmitted Zika infection is that most infected persons remain asymptomatic.

To educate the general public and the aforementioned targeted populations (women of childbearing age, Latino/Hispanic and Caribbean populations, and travelers) regarding Zika's health effects, modes of transmission, and methods of prevention, PDPH developed an education campaign which began in the spring and summer of 2016. While the department had experience in communicating "fight-the-bite" and sexually transmitted disease (STD) prevention messages, Zika brought unique challenges to health messaging. The target population for sexually transmitted Zika had a different demographic and risk-factor profile than the target population for the city's existing STD prevention campaign, and "fight-the-bite" messages did not sufficiently address the daytime biting nature of *Aedes*

(continues)

sp. mosquitoes. Additionally, travel health messages that detailed the risks of infection to pregnant females, delineated risk areas, and clarified travel and laboratory testing guidance needed to be developed and disseminated. Message development, review, and implementation engaged the PDPH's Zika ICS to ensure coordination and consistency across all programs within the health department.

Given the challenges faced in developing a new campaign addressing the complexity of Zika, the changing nature of the epidemic, identification of numerous targeted populations, and limited resources, it was essential that the health department understand the penetration and impact of its education campaign. Evaluation is an integral component of campaign planning, design, and implementation, and findings can be used to understand public needs and behaviors, identify whether public knowledge has increased, and whether specific actions were successfully promoted. Public health professionals can then use the findings to drive adjustments to strategies and tactics, modify efforts of current response activities, and shape activities in the future.

PDPH sought to identify an epidemiological method which facilitated rapid data collection among a representative sample of the targeted community within a rapid time frame and with limited resources. The Community Assessment for Public Health Emergency Response (CASPER), a method used frequently in disaster epidemiology to rapidly collect health information in a representative manner, was thus chosen to perform the evaluation.

Health Education Campaign Components

PDPH implemented its Zika education campaign in summer 2016 (**FIGURE 14-1**). Content focused on travel risks, symptoms, and recommendations for pregnant women; prevention of sexual transmission; mosquito-bite prevention; and standing water reduction. The campaign utilized press releases, mass media (which included television, newspaper, and radio ads), print materials and small media (such as posters in healthcare facilities and airports, fact sheets, and brochures), and digital ads (Google, Facebook, YouTube, Twitter, and Instagram). Health messaging was also deployed on the city's website and public transportation via ads on buses. Community outreach included presentations and in-services to healthcare providers and attending festivals and cultural events throughout the city. Latino populations were also targeted due to expected travel-association of cases recognized in this stage through a radio commercial on La Mega, a Spanish-speaking radio station, and an ad in a local Spanish newspaper. Travel messages were also placed at the Philadelphia International Airport.

Using a Community Assessment as a Campaign Evaluation

As mosquito season waned in September 2016, PDPH made the decision to evaluate the Zika media and education campaign so that future campaigns could be improved in terms of messages and modalities used and resources directed appropriately. The department weighed several methods to conduct the evaluation including online surveys or convenience sample surveys within clinics serving targeted populations. The major limitation with these methods was the lack of a representative sample. This led to the health department selecting the CASPER approach. Although CASPERs are more often performed in the context of an acute public health emergency, the method and approach lends itself well to performing community assessments in a rapid and representative manner. Furthermore, CASPER was

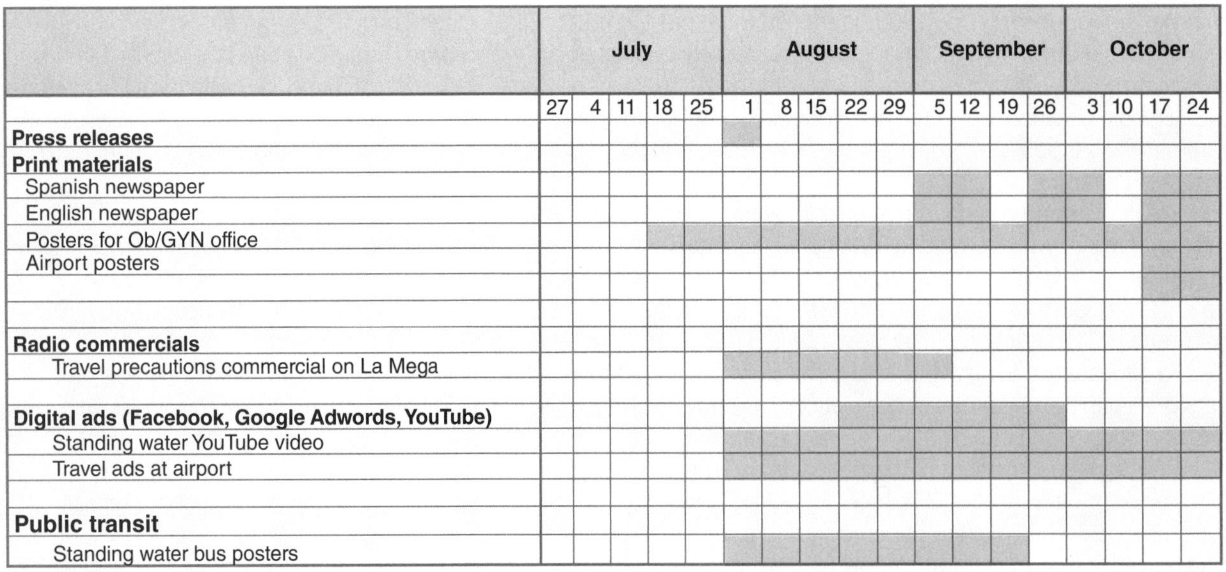

FIGURE 14-1 Timeline of Philadelphia Department of Public Health 2016 health education campaign

a tool that would lend itself well for potential future departmental activities to assess public health needs following a public health emergency, and the agency wanted to better understand what resources would be needed to perform a CASPER in an emergency setting.

There were four objectives which the CASPER sought to address:

1. Evaluate the saturation of our health education campaign
   a. Did the community see the health department's ads? If so, did the messages provide new information, change behavior, or make people think?
2. Identify the most trusted sources of information
   a. Where do members of the public get their information?
3. Understand the knowledge, attitudes, and perceptions regarding Zika in the community
   a. What do Philadelphians think of Zika? What do people know about it? How do they feel about it? Do Philadelphians practice Zika prevention methods?
4. Determine if CASPER is a feasible model to collect information following public health emergencies in Philadelphia

Methods and Data Collection

The CDC's CASPER toolkit was followed for the identification of the sampling frame.[11] Thirty clusters were selected and mapped based on census blocks. Clusters were chosen with an intentional over selection of Hispanic neighborhoods and zip codes with a history of a prevalence of mosquito-borne diseases. Within each cluster, seven housing units were randomly selected for an interview ($n = 210$). A tracking sheet was utilized to denote which houses or units were approached and the outcome of the attempted visit (e.g., no answer, completed questionnaire, refusal, etc.). Data from these tracking sheets were used to calculate response and cooperation rates.

Teams were assigned with the objective to provide diversity in skill sets—mixture of knowledge and experience with Zika, epidemiology methods, and familiarity with field work, as well as ethnicity, gender, and age. Team members were comprised of Division of Disease Control, Environmental Health Services, and Maternal, Child and Family Health staff who underwent training prior to going in the field. Approximately, 50 people went out over a span of 3 days in mid-October. Additional field work was conducted over the span of 2 weeks. There were English and Spanish speakers on most teams, and field staff were provided with the use of a telephone translation service.

The questionnaire consists of five sections (demographic information, media exposure, knowledge regarding Zika, health behaviors and perception of risk, and trusted sources of information). For situations regarding additional follow-up, team members noted the individual's concern and contact information separate from the database and provided this information to the study lead. Campaign exposure was measured through aided recall, and field staff used a handout with visual examples of all the media materials. Staff were also provided with the introduction and consent scripts, printed copies of English and Spanish surveys, a tracking form, the referral form, a wallet card with basic Zika facts and PDPH website, and a one-page fact sheet on Zika prevention. Data from the questionnaire was entered into an MS Access database and subsequently analyzed using univariate procedures in SAS v9.3.

An after-action conference was conducted following the CASPER. It included all active participants and was intended to identify overarching themes, successes, and areas for improvement. Participants evaluated the trainings, field support services, internal protocols, and challenges with following the CASPER methodology. Feedback was captured at this in-person meeting and also via an online survey, using Survey Monkey.

Results

There was an overall completion rate of 64%, which was below the 80% needed to represent the sampling frame. However, sampling did provide a good representation of the targeted community (**TABLE 14-1**). Out of the 135 respondents, 24 (18%) were identified as Hispanic/Latino.

The health department learned that the majority of people (89%) had heard of Zika, and 96% knew Zika could be transmitted by mosquitoes. Conversely, only 54% of respondents were aware of sexual transmission. Incorrect modes of transmission identified were urine or saliva (43%), polluted water (38%), sneeze and cough (27%), and vaccines (13%). Respondents most reported seeing bus ads (37%), posters in doctor's offices (30%), and online ads (16%) (**FIGURE 14-2**). Respondents suggested in-person outreach, television ads, social media, and utilization of community centers as the most effective outreach strategies. Trusted sources of health information include their doctor, the CDC, and health department (**TABLE 14-2**). Respondents also trusted news or media (if it has a local health spokesperson) not just a commercial. Households with a woman of childbearing age were more likely to consider Zika an important health issue. Hispanic respondents were more likely to have concerns about getting Zika in Philadelphia.

(continues)

	Philadelphia City Demographics (Census Information)	CASPER Demographics
TABLE 14-1 CASPER Demographics		
Asian/Pacific Islander	6.3	6 (5%)
Hispanic/Latino	12.3	24 (18%)
White	41	38 (29%)
Black/African American	43.4	61 (46%)
American Indian	0.5	1 (1%)
Other	2.8	2 (2%)

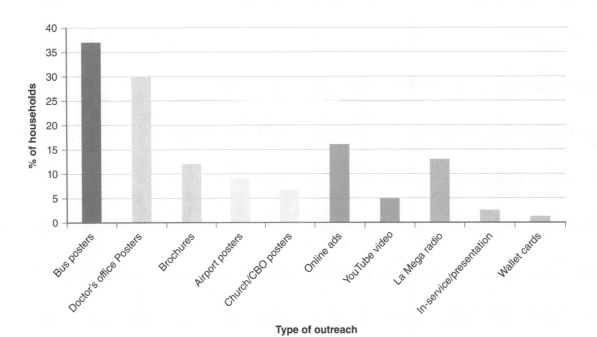

FIGURE 14-2 Bar graph of Zika educational materials

Sources of Health Information	Trust Level 1 (Definitely Do Not Trust) →5 (Definitely Trust)
TABLE 14-2 Trusted Sources of Information	
Doctor	5
Family or friends	3
Local health department	5
Church or community-based organizations	3
Centers for Disease Control and Prevention	5
News media	4
Other Internet sources	3

Discussion

PDPH's first CASPER was successfully planned and carried out over the span of 9 weeks, a relatively short time frame given competing priorities. Approximately, 50 staff members were pooled from different programs, resulting in collaboration across seven programs and three divisions within PDPH. It was noted that the significant number of staff required to perform the CASPER may be impacted during an acute public health emergency and should be considered in future planning. The just-in-time training mechanisms prepared staff well for their role in the field and staff felt comfortable performing their assigned duties, though the intricacies of the CASPER method (particularly sample selection) resulted in some confusion. This activity laid the foundation for future assessments using the CASPER, and tools such as the database, tracking sheet, and check-in rosters can be easily modified and adapted for future events.

Although the response rate was below the threshold needed for a representative sample, information collected during the CASPER identified that the majority of the public had a good understanding of the role of mosquitoes and mosquito bites in Zika transmission, but the majority did not correctly identify sex as a mode of transmission. Health communication materials of greatest penetration included public transportation ads and posters. Materials were considered clear but could not be directly linked to changes in behavior. Lastly, public health agencies were viewed as the most trusted sources of health information.

One limitation to interpreting the results of the CASPER is that the overall completion rate did not meet the threshold needed to represent the sampling frame. This may have been in part due to people not being home for the majority of the hours in the field or being reluctant to complete interviews due to interview fatigue. The cooperation rate, which represents the eligibility and willingness of community to complete the interview, was 40%. The lower it is, the more this sample becomes one of convenience. The contact rate was 39%, which indicated that interview teams had to approach many households to obtain interviews, further causing the sample to become one of convenience.

The CASPER method itself has limitations that may impact these rates, such as a reliance on outdated census data. Another limitation of the methodology is the focus on randomization in both stages of sample selection resulted in an insufficient sample size. The CASPER method also recommends three attempts be made at each household, resulting in long wait times in between attempts. This may be due to the geographic characteristics of Philadelphia, a densely urban area. One suggestion provided at the after-action conference was to do the first stage of selection randomly, but do the second stage of sampling as a convenience sample. More efficient methods should be explored. While the data collected is still of utility, another method, such as convenience sampling, at the second stage of household selection would likely have increased the sample size. Other methods may need to be explored for future assessments to achieve a higher response rate in a manner that still surveys a representative sample of the targeted population.

Advantages of the CASPER approach included enhancing the visibility of the health department and its activities and a venue for having individual discussions and disseminating material directly to community members. This type of outreach provided gratification to a number of staff members, who reported that some interviewees said they had never heard of a city agency coming out in person. Though this CASPER is not a "gold standard" of the method, the information obtained was still useful for refining health education activities. The data, even if not representative, were analyzed as cross-sectional data and provided a baseline level of understanding of the community's knowledge of Zika. On the basis of the CASPER results, the following year's education campaign increased messaging, focusing on the prevention of sexual transmission and the incorporation of basic travel health tips. Public transportation ads and print materials in doctor's offices were also increased.

The Zika epidemic presented a complex, constantly evolving, communication challenge that requires consistent coordination. Well-laid communications plans can help public health officials deal with uncertainty, reduce chaos, and are an essential component of effective emergency response and risk management. Performing an evaluation of a health communications campaign allowed PDPH to better understand what modalities and messages were most successful and also identify gaps in its existing campaign.

Lessons Learned

1. There is a burden to evaluation, and there are always trade-offs, regardless of the evaluation method you choose. Doing a field survey like the CASPER requires a number of trained staff and is time-consuming. In the after-action conference, PDPH discussed a number of other methods, such as phone surveys, that would be less time-consuming. Other methods, however, would not be without challenges. Phone numbers, particularly for cell phone numbers, may be difficult to obtain unless it is an emergency situation, for example.

2. The CASPER was not designed to be a risk communications strategy, but PDPH found that it helped foster good relations with the community. Some interviewees said they had never heard of a city agency coming out in person, and another person said that no one ever asks about the needs of the poor neighborhoods. When asked what the health department could do to improve future education efforts, field staff were told,

(continues)

"This. Exactly what you're doing." Going out in person also gave PDPH staff the chance to link interviewees to other health services and clarify any concerns and misconceptions about Zika.

3. Risk communications needs to go both ways. Far too often, agencies do not conduct program evaluations and do not know whether their messages reach the intended audience. Two-way communication builds trust, which becomes even more critical in an emergency. Ultimately, the mission of public health is to take these lessons learned and integrate emergency response activities into routine functions. This helps preparedness planners build a platform for things to come, and improves response to future outbreaks. PDPH staff members also reported that participating in field data collection helped them better understand the city, which enhances their own planning and projects. Ongoing reciprocal communication is an integral part of the risk management process. Evaluation findings can help agencies revise tactics, channels, spokespeople, and messages.

4. The ads on public transportation were the most visible and, thus, will be prioritized in future risk communications activities. Community outreach will be delved into further for future seasons.

Discussion Questions

1. What are the strengths and limitations of various methods for data collection?
2. The CASPER methodology was adapted to fit the context and needs of a local health agency. Can you think of other ways to adapt it?
3. What makes risk communications difficult?
4. What are some of the challenges to evaluating a risk communications campaign or assessing level of knowledge in a community?

References

1. WHO. *WHO International Health Regulations (IHR) Monitoring Framework: Implementation Status of IHR Core Capabilities, 2010–2016.* Available at: http://gamapserver.who.int/gho/interactive_charts/ihr/monitoring/atlas.html. Accessed January 14, 2017.
2. Ministère de la Santé et de Hygiène Publique. *Guide Technique pour la Surveillance Integrée de la Maladie et la Ripose en Guinée.* 2011.
3. Comité Interministeriel de Lutte contre la grippe aviaire. *Plan National Multi-Sectoriel de Preparation et de Riposte à la Grippe Aviaire.* 2006.
4. WHO. *Origins of the 2014 Ebola Epidemic.* 2015. Available at: http://who.int/csr/disease/ebola/one-year-report/virus-origin/en/. Accessed January 14, 2017.
5. Saéz MA, Weiss S, Nowak K, et al. Investigating the Zoonotic Origin of the West African Ebola Epidemic. *EMBO Molecular Medicine.* 2015;7(1):17–23. doi:10.15252/emmm.201404792.
6. Brooks JC, Pinto M, Gill A, et al. Incident Management Systems and Building Emergency Management Capacity during the 2014–2016 Ebola Epidemic—Liberia, Sierra Leone, and Guinea. *MMWR.* 2016;65(3):28–34.
7. World Bank. *Summary on the Ebola Recovery Plan: Guinea.* April 16, 2015. Available at: http://www.worldbank.org/en/topic/ebola/brief/summary-on-the-ebola-recovery-plan-guinea. Accessed January 14, 2017.
8. WHO. *Hundreds of Contacts Identified and Monitored in New Ebola Flare-up in Guinea.* March 22, 2016. Available at: http://www.who.int/csr/disease/ebola/guinea-flareup-update/en/. Accessed January 14, 2017.
9. Henao-Restrepo AM, Camacho A, Longini IM, et al. Efficacy and Effectiveness of an rVSV-Vectored Vaccine in Preventing Ebola Virus Disease: Final Results from the Guinea Ring Vaccination, Open-Label, Cluster-Randomised Trial (Ebola Ça Suffit!). *The Lancet.* 2017;389(10068):505–518. doi:10.1016/S0140-6736(16)32621-6.
10. Centers for Disease Control and Prevention. *Estimated Range of Aedes albopictus and Aedes aegypti in the United States, 2016.* Available at: https://www.cdc.gov/zika/vector/range.html. Accessed June 2017.
11. Centers for Disease Control and Prevention (CDC). *Community Assessment for Public Health Emergency Response (CASPER) Toolkit.* Second edition. 2012. Available at: https://www.cdc.gov/nceh/hsb/disaster/casper/docs/cleared_casper_toolkit.pdf. Accessed June 2017.

Glossary

Agroterrorism: the threat or use of biological or chemical agents against the agricultural industry or food supply system.

Amerithrax: the most well-known bioterrorism event in the United States; it occurred in the fall of 2001 and involved finely milled anthrax sent through the mail, targeting senators and media outlets.

Attribution assessment: the task of determining who was responsible for a deliberate event.

Australia Group: informal group of countries that creates a list of common export controls for chemical and biological agents and related equipment to harmonize national export control measures.

Biobank: a managed repository of biological material and its associated information that can be accessed for research and other purposes.

Biodefense: measures taken to prevent, detect, respond to, and recover from harm caused by a biological agent.

Biological agent: any microorganism, including bacteria, viruses, fungi, rickettsia and chlamydia, prions, and protozoa, that are capable of causing harm, death, or some disease in a living organism.

Biological warfare: military use of a biological agent by a state to cause death or harm to humans, animals, or plants.

Biological Weapons Convention: international treaty prohibiting the development, production, proliferation, and retention of biological or toxin weapons.

Biorisk: the chance that any type of adverse event involving a biological agent leading to potential harm will occur.

Biosafety: process of maintaining safe conditions to prevent people and the environment from being exposed to hazardous biological agents.

Biosafety level: practices, equipment, and infrastructure associated with safely containing biohazardous materials or agents; levels correspond to actions that must be taken to contain increasingly dangerous agents.

Biosecurity: process to reduce or eliminate the ability of a biological agent to adversely affect human, animal, or plant health; the protection and control of agents to prevent against loss, theft, misuse, or intentional release.

Biosurveillance: any method to detect and monitor a biological incident, disease activity, or threat to health, whether of intentional or natural origin.

Bioterrorism: the threat or use of a biological agent typically by a nonstate actor to cause death or harm to humans, animals, or plants, specifically targeting civilian populations or resources.

Blister agent: type of chemical weapon causing irritation of the skin and mucous membrane.

Blood agent: type of chemical weapon causing seizures and respiratory and cardiac failure in high doses.

CASPER: a method used in disaster epidemiology to rapidly collect health information in a representative manner

Category A, B, and C threat agents: categories assigned to the major known biological threat agents, based on the amount of morbidity and mortality the agents are capable of causing, ease of weaponization, previous history of weaponization, and need for specific response planning.

Chemical warfare: use of chemical substance to intentionally harm or kill humans, plants, or animals.

Chemical Weapons Convention: international treaty banning the use, proliferation, and stockpiling of chemical weapons.

Choking agent: type of chemical weapon causing damage to the lungs, including pulmonary edema and hemorrhage.

Code of conduct: guidelines that organizations and individuals voluntarily agree to abide by, which set standards for behavior.

Communicable disease: a disease transmitted from person to person.

Cooperative Threat Reduction: efforts conducted primarily through the Departments of Defense and State to engage countries to reduce threats, particularly around weapons of mass destruction, biosecurity, and biosurveillance.

Decontamination: the process of eliminating an infectious or toxic agent that may constitute a public health risk from either a living or inanimate surface.

Disaster Risk Reduction: the development and application of policies, strategies, and practices to reduce vulnerabilities and disaster risks throughout society.

Disease: illness or medical condition that presents harm to a living being.

Disease outbreak: an occurrence of disease greater than would otherwise be expected at a particular time and place.

Dual use: research, agents, technologies, equipment, or information that can be used for both legitimate scientific purposes and for malevolent use.

Emergency management: the managerial function charged with creating the framework within which communities reduce vulnerability to hazards and cope with disasters.

Emergency operations center: a central command and control facility responsible for carrying out the principals of emergency preparedness and emergency management or disaster management functions at a strategic level during an emergency.

Emerging infectious disease: an infectious disease that newly appears in a population or that has been known for some time, but rapidly increasing in incidence or geographic range.

EOC-NET: established by the World Health Organization (WHO) in 2012 to help identify and promote best practices and standards for emergency operations centers (EOCs) and provide support for EOC capacity building in WHO member states.

Epidemic: See disease outbreak.

Epidemiology: the study of patterns of health and illness and associated factors at the population level.

Executive Order: a presidential directive with the authority of a law that directs and governs actions by executive officials and agencies.

Federal Emergency Management Agency: the U.S. federal agency responsible for responding to national emergencies, including natural disasters.

Geneva Protocol: international treaty that bans the use of chemical and biological agents in war.

Global Health Security Agenda: multinational initiative to accelerate global progress to prevent, detect, and respond to biological threats.

Global Partnership Program: a program established in 2002 by the United States, Canada, France, United Kingdom, Germany, Japan, Italy, and Russia (the G8) to collaborate on and implement projects around the world to counter weapons of mass destruction proliferation.

Health security: as per the World Health Organization, health security is the activities and intersect of disciplines necessary to minimize the impact of acute public health events on populations, economies, and political stability.

Health status: all aspects of physical and mental health and their manifestations in daily living, including impairment, disability, and handicap.

Health threat: an environmental, biological, chemical, radiological, or physical risk to public health in the context of national or global security.

Healthcare worker: someone whose job involves close contact with patients or patient items, including a variety of professions such as clinicians, therapists, social workers, pharmacists, and other technicians.

Homeland defense: the protection of U.S. territory, populations, and infrastructure against external threats or aggression.

Homeland security: the actions and policies associated with preventing, deterring, responding to, and recovering from aggressions targeted at U.S. territory, populations, and infrastructure.

Homeland Security Exercise and Evaluation Program: provides a capabilities based program that provides a standardized methodology and consistent terminology for designing, developing, conducting, and evaluating an exercise.

Homeland Security Presidential Directive: a directive from the George W. Bush administration's Homeland Security Council that recorded or communicated presidential decisions and policies related to homeland security.

Incidence: number of new cases of illness or disease during a specific period of time in a specific population.

Incident Command System: the standardized approach to the command, control, and coordination of emergency response personnel.

Intelligence Community: the collection of agencies, offices, programs, and bureaus that collect, analyze, and report on intelligence information in support of policymakers across the government.

International Atomic Energy Agency: an international organization, reporting to the U.N. General Assembly and Security Council that promotes the peaceful and safe use of nuclear energy, while inhibiting the intentional, offensive use of nuclear weapons.

International Health Regulations: an international treaty obligating all member states of the World Health Organization to detect, report, and respond to potential public health emergencies of international concern, and improve global health security through international collaboration and communication to detect and contain public health emergencies at the source.

Isolation: separation and restriction of movement of people or animals that are believed to have a communicable disease.

Medical countermeasures: pharmaceutical products and equipment such as drugs, vaccines, and ventilators to both prevent the harmful effects of a biological, chemical, or radiological agent and mitigate the consequences for those who become ill.

Medical intelligence: collection, analysis, and reporting of health threats and issues, including infectious disease threats, environmental health risks, data to support force health protection, and the medical information on individuals with regional and international importance.

National Incident Management System: a document providing for standardized incident management protocols for responding to any type of emergency at all levels of government.

National Preparedness Goal: Federal Emergency Management Agency created this goal with the purpose of making sure that the community to be prepared for all types of disasters and emergencies.

National Response Framework: a broad national plan for preparedness and response to disasters and emergencies.

National Science Advisory Board for Biosecurity: an advisory board to the Secretary of Health and Human Services made up of scientists and ex-officio members from across the federal government; it makes recommendations on criteria for identifying dual use research of concern and provides national guidelines for oversight of dual use research and advises on educational programs, codes of conduct for scientists, guidelines for dissemination of research methodologies and results, and strategies for international dialogues on dual use research.

National security: the actions and policies associated with safeguarding the territorial integrity, existence, and safety of the state.

National Security Council Directives: types of executive orders (with varying names depending on the administration) done with the advice and consent of the National Security Council that have the effect of law.

Nerve agent: a type of chemical weapon that primarily acts on the nervous system, causing seizures and death.

Notifiable disease: a disease that must be reported to a public health authority, either by statute or regulation.

Nuclear Non-Proliferation Treaty: an international treaty to limit the spread of nuclear weapons, encourage disarmament, and foster the right to peacefully use nuclear technology.

Nuclear weapon: an explosive device powered by a nuclear reaction.

Pandemic: an infectious disease that spreads through human populations across a large region, over multiple continents.

Pandemic Influenza Preparedness Framework: adopted in 2011 to promote a new system of equitable access to influenza samples and subsequent benefits, including vaccines.

Personal protective equipment: clothing and equipment that create a barrier between humans and health hazards, such as surgical masks.

Population health: health outcomes of a group of individuals, including the distribution of such outcomes within a group.

Preparedness: the actions and policies associated with preventing, protecting against, responding to, and recovering from a major event.

Preparedness cycle: showing the continued development process of planning, equipping and organizing,

training, exercising, and evaluating/improvement planning.

Prevalence: total number of cases of a disease or illness in the population at a given time.

Public health emergency: an acute event capable of causing large-scale morbidity and mortality, either immediately or over time; these events have the ability to overwhelm normal public health capabilities.

Public Health Emergency of International Concern: a technical term associated with the International Health Regulations (2005), determined through an algorithm and defined as an event that constitutes a public health risk to other nations and potentially requires an internationally coordinated response.

Public health emergency operations center: the facility from which the management of a public health emergency will take place.

Public health preparedness: the actions and policies associated with preventing, protecting against, responding to, and recovering from public health emergencies.

Quarantine: separation and restriction of movement of well people or animals that may have been exposed to an infectious agent.

Radiological event: an explosion or other release of radioactivity.

Select agent: List of biological agents, subject to federal regulations, that may pose a severe threat to public health and security.

SMART: an acronym meaning that each objective that is developed fits within a pattern to allow for measurement and evaluations.

Sphere Project: an initiative created by a group of humanitarian response professions to improve the quality of humanitarian response and hold organizations and individuals accountable to affected populations, donors, and constituents.

Stafford Act: the principal document for U.S. federal authority for assisting states and local governments in responding to any type of disaster.

Strategic National Stockpile: federal stockpile of drugs, vaccines, and medical equipment that can be rapidly deployed to any locality in the country in response to a public health emergency.

Surge capacity: ability of clinical care facilities and laboratories to accommodate a sharp increase in patients and samples during a public health emergency.

Synthetic biology: the design and creation of biological components and systems that do not naturally exist.

Threat and Hazard Identification and Risk Assessment: the process for determining what are the community's greatest threats and hazards and what would the risk be for each of them happening, as well as the potential harm to the community if they did happen; this process helps community planners in determining the priority for planning efforts.

Toxin: poisonous substances produced by living entities.

U.N. Security Council Resolution 1540: resolution obligating U.N. member states to ensure they do not support nonstate actors in their efforts to develop, acquire, possess, or use nuclear, chemical, or biological weapons.

Weapons of mass destruction: weapons that cause large-scale destruction, generally including nuclear, radiological, chemical, and biological weapons; it may also include high-yield explosives.

World Health Organization: the directing and coordinating authority for health within the U.N. system; it is responsible for providing leadership on global health matters, shaping the health research agenda, setting norms, articulating evidence-based policy options, and providing technical support to countries.

Zoonosis: any disease that is transmitted from animal to human.

List of Figures

List of Boxes

List of Tables

Index

Note: Page numbers followed by *b*, *f*, or *t* indicate material in boxes, figures, or tables, respectively.

© f00sion/E+/Getty

Convention on Biological Diversity
(CBD), 109
COOP. *See* Continuity of Operations Plan
(COOP)
Cooperative Threat Reduction (CTR)
programs, 57
coronavirus, 41*f*, 103–104
Council of State and Territorial
Epidemiologists (CSTE), 6
CPG 101. *See* Community Preparedness
Guide 101 (CPG 101)
CRI. *See* Cities Readiness Initiative (CRI)
Crim-Epi, 57, 142
criminal investigation, elements of, 142*f*
CSTE. *See* Council of State and Territorial
Epidemiologists (CSTE)
CTR programs. *See* Cooperative Threat
Reduction (CTR) programs
CWC. *See* Chemical Weapons
Convention (CWC)
CWS. *See* Chemical Warfare Service
(CWS)
cyber-attack, and health effects, 151–152
cyber intelligence (CYBINT), 60
CYBINT. *See* cyber intelligence
(CYBINT)

D

The Dalles, Oregon, 26
delayed-notice events, 116
deliberate use, of biological agents, 23*f*
Demobilization Unit, ICS, 162
Department of Commerce, 58
Department of Defense (DoD)
disease and development
assistance, 43
global disease surveillance
networks, 141
on homeland security, 4
intelligence community members
of, 59*b*
public health emergency programs,
57–58
Department of Energy (DoE), 58, 59*b*
Department of Health and Human
Services (DHHS), 152, 173
for Emergency Support Function
(ESF), 117
expansion of research infrastructure,
104–105
offices and organizations of, 56–57
Public Health Improvement Act, 72
Department of Homeland Security
(DHS), 138
BioWatch, 140–141
expansion of research infrastructure,
104–106
Federal Emergency Management
Administration, 55

formal response process to
disasters, 51
Homeland Security Act of 2002
creating, 53
intelligence community members,
59*b*
Natural Biosurveillance Integration
Center, 140
Office of Health Affairs, 55
production of medical
countermeasures, 111
Department of Interior, 58
Department of Justice, 59*b*
Department of Labor, 58
Department of State (DoS), 58
global disease surveillance
networks, 141
intelligence community
members, 59*b*
Department of Transportation, 58
Department of Treasury, 59*b*
Department of Veteran's Affairs, 59
DHHS. *See* Department of Health and
Human Services (DHHS)
DHS. *See* Department of Homeland
Security (DHS)
diplomacy, 44*b*
9/11 Commission Report findings,
53*b*
director of national intelligence (DNI),
59
disaster assistance, history of federal,
50–51
Disaster Relief Act of 1974, 50
disaster risk, 123, 125
disaster risk reduction (DRR), 123–125
Hyogo Framework, 123, 125
Sendai Framework for, 124*f*, 125
disease cowboys, 108*b*
disease surveillance, 6
DNI. *See* director of national intelligence
(DNI)
Documentation Unit, ICS, 162
DoD. *See* Department of Defense (DoD)
DoE. *See* Department of Energy (DoE)
domestic investigations of suspected BW
use, 143–144
DoS. *See* Department of State (DoS)
drinking water, Bioterrorism Act and,
72
DRR. *See* disaster risk reduction (DRR)
drugs, Bioterrorism Act and, 72
dual-use dilemma, 96–97*b*
oversight of research through Fink
Report, 94–95
overview of, 92–93
for synthetic biology, 99–100
Dual Use Research of Concern (DURC),
92, 96–97*b*
DURC. *See* Dual Use Research of
Concern (DURC)

E

Ebola epidemic
case study of, 182–184
cases and deaths data, 42*f*
in West Africa, 36, 37*b*, 42
ECDC. *See* European Union Center for
Disease Prevention and Control
(ECDC)
economics, global interconnectedness
and spread of disease, 41
education and training
Pandemic and All-Hazards
Preparedness Act, 7*b*
use of biological weapons, 28
EID. *See* emerging infectious disease
(EID)
EIS. *See* Epidemic Intelligence Service (EIS)
emergency management, 6
Emergency Medical Teams (EMTs),
129, 131
emergency operations center (EOC), 155,
167, 175
development, 168–169
Emergency Operations Center Network
(EOC-NET), 170
emergency operations centers (EOCs),
182
Emergency Operations Coordination,
171, 176
Emergency Relief Coordinator (ERC),
126
Emergency Response Framework (ERF),
129
Emergency Support Function Leadership
Group (ESFLG), 117
Emergency Support Functions (ESFs),
64*b*, 66*f*
ESF #8, 65–66, 65*b*
emerging biological agents, 27
emerging infectious disease (EID), 35
global interconnectedness and threat
of, 38–43
EMTs. *See* Emergency Medical Teams
(EMTs)
enhanced biological agents, 27
environmental health services, 167
Environmental Protection Agency (EPA),
58
environmental sniffers, BioWatch,
140–141
EOCs. *See* emergency operations centers
(EOCs)
EPA. *See* Environmental Protection
Agency (EPA)
epi curve, 142, 143*f*
EPI-X notifications. *See* Epidemic
Information Exchange (EPI-X)
notifications
Epidemic Information Exchange (EPI-X)
notifications, 169

United States Agency for International
Development (USAID), 43, 141
United States Army Medical Research
Institute for Infectious Diseases
(USAMRIID), 104, 106
United States Department of Agriculture
(USDA), 57, 105, 106
United States Northern Command
(USNORTHCOM), DoD, 57b
United States Postal Service (USPS), for
medical countermeasures, 78
Uniting and Strengthening America
by Providing Appropriate Tools
Required to Intercept and
Obstruct Terrorism Act, 72
universal task list (UTL), 61
University of Texas Medical Branch
(UTMB), at Galveston, 107–108
UNSCR. *See* United Nation Security
Council Resolution (UNSCR)
USAID. *See* United States Agency for
International Development
(USAID)
USAMRIID. *See* United States Army
Medical Research Institute for
Infectious Diseases (USAMRIID)
USDA. *See* United States Department of
Agriculture (USDA)
USNORTHCOM. *See* United
States Northern Command
(USNORTHCOM)
USPS. *See* United States Postal Service
(USPS)
UTL. *See* universal task list (UTL)
UTMB. *See* University of Texas Medical
Branch (UTMB)

V

VECTOR. *See* State Research Centre
for Virology and Biotechnology
(VECTOR)

vesicants (blister agents), chemical
warfare, 14
viral sovereignty, 82
viruses, as biological agents, 27b

W

War Research Service (WRS), 23
weapons of mass destruction (WMDs),
58
West Africa Ebola Outbreak, 109–110,
111, 113–114. *See also* Ebola
epidemic
WFP. *See* World Food Program (WFP)
WHA. *See* World Health Assembly
(WHA)
WHO. *See* World Health Organization
(WHO)
WMDs. *See* weapons of mass destruction
(WMDs)
work program, 81–82
workforce
affect of HIV/AIDS in sub-Saharan,
42
affect of naturally occurring diseases
on, 34
jobs in public health preparedness,
6–7
Pandemic and All-Hazards
Preparedness Act, 6–7
World at Risk report, 28
World Food Program (WFP), 183
World Health Assembly (WHA)
on destruction of smallpox stockpiles,
115
World Health Organization (WHO)
defining public health security,
33–34
*Framework for a Public Health
Emergency Operations Centre*, 169
global disease surveillance networks,
141

grades of emergencies, 129, 129f,
130–131t
International Health Regulations of
2005, 5
investigating alleged BW use,
144–145
on link between disease and security,
37–38
memorandum of understanding
(MOU), 136b
natural disasters and humanitarian
response, 129–131
on SARS outbreak, 40–41
smallpox destruction debate,
114–115
World War I
biological weapons in, 22
chemical weapons in, 15
WRS. *See* War Research Service (WRS)

Y

Yellow Rain, 24–26, 25f
Yeltsin, Boris, 24, 29
Yersinia pestis, 22, 92t

Z

Zika virus, 42–43, 43f
case study of, 185–190
educational materials, 188f
ZMapp drug, 114